Airway Smooth Muscle: Modulation of Receptors and Response

Editors

Devendra K. Agrawal, Ph.D.

Associate Professor of Medicine, Pharmacology, and Biochemistry
Creighton University School of Medicine
Omaha, Nebraska

Robert G. Townley, M.D.

Professor of Medicine and Chief of Allergic Disease Center
Creighton University School of Medicine
Omaha, Nebraska

CRC Press
Boca Raton   Ann Arbor   Boston

Library of Congress Cataloging-in-Publication Data

Airway smooth muscle: modulation of receptors and response / editors.
 Devendra K. Agrawal, Robert G. Townley.
  p. cm.
 Includes bibliographical references.
 Includes index.
 ISBN 0-8493-5904-X
 1. Respiratory organs—Muscles—Physiology. 2. Smooth muscle-
Physiology. 3. Airway (Medicine)—Physiology. I. Agrawal,
Devendra K. II. Townley, Robert G.
 [DNLM: 1. Muscle, Smooth—physiology. 2. Receptors, Endogenous
Substances—physiology. 3. Respiratory Airflow—physiology.
4. Respiratory Muscles—physiology. WF 102 A2984]
QP121.A574 1990
612.2—dc20
DNLM/DLC
for Library of Congress   90-1825
                                                                            CIP

   Direct all inquiries to CRC Press, Inc., 2000 Corporate Blvd., N.W., Boca Raton, Florida 33431.

© 1990 by CRC Press, Inc.

International Standard Book Number 0-8493-5904-X

Library of Congress Card Number 90-1825
Printed in the United States

PREFACE

Airway smooth-muscle dysfunction is critical in various pulmonary diseases such as chronic bronchitis, cystic fibrosis, and emphysema, and plays a predominant role in bronchial asthma. Airway smooth-muscle tone is controlled by three basic mechanisms: myogenic, neurogenic, and humoral influences. Any disturbance in these mechanisms separately or collectively may affect airway smooth-muscle responsiveness. In recent years, despite a substantial amount of data having been accumulated about these mechanisms, significant evidence points to airway smooth-muscle itself as a major contributor of abnormal physiology in airway diseases.

Asthma is a multifactorial disease. Asthmatics exhibit marked bronchoconstriction in response to a wide variety of stimuli. Mediators released from inflammatory cells may act directly or indirectly on airway smooth muscle. In addition, epithelium is essential for maintaining and modulating airway smooth-muscle tone.

Our goal for this publication is to provide a state-of-the-art summary of airway smooth muscle from a group of experts with multiple disciplines. The text includes morphology, biochemistry, and electrophysiological behavior of airway smooth muscle. Chapters have been included on methodological aspects to measure smooth-muscle function *in vivo* in humans and experimental animals as well as *in vitro* in isolated trachea, bronchi, and lung parenchyma. In addition, there is a discussion of ion channels and their receptors in modulating receptor-response coupling in airway smooth muscle.

In light of the complexity in airway diseases and an exponential growth in research in this area, it is likely that controversies and inadequacies still exist. The authors have been encouraged to critically review the field and express their personal views on such controversies to provoke new ideas and unique perspectives.

We would like to express our sincerest thanks to all the contributing authors for their unfailing efforts and patience during the various stages of preparation of this book. Also, we thank CRC Press for providing guidance and advice in the preparation of this volume.

Devendra K. Agrawal
Robert G. Townley

THE EDITORS

Devendra K. Agrawal, Ph.D., is an Associate Professor of Medicine, Pharmacology, and Biochemistry at Creighton University School of Medicine, Omaha, Nebraska.

Dr. Agrawal received the M.Sc. degree in Chemistry in 1973 and a Ph.D. in Biochemistry in 1978 from Lucknow University, India. He held the appointment as Clinical Biochemist at King George's Medical College, Lucknow, India until 1980. He then joined Professor Edwin E. Daniel's laboratory at McMaster University, Hamilton, Ontario, Canada to pursue further studies in vascular smooth-muscle pharmacology and was awarded a Ph.D. in Medical Sciences in 1984. He was a Postdoctoral Fellow from 1984 to 1985 at the University of British Columbia, Vancouver, Canada, after which he was appointed Assistant Professor in 1985 at Creighton University in the Department of Internal Medicine with a joint appointment in the Department of Pharmacology. He was promoted to the rank of Associate Professor in 1990.

Dr. Agrawal is a member of various distinguished societies. These include the American Academy of Allergy and Immunology, American Association for the Advancement of Science, American Society for Biochemistry and Molecular Biology, American Society for Pharmacology and Experimental Therapeutics, American Thoracic Society, American Lung Association of Nebraska, and the Phi Beta Delta Honor Society for International Scholars.

Dr. Agrawal was awarded a Postdoctoral Fellow from the Canadian Heart Foundation. He was a recipient of the James M. Keck Faculty Development Award, Morris F. Miller Faculty Development Award granted by the Health Future Foundation, Omaha, Nebraska, and the 1990 Young Investigator Award from the Creighton University School of Medicine. He has been the recipient of research grants from the American Lung Association of Nebraska, Health Future Foundation, National Institute of Health, and various pharmaceutical companies.

Dr. Agrawal is the author and co-author of more than 40 papers in peer-reviewed journals. He also contributed review papers or chapters in 10 books. His major research interests have been in the biochemistry and pharmacology of the vascular and airway smooth muscle. Recent research work of Dr. Agrawal is focused on inflammatory cells, their mediators, and their interaction with airway epithelium and airway smooth muscle.

Robert G. Townley, M.D., is Professor of Medicine and Chief of the Allergic Disease Center at the Creighton University School of Medicine in Omaha, Nebraska.

Dr. Townley received his M.D. degree in 1955 from the Creighton University School of Medicine.

Dr. Townley is a member of the New York Academy of Sciences, the American Federation for Clinical Research, the Central Society for Clinical Research, and the American Thoracic Society. He is a fellow of the American College of Chest Physicians and the American Academy of Allergy and Immunology.

He has been the recipient of many honors and awards. Some of these include the Eben J. Carey Award, the Lederle Student Fellowship, President of the Nebraska Thoracic Society, Board of Directors of the Nebraska Thoracic Society, a member of the Presidential Task Force for N.H.L.I. to implement and set priorities of the Kennedy-Rogers Bill for Heart, Lung, and Blood Research, and the 1988 Distinguished Research Career Award from the Creighton University School of Medicine.

Dr. Townley has presented numerous invited lectures at international and national meetings on asthma and allergy. He has published more than 100 research papers. His current research interest involves the mechanisms underlying bronchial hyperreactivity in asthma and implementations of various therapeutic interventions.

CONTRIBUTORS

Devendra K. Agrawal, Ph.D.
Associate Professor
Department of Internal Medicine
Creighton University School of Medicine
Omaha, Nebraska

Krishna P. Agrawal, M.D.
Head
Physiology Department
Institute of Nuclear Medicine and Allied
  Sciences
Delhi, India

Dale Robert Bergren, Ph.D.
Associate Professor of Physiology
Department of Biomedical Sciences
Division of Physiology
Creighton University School of Medicine
Omaha, Nebraska

Againdra K. Bewtra, M.D.
Associate Professor
Department of Internal Medicine
Creighton University School of Medicine
Omaha, Nebraska

J. P. Boyle, Ph.D.
Smooth Muscle Research Group
Department of Physiological Sciences
The University of Manchester
Manchester, England

Naresh Chand, D.V.M., Ph.D.
Associate Director of Pharmacology
Wallace Laboratories
Cranbury, New Jersey

William Diamantis, Ph.D.
Director of Pharmacology
Wallace Laboratories
Cranbury, New Jersey

R. W. Foster, M.B., Ph.D.
Reader in Pharmacology
Smooth Muscle Research Group
Department of Physiological Sciences
The University of Manchester
Manchester, England

Roy G. Goldie, Ph.D.
Senior Research Fellow
Medical Research Council
Department of Pharmacology
University of Western Australia
Perth, Australia

D. M. Good, Ph.D.
Pharmacologist
Medicinal Research Center
SmithKline Beecham Pharmaceuticals
Harlow, England

Douglas W. P. Hay, Ph.D.
Associate Fellow
Department of Pharmacology
SmithKline Beecham Pharmaceuticals
King of Prussia, Pennsylvania

Peter J. Henry, Ph.D.
Research Officer
Department of Pharmacology
University of Western Australia
Perth, Australia

Russell Hopp, D.O.
Associate Professor of Pediatrics
Department of Pediatrics
Creighton University School of Medicine
Omaha, Nebraska

Karmelo M. Lulich, Ph.D.
Lecturer
Department of Pharmacology
University of Western Australia
Perth, Australia

**James W. Paterson, M.B.B.S.,
  A.K.C., F.R.C.P., F.R.A.C.P.**
Professor of Pharmacology
Department of Pharmacology
University of Western Australia
Perth, Australia

Chun Y. Seow, Ph.D.
Department of Medicine
University of Chicago
Chicago, Illinois

Roger C. Small, M.R., Pharm.S., Ph.D.
Senior Lecturer in Pharmacology
Department of Physiological Sciences
The University of Manchester
Manchester, England

R. Duane Sofia, Ph.D.
Vice President
Preclinical Research
Wallace Laboratories
Cranbury, New Jersey

Newman L. Stephens, M.D., F.R.C.P.
Professor
Department of Physiology
University of Manitoba
Winnipeg, Canada

Karen Stuart-Smith, M.D.
Department of Anaesthetics
Victoria Infirmary
Glasgow, Scotland

Theodore J. Torphy, Ph.D.
Director
Department of Pharmacology
SmithKline Beecham Pharmaceuticals
King of Prussia, Pennsylvania

Robertson Towart, Ph.D.
Research Pharmacologist
Department of Research
ZYMA S.A.
Nyon, Switzerland

Robert G. Townley, M.D.
Professor of Medicine
Department of Medicine
Creighton University
Omaha, Nebraska

Paul M. Vanhoutte, M.D., Ph.D.
Professor of Medicine and Pharmacology
Department of Medicine
Baylor College of Medicine
Houston, Texas

Dedicated to Our Wives
Rekha Agrawal and Nancy Townley
and to Our Children

TABLE OF CONTENTS

Chapter 1
Structure of Airway Smooth Muscle 1
Newman L. Stephens

Chapter 2
Biochemical Regulation of Airway Smooth-Muscle Tone: An Overview 39
Theodore J. Torphy and Douglas W. P. Hay

Chapter 3
Airway Smooth Muscle: Electrophysiological Properties and Behavior 69
Roger C. Small, J. P. Boyle, R. W. Foster, and D. M. Good

Chapter 4
Calcium and Potassium Channels in Airway Smooth Muscle 95
Robertson Towart

Chapter 5
Evaluation of Airway Smooth-Muscle Function *In Vitro* 111
Roy G. Goldie, K. M. Lulich, P. J. Henry, and J. W. Paterson

Chapter 6
Epithelium-Derived Relaxing Factor 129
Karen Stuart-Smith and Paul M. Vanhoutte

Chapter 7
In Vivo Measurement of Airway Responses in Experimental Animals 147
Krishna P. Agrawal

Chapter 8
Clinical Methods to Evaluate Airway Reactivity 167
Russell J. Hopp, Againdra K. Bewtra, and Robert G. Townley

Chapter 9
Pulmonary Reflex Effects on Airway Smooth Muscle and Ventilation 181
Dale R. Bergren

Chapter 10
Adrenergic and Cholinergic Receptors and Airway Responsiveness 229
Robert G. Townley and Devendra K. Agrawal

Chapter 11
Airway Histamine Receptors and Their Significance in Allergic Lung Diseases 259
Naresh Chand, W. Diamantis, and R. D. Sofia

Chapter 12
Mechanical Properties of Airway Smooth Muscle 271
Chun Y. Seow

Index 299

Chapter 1

STRUCTURE OF AIRWAY SMOOTH MUSCLE

N. L. Stephens

TABLE OF CONTENTS

I.   Introduction 2
II. The Airways 2
     A.   The Trachea 2
          1.   Dimensions 2
          2.   Tracheal Mucous Membrane; Interaction Between
               Epithelium and Smooth-Muscle Contraction and
               Relaxation 3
          3.   The Tunica Fibrosa Tracheae, Including the Musculus
               Transversus Tracheae 3
     B.   The Bronchial Airways 4
          1.   Bronchial Wall Structure 4
          2.   Layers of the Bronchial Wall 4
          3.   Types of Bronchi 4
          4.   The Mucosa 4
          5.   Mucous Membrane Diverticula 5
          6.   The Muscular Layer 5
     C.   The Terminal Bronchiole 7
     D.   The Respiratory Bronchiole 7
     E.   Parenchymal Smooth Muscle 9

III. Airway Smooth Muscle 10
     A.   Multiunit and Single-Unit Properties of Airway Smooth
          Muscles 13
     B.   Morphology of Airway Smooth Muscle; Muscle Bundles 14
          1.   Microscopic Features 14
     C.   Membranes of Airway Smooth Muscle, Including the Basement
          Membrane 15
          1.   The Sarcolemma 15
          2.   Basement Membrane 17
          3.   Pinocytotic Vesicles 18
          4.   Sarcoplasmic Reticulum 18
          5.   The Excitation-Contraction Coupling (EEC) Apparatus 18
     D.   Intercellular Communications: Gap Junctions, Intermediate
          Junctions, other Connections 21
          1.   Close Appositions 21
          2.   Intermediate Junctions 21
          3.   Gap Junctions or Nexuses 21
               a.   Species Distribution of Gap Junctions 25
     E.   Mitochondria 25
     F.   Golgi Apparatus, Lysosomes 26
     G.   Contractile Apparatus 26
     H.   The Nucleus and Nuclear Membrane 31
     I.   Innervation 31

IV.   Human Airway Smooth Muscle...34

V.   Conclusion..34

Acknowledgments...35

References..35

I. INTRODUCTION

In the last decade, the desire to elucidate the pathogenesis of asthma has seen an astounding increase in airway smooth-muscle research.[1-6] The bulk of this has been devoted to its pharmacology. Study of its structural characteristics has been neglected, apart from a few exceptions.[7-12] More recently, immunohistochemical techniques have been applied to determine the neural location of transmitters and polypeptides.[13-20] Unfortunately, they have not been utilized to determine structural characteristics of the contractile apparatus.

Most recent reports of ultrastructure have dealt almost exclusively with the airway smooth muscle and its innervation. The remainder of the structural components of the airways have been conspicuously neglected. Fortunately, excellent studies of these components were carried out almost half a century ago.[7,8,21-25] Recent reviews[2,3] have almost totally ignored these. The objective of the current review is to present a more comprehensive account of the structure of airways and their musculature.

The first part of this chapter, entitled "The Airways", will deal with the anatomy of the airways and such of their nonmuscular components as are relevant to understanding how airways subserve ventilation. This will also include pulmonary smooth muscle (parenchymal and interstitial)[24,25] not directly related to airways. The second part, entitled "Airway Smooth Muscle", will deal with the ultrastructure of airway smooth muscle proper.

II. THE AIRWAYS

A. THE TRACHEA

1. Dimensions

The trachea, with its incomplete C-shaped cartilage rings, sheet of smooth muscle, and an epithelial cell layer, forms an elastic tube which is delimited by the larynx above and bronchial bifurcation below. On the average it is about 10 cm long and 2 cm wide. It is wider transversely than sagitally. Its dimensions are set by transmural pressure differences and by the cartilage rings which are incomplete dorsally. The pressure differences are in turn controlled by transpulmonary pressure gradients and by contraction of the smooth muscle in the airway.

The innermost lining of the trachea is a mucous membrane, followed by a submucosal region and a tunica fibrosa in which the cartilages and muscles reside, the former being called the paries annulatus and the latter the paries membranaceus. The paries membranaceous forms a sheet joining the incomplete ends of the C-shaped cartilages.

2. Tracheal Mucous Membrane; Interaction Between Epithelium and Smooth-Muscle Contraction and Relaxation

This consists of the epithelial layer, the subjacent basement membrane, and the membrane propria.

The epithelium consists of ciliated epithelium of a pseudostratified columnar type; the cells extend downwards to the basement membrane. Among these cells lie goblet cells, which are smaller in number than the epithelial. The cilia are covered by a serous fluid layer, above which is a mucous layer. They beat in a coordinated fashion, sweeping particles entrapped in the mucous towards the oral cavity, where they are either expectorated or swallowed. The ciliary recovery stroke is made in the serous layer, and hence utilizes less energy than if it were made in the more viscous mucus. The third type of cell present in this layer is the basal or substituting cell, which gives rise to the other two. The nuclei of these various cells lie in six layers, those of the substituting cell layer being circular, while those above are ellipsoidal. Lymphocytes are interspersed throughout clefts that lie among the cells of the epithelial layer. It must be noted that the migrating cells cannot cross the epithelial layer because the clefts are closed off by a cuticular membrane.

The membrana propria is a cellular layer consisting mainly of lymphocytes. Subjacent to it a rich fibrous layer is present. This layer contains capillaries, lymph vessels, and collagenous fibers; glandular ducts transverse it. The submucosa fuses with the perichondrium of the tracheal cartilages. In the paries membranaceous zone the submucosa is more flexible, thus permitting mobility of the mucosa. It is in the submucosa that glands are present. Functional interaction between airway epithelium and smooth-muscle contraction has been discussed in detail at various places in the following chapters.

3. The Tunica Fibrosa Tracheae, Including the Musculus Transversus Tracheae

This is made up of collagen and elastin fibers, and in it lie the cartilages of the paries annulatus. In all, about 20 cartilaginous rings are present. These open dorsally. Each ring is surrounded by a perichondrium, which is thicker on the external aspect of the ring than on the inner. The fibrosa is divided by the cartilages into an outer perichondrium, a middle that connects the cartilages edge to edge, and a thinner inner one which fuses with the inner perichondrium.

The musculus consists of bundles of smooth-muscle cells which run transversely, bridging the ends of the cartilages. Small elastic tendons attach the muscles to the internal perichondrium near the dorsal ends of the cartilages. The muscle cells will be described in greater detail in following sections. The function of the smooth-muscle layer is the subject of controversy and no clear-cut opinion exists.[26] Early workers surmised that the smooth-muscle layer helped reduce the anatomical dead space, and, at relatively low ventilatory frequencies, improved alveolar ventilation. The muscle membrane constitutes about 25% of the tracheal circumference, and, since the muscle can shorten by about 80% (assuming the shortening is isotonic) of its initial length,[27-29] this could result in reduction of the lumen volume by 40%. In disease conditions, such as chronic asthma and bronchitis, thickening of the epithelial layer could, along with muscle contract, produce almost complete closure of the airway.

To what extent the trachea can narrow, either because of smooth-muscle contraction or of passive compressive forces as in a cough, has not been adequately measured. At the moment the glottis opens during coughing the intrathoracic trachea narrows considerably,[30] thus enabling the air to move the mucus cephalad, not only by friction, but also by propelling it.

B. THE BRONCHIAL AIRWAYS

1. Bronchial Wall Structure

For long, the bronchial airways were treated as passive air conduits, but the role of the contained muscle is now being sought. No clear-cut function has been assigned, and the following list is speculative: (1) as mentioned for the trachea, reduction of anatomical dead space with improved alveolar ventilation is one possibility; (2) clearing of the airway by propelling mucus upwards to the mouth and emptying of the mucus glands by a rhythmic massaging action; (3) regulation of regional ventilation.

2. Layers of the Bronchial Wall

The bronchial wall, much like the tracheae, consists of a mucosa, a muscularis, and a cartilage-containing fibrous layer. The layers are stable, and interspersed between them are two more flexible layers, the submucosa and the extramuscularis.

3. Types of Bronchi

The structure of bronchi appears to vary with the size of the bronchi. These are the large, medium, and small bronchi, the last named leading to the bronchioles. The large bronchi are the right and left main, as well as the lower lobe bronchi. The medium are comprised of the upper and middle lobar and the segmental. The remainder of the tree constitutes the small bronchi.

4. The Mucosa

This is made up of the epithelial cell layers, the basement membrane, and the tunica proprium, the last containing blood vessels, lymphatics, and fibers (see Figure 1).

The epithelium resembles that of the trachea with a pseudostratified, ciliated layer three to four cells thick. These are interspersed with clearer goblet cells that are sometimes arranged in pairs as in Figure 2. As the bronchiole is approached there is a reduction of these layers until only a single-layered epithelium remains. Goblet cells increase in number in disease states. The ciliated cells are connected together by a cuticular membrane which prevents flow of fluids into the lumen. Once again, as in the tracheal epithelium, intercellular clefts are present that contain wandering cells such as lymphocytes, polymorphonuclears, and mast cells.[31] There are in addition isolated nonciliated cells with unique superficially located nuclei; the cell cytoplasm bulges toward the lumen.

The last type of cells to be described are those reported by Frohlich[31] as the light cells. These are large, rounded cells, with poorly staining cytoplasm, located particularly at the bronchial division sites with intracellular nerve endings in them. These nerves are believed to be sensory and it is speculated the cells may be chemoreceptors.

In dilated bronchioles, the single-layered epithelium consists of cuboidal cells, but in contracted bronchioles they develop a so-called high cuboidal shape. The numbers of goblet cells are reduced and are absent from the terminal bronchioles. Naturally, no glands are present.

The basement membrane varies from 2 μm thick in bronchioles to 8 μm in larger bronchi. It appears to consist of a network of reticular fibers.

The membrana propria contains blood vessels and lymphatics and is fibrous. These fibers are elastic and lie mainly in the longitudinal axis of the bronchiole (see Figure 3). Circular fibers of the muscularis are clearly seen. These appear to extend into the walls of nearby alveoli.

Mucous membrane glands present in the trachea are especially abundant in medium bronchi, and progressively decrease till they become absent in the bronchioles. The glandular ducts run somewhat transversely. When the smooth muscle contracts it becomes separated from the fibrocartilaginous layer, and the ducts become even more radially oriented.

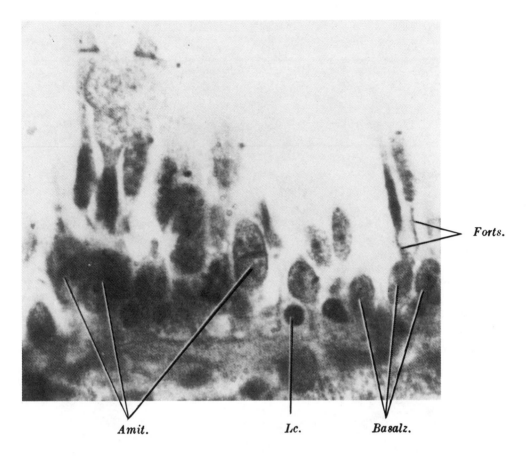

FIGURE 1. Epithelium of the left bronchus. Amit., amitosis; Basalz., basal cells; Lc., lymphocyte; Forts., processes of goblet and ciliated cells extending to the basement membrane. (Magnification × 1000.) (From Hayek, V. H., *The Human Lung*, Hafner Publishing, New York, 1960. With permission.)

5. Mucous Membrane Diverticula

Figure 4 shows diverticular structures in the mucosa. These traverse the submucosa and may even reach into peribronchial tissue. The termination of the diverticulum is surrounded by lymphoid tissue.

6. The Muscular Layer

In the large bronchi, just as in the trachea, the muscle layer extends between the dorsal ends of C-shaped cartilages. In succeeding generations of bronchi the attachment to the cartilage (which itself is beginning to fragment) becomes rapidly attenuated, and, in the small bronchi, the muscle is not directly attached to the cartilaginous plaques. The space between the muscle layer and the fibrocartilage becomes very mobile and has a profuse vascular network in it. It is claimed that when the musculature contracts, the enlargement of the subjacent space causes the vessels to engorge, and this aids in the warming of luminal air.

In the bronchioles the mobility of the muscular layer is once again lost because of the close connection between the elastic structures of the bronchial wall and structures of the alveolar walls.

In large bronchi, muscle bundles run almost transversely. They are not attached to the dorsal ends of the C-shaped cartilages, but to the perichondrium of the internal aspect of the cartilages where they insert by means of small tendons. This attachment of the muscle

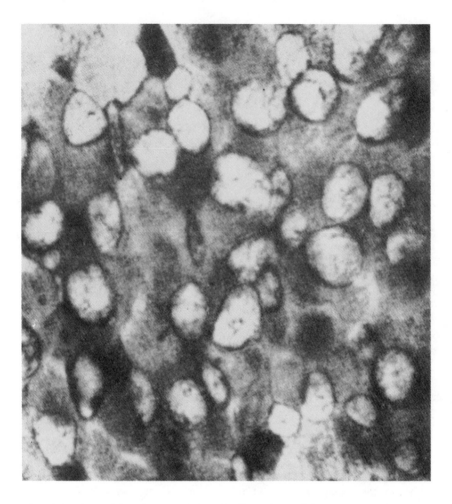

FIGURE 2.   Tangential section through the epithelium of a small bronchus. (Magnification ×
1000.)

shifts progressively more ventrally as one approaches the smaller bronchi, until the bundles
from a closed muscular membrane from which, at the points of bronchial and bronchiolar
bifurcation, small bundles extend to the cartilage. In small bronchi the muscle bundles are
thinner and lie in crisscrossing helical orientations. The helical pitch becomes tighter in the
bronchioles; in this location also the thickness of the muscular layer is at a maximum.

The muscular bundles are supported by sheaths made up of collagen, elastin, and reticular
fibers. Collagen fibers run obliquely across the muscle bundles; the elastic fibers tend to be
more parallel. In the terminal bronchioles, the attachment of the elastic sheath fibers of the
muscle bundles to the alveolar wall tissue results in stretching of the adjacent alveoli when
the muscle contracts. A unique radial arrangement of the alveolar septa then results (see
Figure 5). The unique attachments and arrangements of the bronchial smooth muscle just
described and the placement of the subjacent vascular network suggest some functional
optimization. In 1940 von Hayek[32] speculated that "the venous network evidently represents
a space-occupying plastic cushion which permits a narrowing of the lumen without occa-
sioning an accompanying movement of the fibrous membrane and of the surrounding lung
tissue by the contracting musculature. The marked alterability of the lumen of the small
bronchi through the contraction of the musculature is made possible by the presence of this
venous network".

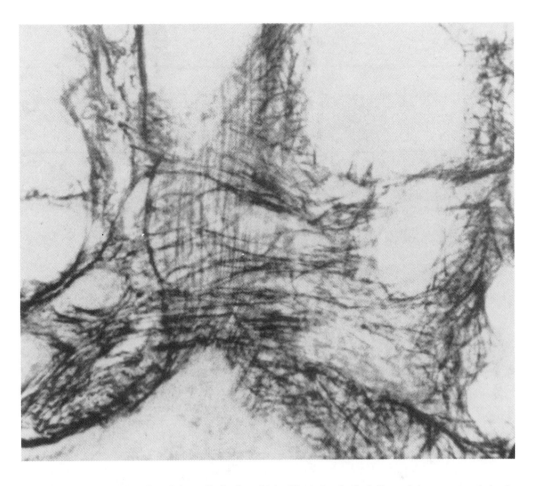

FIGURE 3.   Tangential section of the wall of a bronchiole. Elastic longitudinal fibers of the mucosa and circular fibers of the muscularis, the latter extending into neighboring alveoli. (Magnification × 120.) (From Hayek, V. H., *The Human Lung*, Hafner Publishing, New York, 1960. With permission.)

C. THE TERMINAL BRONCHIOLE

This succeeds the small bronchi which still are lined with cuboidal epithelium. Some of the lining cells are ciliated, and between the cuboidal cells a different type of cell is seen. This is also present in the respiratory bronchiole and will be dealt with later.

D. THE RESPIRATORY BRONCHIOLE

The terminal bronchioles are succeeded by respiratory bronchioles which, of course, bear alveoli. In between the openings of these walls, cuboidal epithelium is no longer present. Altogether, eight respiratory bronchioles arise by two sets of divisions. One can thus talk of respiratory bronchioles of the first, second, and third order, the last leading to alveolar ducts. The total length of the respiratory bronchioles is about 2.5 mm. Their average luminal area is 0.14 mm².

In the respiratory bronchioles, between the alveoli that project outward from the airway, there are ring-like projecting ridges or diaphragms. In these, substantial ring-like aggregations of smooth-muscle fibers are present (see Figure 6) that appear to almost totally encircle the respiratory bronchiole.

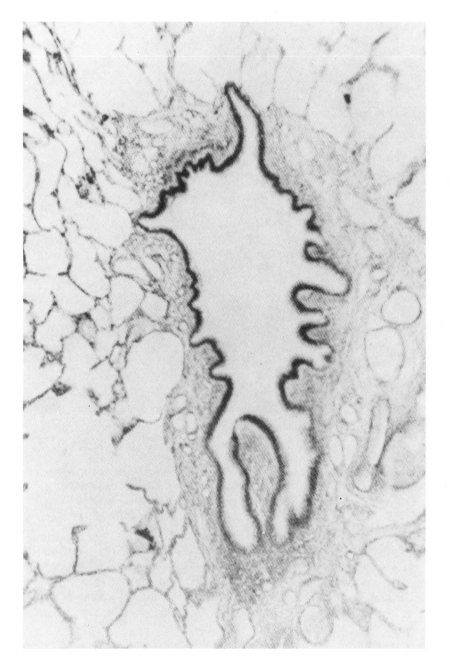

FIGURE 4.   Cross section of a bronchus with diverticula protruding through the muscularis, surrounded on the right by lymphoid tissue; extending on the left to the alveoli. (Magnification × 40.) (From Hayek, V. H., *The Human Lung*, Hafner Publishing, New York, 1960. With permission.)

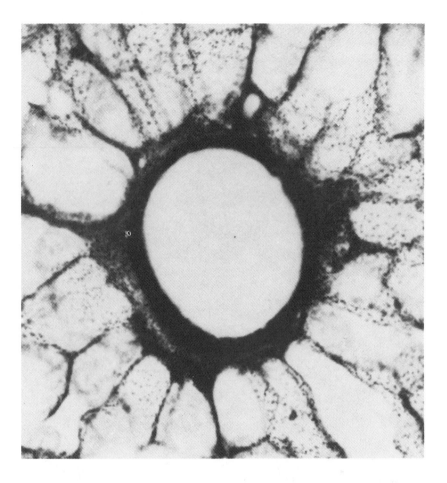

FIGURE 5. Bronchiole, moderately contracted; exact cross section with radial arrangement of the contiguous alveolar septa. (Magnification × 60.) (From Hayek, V. H., *The Human Lung*, Hafner Publishing, New York, 1960. With permission.)

E. PARENCHYMAL SMOOTH MUSCLE

The presence of smooth muscle truly parenchymal (interstitial) in origin has been postulated by Baltisberger,[24] but has also been a controversial issue. von Hayek[33] believes that the muscle is merely a local extension of respiratory bronchiolar smooth muscle into adjacent alveoli. Figure 7 shows muscle entrance rings of the alveoli that really occupy intervals between alveolar mouths, which are likely the source of the so-called interstitial muscle. Baltisberger[24] also described collections of subpleural smooth muscle whose function is not really known. A second source is bundles that radiate from the bronchioles to a greater extent than the two just described. Figure 8 shows that these can actually traverse several alveoli. The function of these muscles is not known. However, their abundance, as they extend outwards from respiratory bronchioles and alveolar entrance orifices, is quite striking, and, according to Baltisberger, "throughout the vicinity of the alveolar ducts not a cubic millimeter of lung tissue is free of muscle, thus enabling narrowing of alveoli in large areas of the lung. This has led to the notion of contraction atelectasis".

In recent times, Kapanci et al.[34,35] have reported that the parenchyma of normal mammalian lung contains a substantial population of contractile, filament-laden cells that they termed "contractile interstitial cells". It is not clear whether or not these are any of the parenchymal muscle groups reported by Baltisberger.[24] These interstitial cells are said to contribute contractile capability to the lung parenchyma, perhaps by modulating elastic recoil

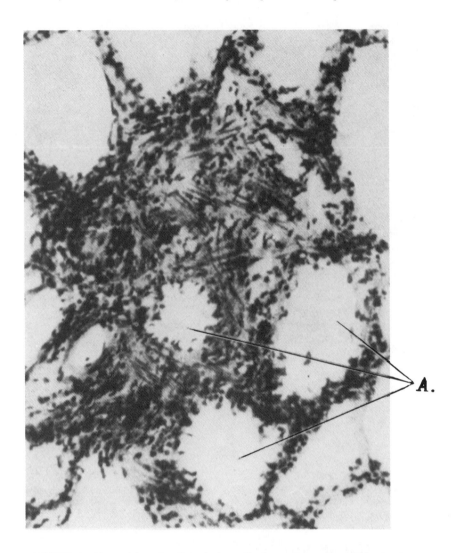

FIGURE 6.   Tangential section through the wall of a respiratory bronchiole showing muscular entrance rings of the alveoli (A.). (Magnification × 140.) (From Hayek, V. H., *The Human Lung*, Hafner Publishing, New York, 1960. With permission.)

and by fine tuning of the match between ventilation and perfusion. Low et al.[36] and Evans et al.[37] have analyzed the type and quantity of actin present in the lung and suggested the presence of nonmuscle-type myosin may be responsible for the contractility of the interstitial cells. Low et al.[36] have also attempted to study what happens to these actions in an Allomycin-induced model of lung fibrosis. They found that normalized actin content remained normal, and there was no change in actin types. Concomitantly, it was found that the fibrotic areas contained increased amounts of the cytoskeleton protein desmin. Possible explanations are that, even though actin content is not increased, there may be an increase in the degree of polymerization of actin in interstitial cells.

III. AIRWAY SMOOTH MUSCLE

While there is considerable doubt as to what the function of airway smooth muscle is *in vivo* under physiological circumstances and therefore of its role in controlling ventilation, there is no doubt about its role in the development of the respiratory distress of asthma. It

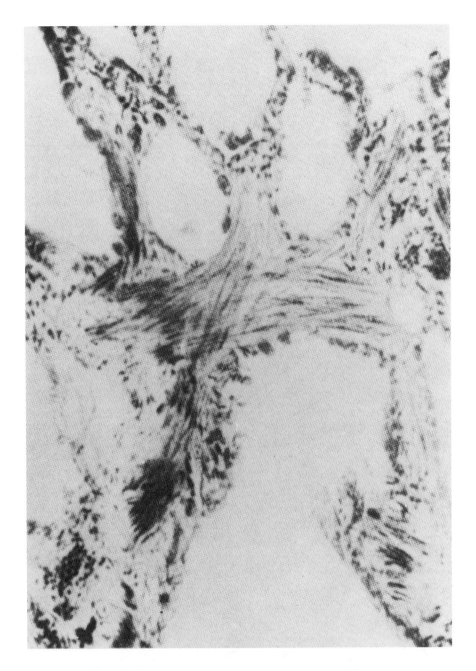

FIGURE 7. Tangential section through the wall of an alveolar duct. Crossing of a longitudinal bundle with a transverse bundle. (Magnification × 140.) (From Hayek, V. H., *The Human Lung*, Hafner Publishing, New York, 1960. With permission.)

is this factor, coupled with the fact that the most prevalent respiratory disorder today is asthma, that has led to the burgeoning interest in airway smooth-muscle research.

The focus in the field has been overwhelmingly on bronchial hyperreactivity with emphasis on inflammatory changes in the mural tissues. Study of the structure and ultrastructure has been neglected and, compared to what was done almost 40 years ago (described in the preceding section), is very little[12,13,28,34,38,39] and latterly centered on immunohistological studies of innervation.[5,6]

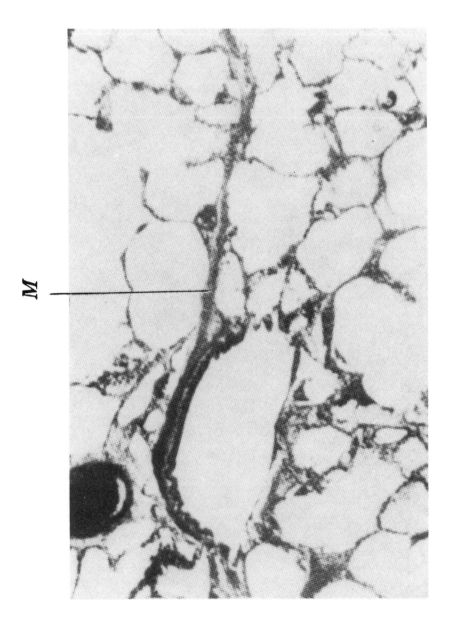

M

FIGURE 8.   Cross section of a respiratory bronchiole with radiating muscle bundle (M). (Approximate magnification × 50.) (From Hayek, V. H., *The Human Lung*, Hafner Publishing, New York, 1960. With permission.)

Histological studies, both quantitative and qualitative, are needed of airway smooth muscle from airways ranging from the trachea to the respiratory bronchioles (because it is clear that the early asthmatic attack involves central airways while the late involves peripheral — less than 1-mm-diameter — airways) and in all those animal species that have been used as models of allergic bronchoconstriction. Studies at different stages of lung development are needed, as the manifestations of asthma vary with age and it is now established that the responsiveness of airway smooth muscle to agonists and antagonists is very age dependent.

Lastly, the most pressing need is to carry out histological studies of smooth muscle from human airways, both healthy and asthmatic. This unexpectedly has turned out to be more difficult than envisaged.

A. MULTIUNIT AND SINGLE-UNIT PROPERTIES OF AIRWAY SMOOTH MUSCLES

While skeletal muscles are divided into fast and slow types, smooth muscles are classified as multiunit and single unit. As their mechanical and electrical properties are dissimilar it becomes necessary to describe their characteristics.

Burnstock[40] has stated that multiunit smooth muscles are so called because they consist of many individual nerve-muscle units, and in this way resemble skeletal muscle. Intercellular gap junctions are few, as activation of individual cells is ensured by the rich innervation. Examples of multiunit smooth muscle are the larger blood vessels and the trachea and central airways. These muscle cells do not develop action potentials and generally possess a non-oscillating resting membrane. No action potentials are seen and a myogenic response is not elicitable.

Single-unit muscle is quite different from multiunit. It has a sparse innervation, and many gap junctions are present between cells. It is this that allows rapid propagation of depolarization from cell to cell with some cells acting as pacemakers and others as pace followers. The resting membrane potential shows an oscillatory rhythm. Action potentials are also seen. These may occur at the peaks of the oscillations, although this is not always so. The action potentials do not overshoot to the same extent as skeletal muscle. They are decrementally conducted. Single-unit smooth muscles demonstrate a strong myogenic response. Examples of such muscles are the intestines, the arterioles, the ureters, and the uterus at term.

In the vascular system the large vessels are of multiunit type, while the small arterioles are of the single-unit type. It may be, by analogy, that small bronchioles are also of single-unit type.

Canine tracheal smooth muscle belongs to an intermediate category. It does not display any action potentials, does not have an oscillating resting membrane potential, nor does it possess as rich an innervation as multiunit muscle should have. On the other hand, it has more gap junctions[41] than a multiunit perparation.

These three categories of single-, intermediate-, and multiunit types are not fixed, and it is well known that the nonpregnant uterus which has multiunit characteristics converts to a single-unit type of smooth muscle as it approaches full term and labor. This conversion should aid the process of labor and parturition. Furthermore, Stephens et al.[42] and Kroeger and Stephens[43] have shown that treatment with tetraethylammonium bromide can induce single-unit characteristics in intermediate-unit type tracheal smooth muscle. Finally, Akasaka et al.[44] have shown, with the aid of an extracellular electrode, that in normal humans very little spontaneous, electrically spiking activity is seen when records are made by endoscopic insertion of the electrode. In asthmatics during an attack, however, a tremendous increase in spike activity is seen. All the above observations have led Macklem[44a] to postulate that the development of asthma in humans is really the conversion of the electromechanical properties of airway smooth muscle from intermediate-unit to single-unit type. Our own interpretation is that the muscle in healthy human airways is of single unit as some spiking activity is present, but with onset of asthma this becomes accentuated, possibly due to increased membrane excitability and a more rapid generator potential.

B. MORPHOLOGY OF AIRWAY SMOOTH MUSCLE; MUSCLE BUNDLES

Macroscopic features have been already partly described in Section A above. It is worth reiterating that all the fibers of the trachealis are arranged parallel to each other and are transverse in direction with respect to the longitudinal axis of the trachea. The trachealis or *musculus transversus tracheae*, which is a constituent of the *paries membranaceous*, consists of a unified layer of thick bundles that branch little. In the canine trachea the sheet is about 50 to 100 cells thick. According to Luschka[21] bundles of muscle fibers extend from the trachealis and insert into the ventral wall of the esophagus. The bronchial artery provides the blood supply to the tracheae and bronchial smooth muscle. It is also possible that the muscle obtains oxygen from the lumen by direct diffusion.

The muscle bundles appear to be made up of parallel muscle fibers and are encased in a loose network of collagen and elastin fibers that spiral with a wide pitch around the bundles.

1. Microscopic Features

An electron micrograph of canine trachealis fixed at rest is seen in Figure 9. This rather limited longitudinal section shows that the cells are indeed parallel to each other. Examination of several random sections confirms that the cells maintain their parallel orientation. The figure also shows that the intercellular space is small and contains collagen fibrils (CF). The space between the bundles of cells is much larger and will be described later. Morphometric studies have shown[42] that 75% of the tracheal strip is made up of muscle cells. This has been confirmed by estimates of collagen and noncollagen protein[45] in the strip. The parallel cell orientation and the predominance of smooth-muscle cells in the strip render the tracheal smooth-muscle preparation ideal for mechanical and biochemical studies.

The very smooth sarcolemma of the resting cell is noteworthy, as it changes markedly with activation.

Studies conducted by Stephens and Kroeger[46] and by Suzuki et al.[47] indicate the muscle cells are fusiform in shape and possess a central, cigar-shaped nucleus. They are about 5 μm in width at mid-nuclear level and range from 500 to 1000 μm in length. The ends of the cell are not sharp as conventionally thought, but splay out into irregular processes as described by Gabella[48] and Stephens and Kroeger.[46]

The general fibrillar gray areas of the cell seen in Figure 9 are due to actin (A) filaments. Dense bodies (DB) are seen scattered, seemingly randomly, throughout the cytoplasm. Electron-dense bands are also seen in the sarcolemma that are analogies of the dense bodies and are called dense bands. Mitochondria (Mit), pinocytotic vesicles (PV), and myelin swirls (MS) are also seen.

In Figure 10, a lower-power micrograph than that of Figure 9 is seen. The picture is a montage of several sections. It is taken from the same trachea and has been fixed at the peak of an isometric contraction. Part of a bundle of muscle fibers is seen. At the top, the interfascicular space is identifiable. Its width is about three to five cell diameters. Part of a mast cell with its typical granules is visible, and immediately below it are two fibroblasts. The space generally contains collagen and elastin fibrils; they are not well seen here and will be described later. It also contains blood vessels and nerve terminals. While the sarcolemma is perfectly smooth in the resting muscle, in the isometrically contracted one it is highly crenated. Nuclei are seen in several cells and show the twisted configuration typical of contracted cells.

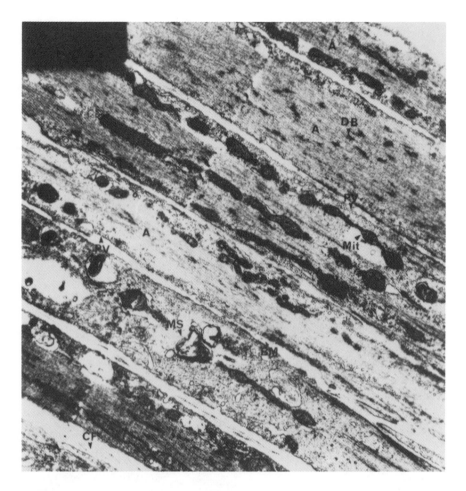

FIGURE 9. Electron micrograph of a longitudinal section of canine tracheal smooth muscle. A, actin filaments; BM, basement membrane; Mit, mitochondria (these are long and serpiginous); CF, collagen fibrils; PV, pinocytotic vesicles; MS, myelin swirls; DB, dense bodies, are also seen. (Magnification × 16,500.) (From Nadel, J. A., *Physiology and Pharmacology of the Airways*, Marcel Dekker, New York, 1980. With permission.)

C. MEMBRANES OF AIRWAY SMOOTH MUSCLE, INCLUDING THE BASEMENT MEMBRANE

1. The Sarcolemma

This consists of a biomolecular lipid leaflet much like that found in all cells. It has the typical five- or seven-layered "tram-line" appearance. The sarcolemma is well defined in Figure 11 and the tram lines are identifiable. At several locations on the sarcolemma electron-dense bands are seen. These are the dense bands previously mentioned that form attachment sites for actin filaments. Immunohistochemical techniques have demonstrated a high α-actinin content in these bands. The attachment of actin to the α-actinin is mediated by vinculin, a cytoskeletal protein. The cytoplasmic dense bodies have a similar structure to the dense bands. Somlyo et al.[49] have shown that actin filaments traverse the dense bodies and demonstrated polar reversal of myosin head binding sites on either side of the body. The structural and biochemical similarity of the bodies to the bands of striated muscle and the polar reversal strongly suggest that the dense bodies are Z analogs in smooth muscle. Desmin filaments are also seen in the region of the dense bodies. They arc from dense band to dense band and may serve to mechanically stabilize them. In skeletal muscle, desmin

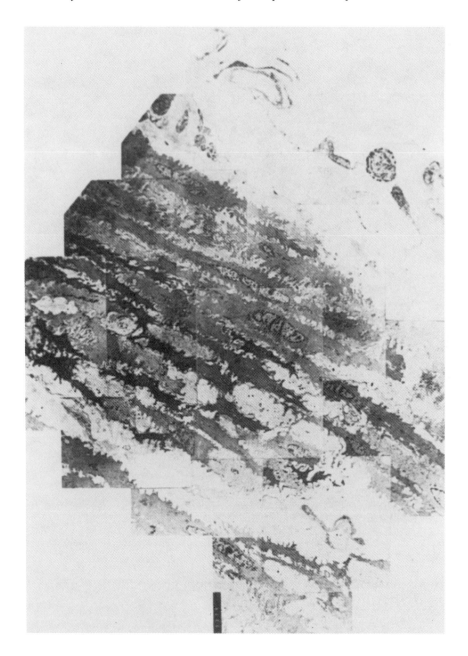

FIGURE 10. Montage of a single bundle of isometrically contracted canine tracheal smooth-muscle cells, reconstructed from low-power electron micrographs. The perifasicular space above the muscle cells contains collagen, a vessel, several fibroblasts, and a mast cell typified by its dark granules. This section shows light and dark cells that are often seen in smooth-muscle sections. The outlines of the light cells suggest they are swollen. The crenate cell outlines of the dark cells, which are in the majority, and the twisted shape of the centrally placed nuclei indicate the cells are contracted. The thick, rectangular calibration box represents a length of 10 μm. (Magnification × 4000.)

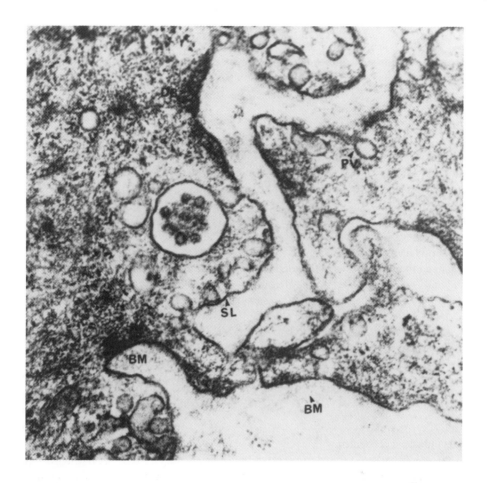

FIGURE 11. Electron micrograph of a transverse section of canine tracheal smooth muscle. The lacy basement membrane (BM) and the "railway track" membranes of the sarcolemma (SL) and pinocytotic vessels (PV) are clearly seen. Sarcolemmal dense bodies (DBS) are present. (Magnification × 75,000.) (From Nadel, J. A., *Physiology and Pharmacology of the Airways,* Marcel Dekker, New York, 1980. With permission.)

filaments also link adjacent Z bands.[50] These bodies will be discussed later in connection with the contractile apparatus.

Sarcolemmal dense bands are maximally present on the tapering ends of the cell. They occupy a minimum area in the perinuclear sarcolemma and progressively increase in extent towards the cell ends. The terminal 10% of the cell sarcolemma may be completely made up of dense bands. The ends of the tapering smooth muscles narrow down acutely, but then widen out with blunted processes. These are lined with a sarcolemma which is totally electron dense material. The basement membrane over it is condensed, and collagen and elastin fibrils run into it. This specialization continues to the end of the next cell and thus creates a strong mechanism for transmitting force axially from one cell to the next.

2. Basement Membrane

This is present around all airway smooth-muscle cells and is clearly seen in Figure 11. Its distribution is irregular and it appears to be separated from the sarcolemma by an irregular, clear interspace. Though not shown in this figure, external to the basement membrane, amorphous and fibrillar elastin and collagen fibrils fuse with the basement membrane. In the region of the dense bands the basement membrane appears condensed. In a contracted cell the troughs of the undulations are the site for the dense bands and organelles are not usually present in this region. It is of course into the dense bands that the thin filaments are inserted. In the adjacent outpouchings of the membrane, dense bands are much less and organelles more numerous. In Figure 11 the pinocytotic vesicles are mainly located in these outpouchings.

3. Pinocytotic Vesicles

Also called caveolae, pinocytotic vesicles are small, flask-shaped invaginations of the sarcolemma. In longitudinal sections (see Figure 11) they seem to be quite separate from the sarcolemma. In reality they always communicate with the extracellular space as evidenced by their filling with tracers such as colloidal lanthanum, ferritin, and peroxidase introduced into the extracellular space. In Figure 11 communications with the sarcolemma are seen. Pinocytotic vesicles are lined with a continuation of the sarcolemma and the basement membrane is carried into the vesicular lumina. At the neck of the vesicles the basement membrane is electron dense. Gabella[48] has reported that in the guinea pig taenia coli they are arranged in parallel rows in the longitudinal axis of the cell; they are interposed between dense bands. He has also estimated that there are approximately 170,000 caveolae in each cell and they serve to increase effective sarcolemmal area by 70%. Pinocytotic (or micro-pinocytotic) vesicles are found in the epithelium and are smaller than those of smooth-muscle cells. Freeze-fracture preparations show a ring of intramembranous particles around their ostia; these may be specific for smooth muscles. It has been speculated that they may serve as stretch receptors.

A few coated pits and coated vesicles are seen in smooth muscle, but appear to differ from pinocytotic vesicles. The coated pits suggest that limited micropinocytosis may be possible.

4. Sarcoplasmic Reticulum

The smooth-muscle sarcoplasmic reticulum appears very rudimentary when compared to the rich and complex structure seen in striated muscle. However, the width of the smooth-muscle cells is only 5% of that of the striated, which suggests a rich supply of sarcoplasmic reticulum is not needed for the former. The amount of sarcoplasmic reticulum present in smooth muscle makes up about 2 to 5% of the total cell volume. It has been suggested that the amount of sarcoplasmic reticulum present in smooth muscle is enough to provide for the needs of excitation-contraction coupling.[59] While in striated muscle more reticulum is seen in fast muscles, in smooth muscle the amount of reticulum seems to depend on the extent to which the muscle relies on intracellular calcium for contraction. Multiunit and intermediate types (trachealis, for example) have more reticulum than single-unit muscle (taenia coli). Figure 12 shows, in a transverse section, a relatively rich supply of sarcoplasmic reticulum in the guinea pig sphincter pupillae.

The discussion up to this point implies the sarcoplasmic reticulum is the major source[62-64] and sink for for intracellular calcium stores. Such indeed is the case, at least in guinea pig smooth muscle. Microsomes of airway smooth muscles have also been shown to actively assimilate Ca^{2+}.[65-67] Calcium oxalate precipitates have been localized in the reticulum. Furthermore, sarcolemmal microsomes have been prepared from smooth muscle and shown to take up and bind calcium in a specific way. Alterations in calcium sequestering function have been reported in sarcolemmal preparations from hypertensive vascular smooth muscle.

5. The Excitation-Contraction Coupling (ECC) Apparatus

In smooth muscle the ECC is not so well defined and structured as in striated muscle, and while considerable work has been carried out, we still do not know what the complete smooth-muscle ECC pathway is, in structural terms. It has been suggested that collections

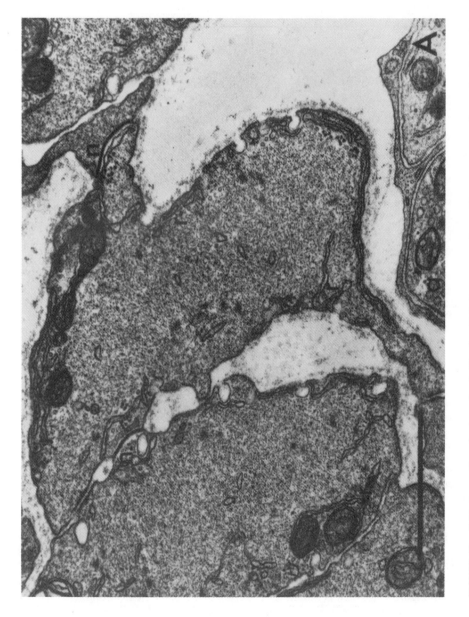

FIGURE 12. Sphincter pupillae of guinea pig. A, Muscle cells in transverse section, with numerous sacs of sarcoplasmic reticulum (r); n, nexus; a, axon. Scale: 1 μm. (From Bulbring, E. and Shuba, M. P., Eds., *Physiology of Smooth Muscle*, Raven Press, New York, 1976. With permission.)

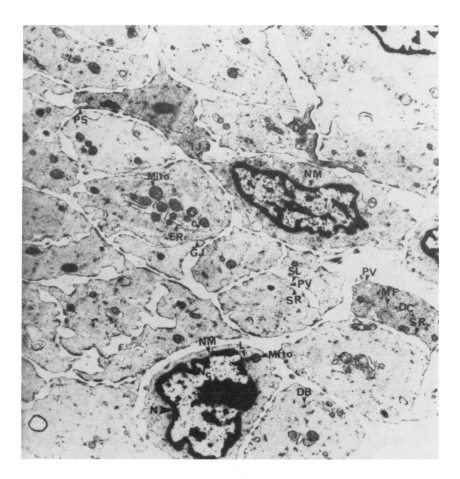

FIGURE 13.   Electron micrograph of a transverse section of canine tracheal smooth muscle. An excitation-contraction coupling apparatus is seen; it is delineated by the three closely grouped arrowheads labeled SL (sarcolemma), PV (pinocytotic vesicle), and SR (sarcoplasmic reticulum, which appears tubular). Many cells show closely apposed junctions, for example, the dark cell in the top right quadrant of the figure. In addition, intermediate cell junctions (IJ) are seen. Peg and socket junctions (PS) are also seen. The participating membranes of this type of junction are in close apposition (with encased electron density) only for limited extents of the junctions. The cell at the bottom shows a nucleus (N) with a nucleolus (NC). Close to the perinuclear membranes (NM), a small, circular structure is seen with homogeneous gray contents. This may be a lysosome (L), which is in contact with a mitochondrion (Mito). Rough endoplasmic reticulum (ER) is also seen. Several dark cells (DC) are present. In all of them, what appear to be thick filaments (MF), cut in transverse section, are seen. These cells also show pinocytotic vessels (PV). Numerous dense bodies (DB) are seen in all cells, scattered randomly. (Magnification × 1500.) (From Nadel, J. A., *Physiology and Pharmacology of the Airway,* Marcel Dekker, New York, 1980. With permission.)

of pinocytotic vesicles, sarcoplasmic reticulum, and mitochondria can often be found near the sarcolemma. Their proximity to each other suggests they could be acting as an ECC apparatus. In Figure 14, which is a transverse section of an isometrically contracted guinea pig taenia coli, numerous sarcoplasmic reticular sacs are seen. The uppermost cell in the figure shows reticulum very close to the sarcolemma and to a pinocytotic vesicle. Where the reticulum approaches the sarcolemma, electron densities akin to those of the striated muscle triads are seen, which strengthens the ECC apparatus analogy.

Such structures have also been found in airway smooth muscle. Figure 13 depicts a transverse section of canine tracheal smooth muscle. In the middle of the picture an aggregation of sarcolemma (SL), sarcoplasmic reticulum (SR), and pinocytotic vesicle (PV) is present that could constitute an ECC apparatus.

D. INTERCELLULAR COMMUNICATIONS: GAP JUNCTIONS, INTERMEDIATE JUNCTIONS, OTHER CONNECTIONS

Intercellular communications in smooth muscle serve three functions. First, they serve as means of electrical communication between cells and facilitate propagation. The special type of junctions that do this are known as nexuses or gap junctions. Second, they serve as a means of transmission of chemical communications between cells; again it is the gap junctions that subserve this function. Third, they facilitate transmission of mechanical forces.

Cell-to-cell communications are of three types: close appositions, intermediate junctions, and gap junctions.

1. Close Appositions

In these the gap between the membranes of the participating cells is 20 to 30 nm wide. The membranes are sometimes arranged in a peg and socket configuration. See Figure 13, which shows a peg and socket (labeled PS) communication between two cells. The lining membranes of these junctions may show densities much like those of intermediate junctions. Occasionally the junctions may be of the nexus type as shown in Figure 13. It has been noted that peg and socket junctions are more often seen in relaxed muscle. A particularly good example of a peg and socket junction is seen in Figure 14. The intercellular gap measures 15 to 20 nm and the electron-dense material on the cytoplasmic face of the membrane is not associated with actin filaments, but with amorphous sarcoplasm. These junctions are very variable in size and shape, some seeming to mushroom into the receptive cell, others forming finger-shaped insertions.

2. Intermediate Junctions

These are characterized by electron-dense material on the cytoplasmic side of both membranes as reported by Gabella.[48] An example is shown in Figure 15. A gap junction is identified and labeled GJ. Just above and to the right of it a typical intermediate junction is seen. The intercellular gap is 30 to 40 nm wide and is thus much larger than that of a gap junction. The intermediate junction shows a band of dense material in its center; it is continuous with the basement membranes of the participating cells and seems to have a periodicity. Typically also the junction appears to be made by two sarcolemmal dense bands in participating cells, approaching each other. The junction may be equal in length to that of the dense bands, though usually it is somewhat smaller. In freeze-fracture preparations the membrane at these sites shows no specialization, and if anything a reduced number of intramembrane particles are seen.

3. Gap Junctions or Nexuses

These are perhaps the most important of the three and have been the subject of considerable research. These are areas of apposition of sarcolemmal membranes that are closer than those of the intermediate junctions. An example from the trachealis is shown in Figure 15, where it is labeled GJ. It must be pointed out that a gap junction can only be clearly recognized when the micrograph is of high magnification and a tilt stage has been used to explore the maximal dimensions of the gap. The gap is 2 to 3 nm in width and is composed of arrays of membrane proteins termed connexons, which, when open, provide intercellular channels. They are low-impedance pathways for cell to cell propagation of electrical activity. They are capable of passing molecules ranging from 800 to 1200 Da in molecular weight.[51,52] Daniel[53] has undertaken several careful studies of gap junctions. Figure 16 (panels A and B) is taken from one of his reports. It represents the electron microphotograph of a freeze-fractured smooth-muscle cell membrane. Each of the hillocks is evidently a single connexon[54] left after the fracture.

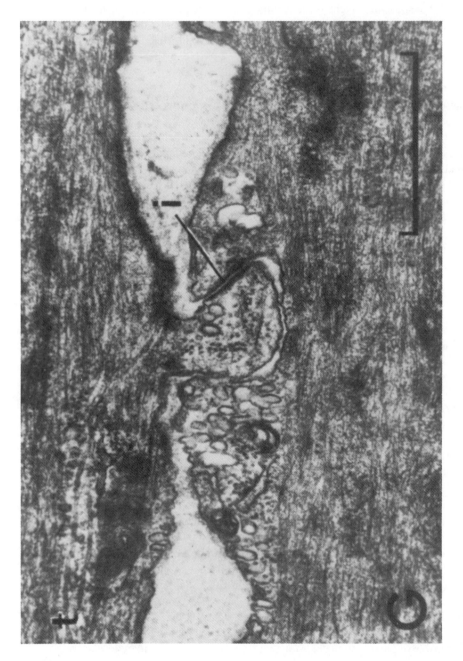

FIGURE 14.   Guinea pig taenia coli in longitudinal section. Cytoplasmic process of a muscle cell invaginating the surface of a neighboring cell. Between the two there is an intermediate junction (i). Microtubules (t) are seen in one of the two cells. Bar = 1 μm. (From Gabella, G., *Br. Med. Bull.*, 35, 213, 1979. With permission.)

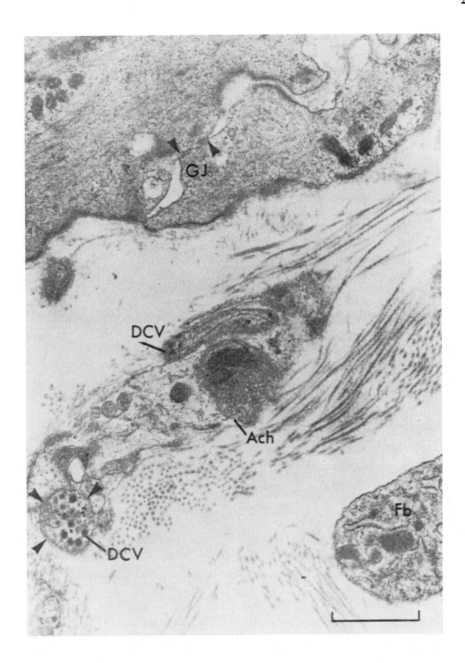

FIGURE 15. Electron micrograph of longitudinal sections of canine tracheal smooth muscle. GJ, gap junction; DC, dense cored vesicle; Ach, acetylcholine containing vesicles; Fb, fibroblast. (Magnification × 26,000.) (From Stephens, N. L., in *Asthma: Basic Mechanisms and Clinical Management*, Barnes, P. J., Rodger, I. W., and Thomson, N. C., Eds., Academic Press, NY, 1988, 11. With permission.)

The electrical conductance at the gap junction can be reduced by a drop in local pH. Whether this is a direct effect or due to increased ionization of calcium is not known. Certainly it is known that increased calcium concentration can reduce electrical conductance. It is also known that catecholamines, prostaglandin E_1 (PGE_1), and cyclic-AMP may enhance electrical conductance. A caveat must be entered to the effect that the presence of gap junctions does not, *a priori*, establish electrical continuity, and several investigators have

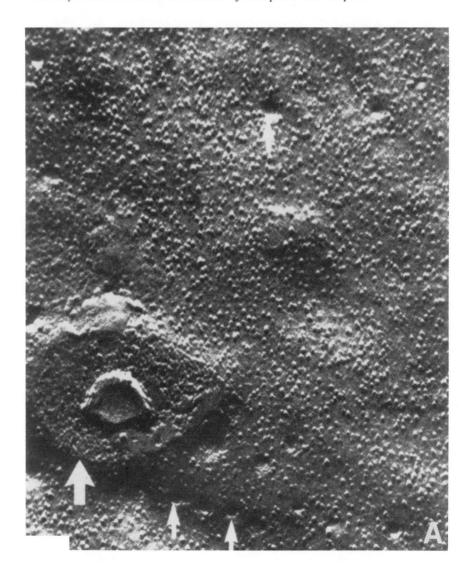

A

FIGURE 16.   Panels A and B. Two large gap junctions (large arrow) in parturient rat myometrium seen in freeze-fracture replicas of the PFC fracture face (protoplasmic face) of the cell·membrane. Note numerous necks of caveolae and membrane particles (small arrows). It is clear that not all membrane particles or small assemblies of particles can be identified as connexons. (From Garfield, R. E., Merrett, D., and Grover, A. K., *Am. J. Physiol.*, 239, C217, 1980. With permission.)

reported increased gap junctions with no change in electrical propagation. Gap junctions are known to increase in the near-term uterus, but are not the cause of increased electrical and mechanical activity, as these in fact precede the appearance of new junctions.

Studies by Stephens and Kroeger[46] and Kannan and Daniel[41] have shown that rhythmic mechanical and electrical activity can be induced within 10 min of the application of potassium conductance blockers such as tetraethylammonium chloride and 4-aminopyridine. This is associated (though perhaps not causally for the reasons just stated) with the induction of new gap junctions. The mechanism for this is not clear. Some have felt that it was not dependent on *de novo* synthesis of protein.[53] Others have implicated[55] protein synthesis, as the addition of cyclohexamide or actinomycin D inhibited the incorporation of [^{3}H] leucine into TCA-precipitable proteins and prevented gap junction formation.

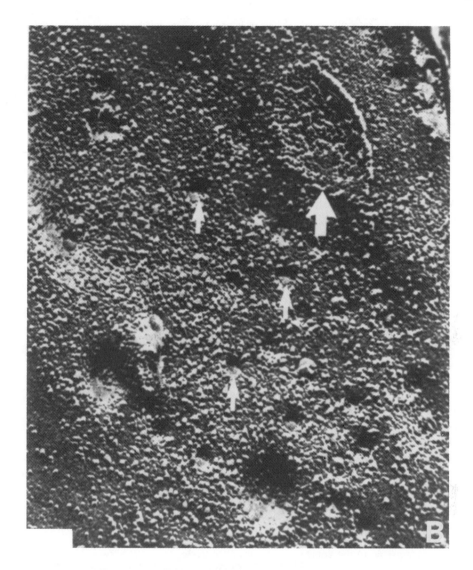

FIGURE 16B.

a. Species Distribution of Gap Junctions

Richardson and Ferguson[56] and Daniel et al.[57] have reported the presence of gap junctions in high density in human tracheal and first- and second-order bronchial smooth-muscle membrane. As one progresses down the airways, fewer gap junctions are found. In dogs, Daniel finds there is no diminution in gap junction density in the smaller bronchi. Bovine trachea appears to be of intermediate type, while the guinea pig trachea[58] differs almost radically in possessing rich innervation, but a paucity of gap junctions, and is thus more like a multiunit smooth muscle.

E. MITOCHONDRIA

These are of interest from two points of view. One is relatively minor and is centered on the question of the extent to which mitochondria are sources and sinks of calcium for ECC in smooth muscle. The current position seems to be that though they can undoubtedly take up calcium and in the process uncouple electron transport from oxidative phosphory-lation, this is only seen when Ca^{2+} levels are extremely high. Mitochondrial sequestration of calcium is therefore only seen under pathological conditions and plays a minor role under physiological conditions. The likelihood that the mitochondria are sources of calcium is very small.

The second point of view relates to energetics. It is well recognized that the role of oxidative phosphorylation in oxidative ATP production is much less important than in striated (specially slow) muscle. Nevertheless, because oxidation yields almost 12 to 18 times as much ATP as that produced by glycolysis, its role is not negligible.

Figure 17 shows an electron micrograph of a longitudinal section of canine tracheal smooth muscle. Two fairly large clusters of mitochondria are seen in adjacent cells. Mitochondria are reported to be located typically at the poles of the nucleus. However, this is not always so, and in about 30% of cells the mitochondria may be located elsewhere in the cytoplasm adjacent to the sarcolemma as shown in the upper cell in this figure. This cell also shows the close relationship between pinocytotic vesicles and mitochondria. One of the mitochondria is unusually long and serpiginous. Such mitochondria are seen in the frog sartorius muscle and hardly ever in smooth muscle. Sarcoplasmic reticular elements (SR) are also seen. Trachealis mitochondrial general shapes and dimensions are similar to those of hamster skeletal muscle. Those with clear pale interiors are large, and are probably the seat of swelling. The remainder are more electron dense and show normal cristae. From their general appearance they would be classified as belonging to Hackenbrock's[68] orthodox type. These are essentially inactive mitochondria that are not producing ATP, undoubtedly due to the fact that in fixing the tissue it became anoxic with resultant cessation of electron transport.

Actively respiring mitochondria are difficult to see in sectioned tissues unless fixation was carried out with oxygenated glutoaldehyde solution. The resting non-ATP-producing states (so-called state IV) and the active state (state III) can be easily demonstrated in isolated mitochondria. Figure 18 shows mitochondria isolated from canine tracheal smooth muscle[69] and fixed in state III. These are in what Hackenbrock has called "condensed state".

Our studies[69] have shown that tracheal smooth-muscle mitochondria phosphorylate oxidatively as well as those from skeletal muscle. Their ADP:0 ratios and respiratory control ratios (RCR) are similar. However, the major difference is that the amount of mitochondrial protein present per gram wet weight of muscle is only 10% of that in skeletal muscle, hence the phosphorylation capacity (amount of ATP synthesized oxidatively per unit wet weight of muscle) is only 10% of that in skeletal muscle. This leads to the conclusion that glycolysis plays a greater role in the energetics of smooth muscle.

There is another very important feature of smooth-muscle energetics. Paul[70] has shown that energy production in vascular smooth muscle is compartmentalized. It appears that ATP produced glycolytically is used to supply energy for membrane ionic pump function, while that produced oxidatively is used by the contractile apparatus.

F. GOLGI APPARATUS, LYSOSOMES

Figure 19 shows a Golgi body, adjacent to the nucleus of a tracheal smooth-muslce cell. It presents the typical features of Golgi apparatus in showing a series of vacuoles and saccules. They are seen in both the smooth-muscle cells and the epithelial cells.

Lysosomal bodies have not been found by us in normal tracheal smooth-muscle cells, except for the rare muscle cell. Paul et al.[71] have found considerable numbers of lysosomes in aortic smooth-muscle cells taken from chronically hypoxic piglets.

G. CONTRACTILE APPARATUS

This consists of contractile proteins, actin and myosin, which are organized into thin and thick filaments, respectively. There is also a regulatory protein system consisting of tropomyosin, which is associated with the actin filament. The second and more important

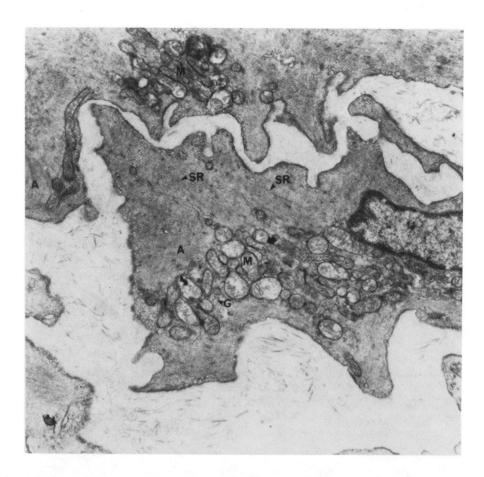

FIGURE 17. Electron micrograph of a longitudinal section of canine tracheal smooth muscle. Mitochondria (M) are seen arranged in clumps. Tubular sarcoplasmic reticular (SR) elements are clearly seen
also. The cell is isotonically contracted, and undulating bundles of actin filaments (A) are seen. Glycogen
(G) granules are present. (Magnification × 8100.) (From Stephens et al., *Physiology and Pharmacology
of the Airways,* Nadel, J. A., Ed., Marcel Dekker, New York, 1980. With permission.)

component of the regulatory system is the myosin light chain (mol wt 20,000 Da), which
resides in the globular head of the myosin molecule. It is phosphorylation of this chain via
a specific myosin light-chain kinase enzyme system that activates the myosin ATPase. The
regulatory components are not seen in the usual light and electron micrographs.

Finally, there is an intermediate filamentary or cytoskeletal system consisting of 10-nm
thick filaments. As thin filaments are about 5 nm in diameter and thick filaments are 15 nm
thick, one can see that the 10-nm filaments are intermediate; this is the basis of the terminology used.

Airway smooth muscle is so called because, like all other smooth muscles, it does not
present a regularly repeating sarcomere pattern of light and dark bands. In electron micrographs, while thin actin filaments are clearly seen filling the entire cytoplasm, the thick
myosin filaments (the major components of the dark bands) are very seldom visualized.

In low-power electron micrographs, actin filaments generally constitute the gray color-
ation of the cytoplasm. At somewhat higher power (Figure 9), in longitudinal sections, the
thin filaments (A) are clearly seen, as for example, in the second and third cells from the
top. The picture also shows dense bodies (DB) scattered across the cytoplasm; actin filaments
appear to run through the bodies. This is typical and responsible for the idea that the dense

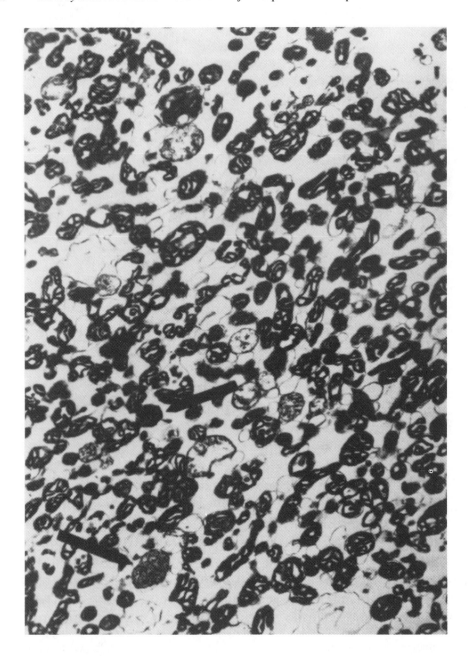

FIGURE 18.   Electron microscopy of mitochondria from canine trachealis smooth muscle. Material from pellet fixed in buffered osmium tetroxide (pH 7.4) and embedded in epoxy. (Magnification × 11,300.) (From Stephens, N. L. and Wrogemann, K., *Am. J. Physiol.*, 219, 1796, 1970. With permission.)

bodies are Z-disc analogs. Somlyo et al.[72] have shown by ''decorating'' actin filaments with myosin heads in a smooth-muscle cell that polar reversal of the myosin binding sites occurs across the dense body.

While the dense bodies appear randomly distributed, this is not so. Using α-actinin (a prominent component of Z-bands, dense bodies, and dense bands) fluorescent antibodies, Fay and Fogarty[73] have obtained improved visualization of the dense bands. With computer-aided imaging techniques, they deduced that these bands are fairly regularly arrayed and

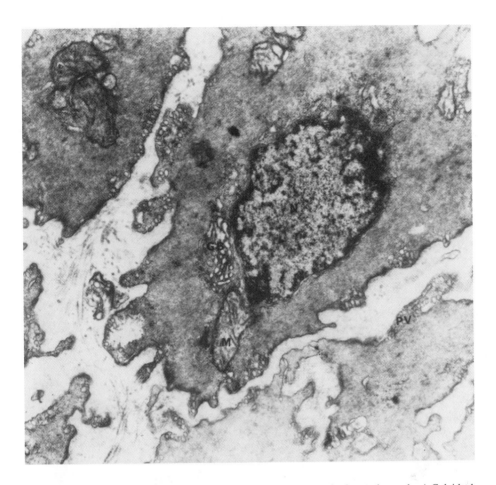

FIGURE 19. Electron micrograph of a transverse section of canine tracheal smooth muscle. A Golgi body (GB) is seen. In addition, this cell is a good example of the localization of pinocytotic vesicles (PV) to the cytoplasm in the sarcolemmal outpouchings; N, nucleus; PV, pinocytotic vesicles; M, mitochondrion. (Magnification × 18,000.) (From Stephens et al., *Physiology and Pharmacology of the Airway*, Nadel, J. A., Ed., Marcel Dekker, New York, 1980, 31. With permission.)

could be delimiting the boundaries of a "sarcomere". Measurements revealed the "sarcomere" length, as computed by the mean center to center distance between stained dense bodies, to be 2.2 ± 0.1 μm (SE). In pictures obtained from cells fixed while contracting in response to acetylcholine, the mean distance was reduced to 1.4 ± 0.1 μm (SE). From the behavior one could infer that the rest length of the sarcomere was 2.2 μm, and this shortened to 1.4 μm. This provided support for the idea that the sliding filament theory of contraction could be applied to smooth muscle also.

The further inference that the sliding of filaments is due to a cross-bridge mechanism was provided some support by electron micrographs of portal venous smooth muscle published by Somlyo et al.[72] See Figure 20, which was taken from their publication. Actin filaments are clearly visible, running parallel to each other and traversing the dense bodies (db). In between the thin filaments, thick filaments of varying length are seen. As in striated muscle, these thin and thick filaments are parallel to each other. Cross bridges can be seen extending from the thick filaments to the thin. Transversely arcing filaments are also seen that can be shown to run from dense band to dense band. These are the 10-nm intermediate filaments and consist of desmin, a cytoskeletal protein. Their role is speculated to be to stabilize the sarcomere by linking the dense bands. Such desmin links between Z-bands in

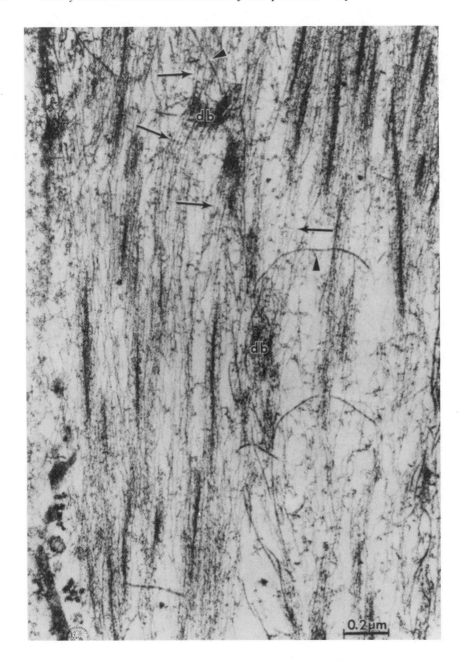

FIGURE 20.   Longitudinal section of a portal vein smooth-muscle cell briefly skinned with saponin and fixed in the presence of tannic acid. Actin filaments (small arrows) insert on both sides of the dense bodies (dbs) and run to the myosin filaments. The 10-nm filaments (arrowheads) are closely associated and surround the dense bodies (see db on the right). The 10-μm filaments connect the dense bodies rather than running parallel to the sarcomere unit. (From Somlyo, A. V., Bond, M., Berner, P. F., Ashton, F. T., Holtzer, H., and Somlyo, A. P., in *Smooth Muscle Contraction,* Stephens, N. L., Ed., Marcel Dekker, New York, 1984, 1. With permission.)

contiguous myofibrils are also seen in skeletal muscle. Desmin is the predominant cytoskeletal protein in intestinal tract smooth muscle. In vascular smooth muscle several cells stain with both desmin and vimentin antibodies. Furthermore, as reported by Somlyo, desmin is found predominantly in the rabbit renal vein and artery, while vimentin is found in the rabbit renal artery, vein, abdominal artery, and the main pulmonary artery. Another view is that different cytoskeletal proteins are found in different phases of growth, with vimentin being the developmental and desmin, the definitive.

The ratio of thin to thick filaments in smooth muscle is about 15:1 in rabbit portal vein. The ratio has not yet been quantified for tracheal smooth muscle.

Myosin is present in much smaller quantities in smooth muscle than in striated muscle, and in electron micrographs thick myosin filaments are not usually seen. However, when special precautions are taken they are seen in large numbers. The total myosin content is only one fifth of that of skeletal muscle, so how the smooth muscle can develop as much force as the skeletal muscle is not really understood. One possibility is that as the cycling rate of smooth muscle at the plateau of the isometric myogram is so low, actin-myosin contact time is greater than in skeletal muscle, thus allowing for greater force development.

Myosin has been extracted from smooth muscle and thick filaments made from it *in vitro*. These filaments qualitatively resemble those from striated muscle. They have tapering ends[74] and demonstrate the presence of globular beads that form cross bridges with actin, which has already been discussed. The mean length of the thick myosin filament is 2.2 μm, which is longer than the myosin filament of striated muscle. No bare area seems to exist. Because of these considerations there would be more cross bridges per half sarcomere in smooth muscle, which would partly explain the relatively greater strength of smooth muscle vis-a-vis the striated muscle. X-ray diffraction studies of smooth muscle have disclosed a 14.3 meridional reflection indicative of the presence of cross bridges as in striated muscle. Very little work has been carried out dealing with the structural properties of actin and myosin in airway smooth muscle. Figure 21 shows the presence of thick filaments in canine tracheal smooth muscle. Though the mechanical properties of airway smooth muscle indicate that the sliding filament model of contraction must be operative in airway smooth muscle, X-ray diffraction and appropriate electron micrographic studies have not been carried out.

H. THE NUCLEUS AND NUCLEAR MEMBRANE

In light microscopic pictures of smooth muscle the central cigar-shaped nucleus is typical. Figure 22 shows a longitudinal section of canine tracheal smooth muscle. The typical nuclei are seen running parallel to each other, suggesting that the cells are also parallel to each other.

Generally, Golgi bodies and mitochondria are situated at the nuclear poles, though this is not invariably so for mitochondria, as was pointed out before.

Nuclear detail is better in electron micrographs. Figure 23 shows a nucleus in the tangential section. The double-layered nuclear membrane is seen, as are occasional membrane pores. At rest the nuclear outline is smooth. During contraction the nucleus appears twisted (see Figure 9) with clefts cutting into the nuclear chromatin. The latter is darkly stained and collected mainly around the nuclear rim. One or two nucleoli are usually present in airway smooth-muscle cells (Figure 13). Studies in other cells have shown they contain RNA. The nucleolus is felt to be a link between the nucleus and the cytoplasm. Granules within the nucleonema of the nucleolus may be newly synthesized, ribosomal subunits.

I. INNERVATION

The major motor nerve of the upper airways of all mammalian species is the vagus with its chief, though not only, transmitter being acetylcholine. The status of the inhibitory system, the adrenergic, is not clear, and in humans there appear to be no adrenergic nerves. Adrenoreceptors are present and account for the remarkable relief afforded to asthmatics by noradrenaline and noradrenaline-like compounds.[72]

In recent times nonadrenergic, noncholinergic inhibitory (putative transmitter vasoactive intestinal polypeptide [VIP]) and excitatory nerves (putative transmitter substance P) have

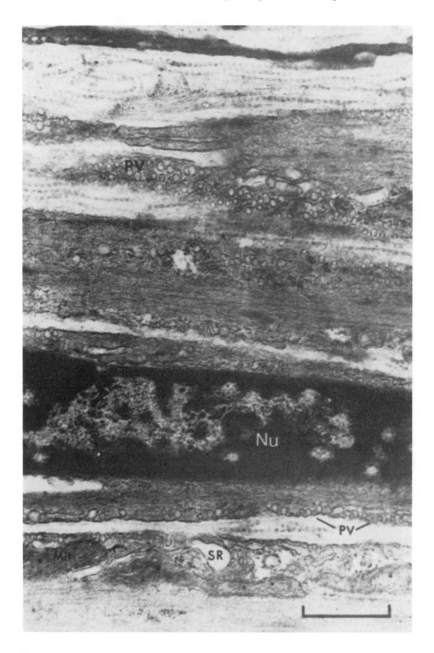

FIGURE 21.   Electron micrograph of a longitudinal section of relaxed canine tracheal smooth-muscle cells. The calibration bar is 2 μm long. Nu, nucleus; PV, pinocytotic vesicles; SR, sarcoplasmic reticulum; Mit, mitochondria. At the top of the section longitudinal collagen fibers are seen. The second and third cells from the top show myosin filaments. (From Stephens, N. L., *Asthma: Basic Mechanisms and Clinical Management,* Barnes P. J., Rodger, I. W., and Thomson, N. C., Eds., Academic Press, NY, 1988. With permission.)

been identified. In humans, perhaps the VIP system is the major relaxant system.

An ever increasing number of transmitters and peptides have been identified and the actions of the latter studied.[78]

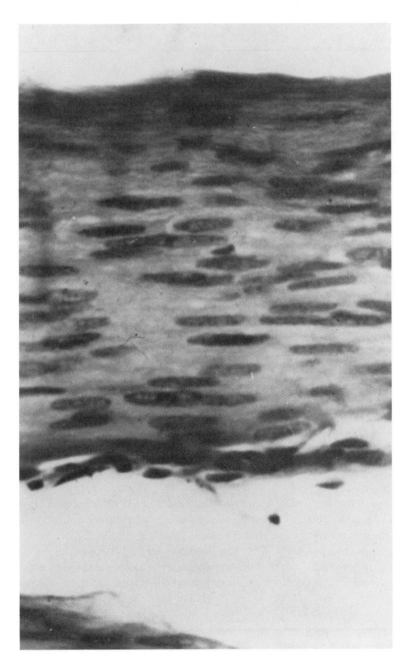

FIGURE 22. Light microscopy of canine tracheal smooth muscle. Section stained with hematoxylin and eosin. (Magnification × 800.) (From Stephens et al. in *Physiology and Pharmacology of the Airways*, Nadel, J. A., Ed., Marcel Dekker, NY, 1980, 31. With permission.)

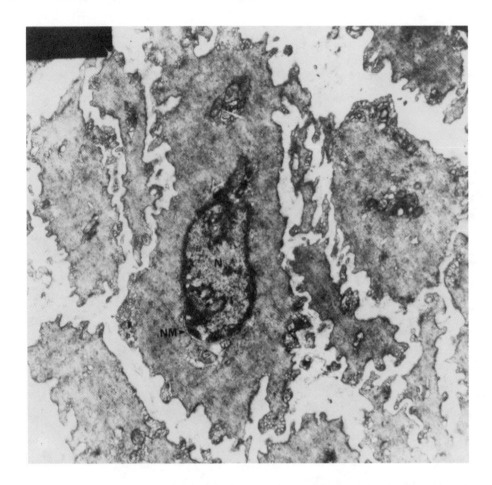

FIGURE 23.   Electron micrograph of a tangential section of a partially contracted tracheal smooth-muscle cell. N, nucleus; NM, nuclear membrane. (Magnification × 18,000.)

IV. HUMAN AIRWAY SMOOTH MUSCLE

Studies in this area need to be carried out urgently, certainly in greater number than heretofore. The major problem is in obtaining adequate amounts of suitable tissue. This is particularly true for tissue from asthmatic subjects. Most tissues are postmortem and show postmortem changes. Material obtained at surgery is generally from cancer patients who have been erstwhile cigarette smokers and whose airways are not really healthy.

In airway smooth muscle from humans[79,80] gap junctions are numerous in the central airways. As one proceeds down the airways their numbers diminish. Motor control in central airways is mainly cholinergic. The smaller airways respond predominantly to histamine and leukotrienes. Human airways possess adrenoreceptors, but these are not neurogenically controlled. The noncholinergic, adrenergic nervous system is the major relaxant in human airways. With respect to the morphology of smooth-muscle cells, their nuclei and organelles, human muscle resembles that from vertebrate airway smooth muscle.

V. CONCLUSION

In this review an attempt has been made to present the macroscopic and microscopic characteristics of the various tissues making up the airways. In addition to this, airway smooth muscle has been dealt with in detail. The changes in muscle structure that occur in models of early allergic bronchospasm have been delineated. They related mainly to density of gap junction distribution. In chronic disease, hypertrophy of smooth muscle, reduplication of epithelial cells, increase in goblet cells, and infiltration with lymphocytes and eosinophils are seen.

Work needs to be carried out using the more modern immunohistochemical techniques to define the structural properties of the contractile apparatus and the cytoskeletal, as these may provide insights into the pathogenesis of asthma.

ACKNOWLEDGMENTS

Thanks are due to Betty Moodie for expert assistance with typing. This study was supported by an operating grant from the American Council for Tobacco Research.

REFERENCES

1. **Stein, M.,** *New Directions in Asthma,* American College of Chest Physicians, Park Ridge, IL, 1975.
2. **Nadel, J. A., Ed.,** *Physiology and Pharmacology of the Airway,* Marcel Dekker, New York, 1980.
3. **Hargreave, F. E.,** *Airway Reactivity,* Astra Pharmaceuticals, Mississauga, Ontario, 1980.
4. **Jenne, J. W. and Murphy, S.,** *Drug Therapy for Asthma — Research and Clinical Practice,* Marcel Dekker, New York, 1987.
5. **Kaliner, M. J. and Barnes, P. J.,** *The Airways Neural Control in Health and Disease,* Marcel Dekker, New York, 1988.
6. **Barnes, P. J., Rodger, I. W., and Thomson, N. C., Eds.,** *Asthma: Basic Mechanisms and Clinical Management,* Academic Press, New York, 1988.
7. **Hayek, V. H.,** The Human Lung, *Hafner Publishing,* New York, 1960.
8. **Krahl, V. E.,** Anatomy of the mammalian lung, *Handbook of Physiology,* Vol. I, Fenn, W. O. and Rahn, H., Eds., American Physiology Society, Washington, D.C., 213.
9. **Weibel, E. R.,** *Morphometry of the Human Lung,* Springer-Verlag, Berlin, 1963.
10. **Weibel, E. R. and Gomez, D. M.,** A principle for counting tissue structures on random sections, *J. Appl. Physiol.,* 17, 393, 1962.
11. **Silva, D. G. and Ross, G.,** Ultrastructural and fluorescence histochemical studies on the innervation of the tracheo-bronchial muscle of normal cells and cats treated with 6-hydroxydopamine, *J. Ultrastruct. Res.,* 47, 310, 1976.
12. **Kirkpatrick, C. T.,** Excitation and contraction in bovine tracheal smooth muscle, *J. Physiol. (London),* 244, 263, 1975.
13. **Laitinen, A., Partanen, M., Hervonen, A., Pelto-Huikko, M., and Laitinen, L. A.,** VIP-like immunoreactive nerves in human respiratory tract, *Histochemistry,* 82, 313, 1985.
14. **Pack, R. J. and Richardson, P. S.,** The adrenergic innervation of the human bronchus: a light and electron microscopic study, *J. Anat.,* 138, 493, 1984.
15. **Murlas, C., Nadel, J. A., and Roberts, Jon,** The muscarinic receptors of airway smooth muscle: their characterization *in vitro, J. Appl. Physiol.,* 52, 1084, 1982.
16. **Barnes, P. J., Basbaum, C. B., and Nadel, J. A.,** Autoradiographic localization of autonomic receptors in airway smooth muscle: marked differences between large and small airways, *Am. Rev. Respir. Dis.,* 127, 758, 1983.
17. **Wharton, J., Polak, J. M., Bloom, S. R., Aurill, J., Brown, M. R., and Pearse, A. G. E.,** Substance P-like immunoreactive nerves in mammalian lung, *Invest. Cell Pathol.,* 2, 310, 1979.
18. **Cadieux, A., Springall, D. R., Mulderry, P. K., Rosrigo, J., Ghater, M. A., Terengli, K., Bloom, S.R., and Polak, J. M.,** Occurrence, distribution and ontogeny of CGRP-immunoreactivity in the rat lower respiratory tract: effect of capsaicin treatment and surgical denervations, *Neuroscience,* 19, 605, 1986.
19. **Cheung, A., Polak, J. M., Bauer, F. E., Cadiaix, A., Christofides, N., Springall, D. R., and Bloom, S. R.,** Distribution of galanin immunoreactivity in the respiratory tract of pig, guinea pig, rat and dog, *Thorax,* 40, 889, 1985.
20. **Springall, D. R., Bloom, S. R., and Polak, J. M.,** Distribution, nature and origin of peptide-containing nerves in mammalian airways in *The Airways: Neural Control in Health and Disease,* Kaliner, M. A. and Barnes, P. J., Eds., Marcel Dekker, New York, 1988, 299.

21. **Luschka, H.,** Anatomic des menschen, Vol. 1, *Abt. Z, Tubingen,* 1863.
22. **Schaffer, J.,** Das Epithelgewebe, in *Handbuch der mikroskopeschen, Anatomie des Menschen,* Vol. 2, Chap. 1, 1927.
23. **Macklin, C. C.,** Functional aspects of bronchial muscle and elastic tissue, *Arch. Surg.,* 19, 1212, 1929.
24. **Baltisberger, W.,** Über die glatte Muskulatur der menschlichen Lunge, *Z. Anat. Entwicklungsgesch.,* 61, 249, 1921.
25. **Hayek, H. V.,** Muskulatur der Bronchi und Bronchioli, *Wien. Klin. Wochenschr.,* 114, 1948.
26. **Otis, A. B.,** A perspective of respiratory mechanisms, *J. Appl. Physiol.,* 54, 1183, 1983.
27. **Macklem, P. and Engel, L. A.,** The physiological role of airways smooth muscle constriction, *Postgrad. Med. J. Suppl. 1,* 51, 45, 1975.
28. **Stephens, N. L., Kroeger, E. A., and Mehta, J. P.,** Force-velocity characteristics of respiratory airway smooth muscle, *J. Appl. Physiol.,* 26, 685, 1969.
29. **Stephens, N. L. and Van Niekerk, W.,** Isometric and isotonic contractions in airway smooth muscle, *Can. J. Physiol. Pharmacol.,* 55, 833, 1977.
30. **Brunings, W.,** Direkte Lanyngoskopie: Wiesbaden, 1910, in *The Human Lung,* Von Hayek, H., Ed., Hafner, New York, 1960, 344.
31. **Frohlich, F.,** Die "Helle Zelle" der Chemo-receptoren, *Frank. Z. Pathol.,* 60, 517, 1949.
32. **von Hayek, H. V.,** "Über einen Kurzschluss Kreislauf (arterio-venil Anastomosen) in den Menschlichen Lunge, *Ztselin. Anat. Entkoklsg.,* 110, 412, 1940.
33. **von Hayek, H. V.,** Reaktive Formveranderungen, *Z. Anat. Entwicklungsgesch.,* 115, 436, 1951.
34. **Kapanci, Y., Costabella, P. M., and Gabbiani, G.,** Location and function of contractile interstitial cells of the lungs, in *Lung Cells in Disease,* Bouhuys, A., Ed., Elsevier/North-Holland, Amsterdam, 1977, 69.
35. **Kapanci, Y., Assimacopoulus, A., Ire, C., Zwahlen, A., and Gabbiani, G.,** "Contractile interstitial cells" in pulmonary alveolar septa: a possible regulator of ventilation/perfusion ratio?, *J. Cell Biol.,* 60, 375, 2974.
36. **Low, R. B., Woodcock-Mitchell, J., Abeher, P. M., Evans, J. N., and Adler, K. B.,** Contractile proteins of the lung, *Curr. Probl. Clin. Biochem.,* 13, 149, 1983.
37. **Evans, J. N., Kelley, J., Low, R. B., and Adler, K. B.,** Increased contractility of isolated lung parenchyma in an animal model of pulmonary fibrosis induced by Allomycin, *Am. Rev. Respir. Dis.,* 125, 89, 1982.
38. **Richardson, J. B. and Beland, J.,** Nonadrenergic inhibitory system in human airways, *J. Appl. Physiol.,* 41, 764, 1976.
39. **Daniel, E. E., Daniel, V. L., Duchon, G., Garfield, R. S., Nicholas, M., Malhotra, S. K., and Oki, M.,** Is the nexus necessary for cell-to-cell coupling of smooth muscle, *J. Membr. Biol.,* 28, 207, 1976.
40. **Burnstock, G.,** Structure of smooth muscle and its innervation, in *Smooth Muscle,* Bulbring, E., Brading, A. F., Jones, A. N., and Tomita, T., Eds., Edward Arnold, London, 1970, 1.
41. **Kannan, M. S. and Daniel, E. E.,** Structural and functional study of control of canine tracheal smooth muscle, *Am. J. Physiol.,* 238, (Cell Physiol. 7), C27-C33, 1980.
42. **Stephens, N. L., Kroeger, E. A., and Kromer, U.,** Induction of myogenic response in tonic airway smooth muscle by tetraethylammonium, *Am. J. Physiol.,* 228, 628, 1975.
43. **Kroeger, E. A. and Stephens, N. L.,** Effect of TEA on tonic airway smooth muscle: initiation of phasic electrical activity, *Am. J. Physiol.,* 228, 633, 1975.
44. **Akasaka, K., Konno, K., Ono, Y., Mue, S., Abe, C., Kumagai, M., and Tse, T.,** A new electrode for electromyographic study of bronchial smooth muscle, *Tohoku J. Exp. Med.,* 117, 49, 1975.
44a. **Macklem, P.,** personal communication.
45. **Stephens, N. L. and Wrogemann, K.,** Oxidative phosphorylation in smooth muscle, *Am. J. Physiol.,* 219, 1796, 1970.
46. **Stephens, N. L. and Kroeger, E. A.,** Ultrastructure, biophysics and biochemistry of airway smooth muscle, *Physiology and Pharmacology of the Airways,* Nadel, J. A., Ed., Marcel Dekker, New York, 1980, 36.
47. **Suzuki, H., Morita, K., and Kuriyama, H.,** Innervation and properties of the smooth muscle of the dog trachea, *Jpn. J. Physiol.,* 26, 303, 1976.
48. **Gabella, G.,** Smooth muscle cell junctions and structural aspects of contraction, *Br. Med. Bull.,* 35(3), 212, 1979.
49. **Somlyo, A. V., Bond, M., Berner, P. F., Ashton, F. T., Holtzer, H., and Somlyo, A. P.,** The contractile apparatus: an update, in *Smooth Muscle Contraction,* Stephens, N. L., Ed., Marcel Dekker, New York, 1984, 1.
50. **Wang, K. and Ramirez-Mitchell, R.,** A network of transverse and longitudinal intermediate filaments is associated with sarcomeres of adult vertebrate skeletal muscle, *J. Cell. Biol.,* 96, 562, 1983.
51. **Flagg-Newton, J.,** The permeability of the cell-to-cell membrane channel and its regulation in mammalian cell junction, *In Vitro,* 16, 1043, 1980.
52. **Flagg-Newton, J. and Loewenstein, W. R.,** Experimental depression of junctional permeability in mammalian cell culture, *J. Membr. Biol.,* 50, 65, 1979.

53. **Daniel, E. E.,** Control of airway smooth muscle, in *The Airways Neural Control in Health and Disease,* Kaliner, M. A. and Barnes, P. J., Eds., Marcel Dekker, New York, 1988, 485.

54. **Revel, J. P., Nicholson, B. J., and Yancy, S. B.,** Chemistry of gap junction, *Annu. Rev. Physiol.,* 49, 263, 1985.

55. **Garfield, R. E., Merrett, D., and Grover, A. K.,** Gap junction formation and regulation in myometrium, *Am. J. Physiol.,* 239 (Cell Physiol. 8), C217, 1980.

56. **Richardson, J. B. and Ferguson, C. C.,** Neuromuscular structure and function in the airways, *Fed. Proc., Fed. Am. Soc. Exp. Biol.,* 38, 202, 1980.

57. **Daniel, E. E., Kannan, M. S., Davis, C., and Posey-Daniel, V.,** Ultrastructural studies on the neuromuscular control of human tracheal and bronchial muscle, *Respir. Physiol.,* in press.

57a. **Daniel, E. E.,** unpublished observations.

58. **Hoyes, A. D. and Barber, P.,** Innervation of the trachealis muscle in the guinea pig, *J. Anat.,* 130, 789, 1980.

59. **Devine, C. E., Somlyo, A. V., and Somlyo, A. P.,** Sarcoplasmic reticulum and excitation-contraction coupling in mammalian smooth muscle, *J. Cell. Biol.,* 52, 690, 1972.

60. **Somlyo, A. P., Smolyo, A. V., and Shuman, H.,** Electron probe analysis of vascular smooth muscle composition of mitochondria, nuclei and cytoplasm, *J. Cell Biol.,* 67, 316, 1980.

61. **Raeymackers, L. and Hasselbach, W.,** Ca^{2+} uptake, Ca^{2+}-ATPase activity, phosphoprotein formation and phosphate turnover in a microsomal fraction of smooth muscle, *Eur. J. Biochem.,* 116, 373, 1981.

62. **Bond, M., Kitazawa, T., Shuman, H., Somlyo, A. P., and Somlyo, A. V.,** Calcium release from and recycling by the sarcoplasmic reticulum in guinea pig smooth muscle, *J. Physiol.,* 355, 677, 1984.

63. **Kowarski, D., Shuman, H., Somlyo, A. P., and Somlyo, S. V.,** Calcium release by noradrenaline from central sarcoplasmic reticulum in rabbit main pulmonary artery smooth muscle, *J. Physiol.,* 366, 153, 1985.

64. **Somlyo, A. P., Somlyo, A. V., Kitazawa, T., Bond, M., Shuman, H., and Kowarski, D.,** Ultrastructure, function and composition of smooth muscle, *Ann. Biomed. Eng.,* 2, 579, 1983.

65. **Grover, A. K., Kannan, M. S., and Daniel, E. E.,** Canine trachealis membrane fractionation and characterization, *Cell Calcium,* 1, 135, 1980.

66. **Hogaboom, G. K. and Fedan, J. S.,** Calmodulin stimulation of calcium uptake and $(Ca^{2+}-Mg^{2+})$-ATPase activities in microsomes from canine tracheal smooth muscle, *Biochem. Biophys. Res. Commun.,* 99, 737, 1981.

67. **Sands, H. and Mascali, J.,** Effects of cyclic AMP and of protein kinase on the calcium uptake by various tracheal smooth muscle organelles, *Arch. Int. Pharmacodyn. Ther.,* 236, 180, 1978.

68. **Hackenbrock, C. R.,** Ultrastructurally linked basis for metabolically linked mechanical activity in mitochondria. I. Reversible ultrastructural changes with change in metabolic steady state in isolated liver mitochondria, *J. Cell Biol.,* 30, 269, 1966.

69. **Stephens, N. L. and Wrogemann, K.,** Oxidative phosphorylation in smooth muscle, *Am. J. Physiol.,* 219, 1796, 1970.

70. **Paul, R. J.,** Chemical energetics of vascular smooth muscle in *Handbook of Physiology,* Sec 2, Vol. II, Bohr, D. F., Somlyo, A. P., and Sparks, H. V., Jr., Eds., 1980, 201.

71. **Paul, R. J., Bauer, M., and Pease, D.,** Vascular smooth muscle: aerobic glycolysis linked to sodium and potassium transport processes, *Science,* 206, 1414, 1979.

72. **Somlyo, A. V., Bond, M., Berner, P. F., Ashton, F. T., Holtzer, H., and Somlyo, A. P.,** The contractile apparatus of smooth muscle: an update: in *Smooth Muscle Contraction,* Stephens, N. L., Eds., Marcel Dekker, New York, 1984, 1.

73. **Fay, F. S. and Fogarty, K.,** The organization of the contractile apparatus in single isolated smooth muscle cells, in *Smooth Muscle Contractions,* Stephens, N. L., Ed., Marcel Dekker, New York, 1984, 75.

74. **Ashton, F. T., Somlyo, A. V., and Somlyo, A. P.,** The contractile apparatus of vascular smooth muscle: intermediate high voltage stereo electron microscopy, *J. Mol. Biol.,* 98, 17, 1975.

75. **Shoenberg, C. F. and Hazelgrove, J. C.,** Filaments and ribbons in vertebrate muscle, *Nature,* 249, 152, 1974.

76. **Lowy, J., Poulsen, F. R., and Vibert, P. J.,** Myosin filaments in vertebrate muscle, *Nature,* 225, 1053, 1970.

77. **Daniel, E. E., Davis, C., Jones, T., and Kannan, M. S.,** Control of airway smooth muscle, in *Airway Reactivity,* Hargreave, F. E., Ed., Astra Pharmaceuticals, Mississagua, Ontario, 1980, 80.

78. **Barnes, P. J.,** State of art: neural control of human airways in health and disease, *Am. Rev. Respir. Dis.,* 134, 1289, 1986.

79. **Richardson, J. B. and Ferguson, C. C.,** Neuromuscular structure and function in the airways, *Fed. Proc., Fed. Am. Soc. Exp. Biol.,* 38, 202, 1980.

80. **Daniel, E. E., Davis, C., Jones, W. R., and Kannan, M. S.,** Control of airway smooth muscle, in *Airway Reactivity,* Hargreave, F. R., Ed., Astra Pharmaceuticals, Mississauga, Ontario, 1980, 80.

Chapter 2

BIOCHEMICAL REGULATION OF AIRWAY SMOOTH-MUSCLE TONE: AN OVERVIEW

Theodore J. Torphy and Douglas W. P. Hay

TABLE OF CONTENTS

I. Introduction 40

II. Contraction 40
    A.   Regulation and Function of Contractile Proteins 40
        1.   Calcium 40
        2.   Initiation of Contraction 41
        3.   Maintenance of Steady-State Tone: the ''Latch Bridge'' 42
        4.   Mechanisms of Latch Bridge Formation 43
        5.   Inconsistencies in the Proposed Model 44
    B.   Signal Transduction 44
        1.   Receptor/G-Protein Coupling 45
        2.   Phosphatidylinositol Turnover: IP_3 Formation 46
        3.   Phosphatidylinositol Turnover: DAG Formation and PKC Activation 47
        4.   Calcium Sources 49

III. Cyclic Nucleotide-Mediated Relaxation 50
    A.   Cyclic AMP 51
        1.   Signal Transduction 51
        2.   Cyclic AMP-Dependent Protein Kinase 51
        3.   Functional Effects 53
    B.   Cyclic GMP 54
        1.   Signal Transduction 54
        2.   Cyclic GMP-Dependent Protein Kinase 55
        3.   Functional Effects 55
    C.   Cyclic Nucleotide Phosphodiesterases 56

IV. Integration of Contractile and Relaxant Pathways 57
    A.   Background 57
    B.   Functional Antagonism 57
        1.   Definition 57
        2.   Description 58
        3.   Order of Addition: Prevention vs. Reversal of Contraction 58
        4.   Underlying Mechanisms of Functional Antagonism 59

V. Conclusion 60

References 60

I. INTRODUCTION

Historically, much of our knowledge concerning the biochemical regulation of airway smooth-muscle tone was inferred from studies conducted with other tissues, primarily vascular smooth muscle. Over the last several years, however, there has been a dramatic increase in the number of studies examining the molecular processes that regulate the function of airway smooth muscle *per se*. The results of these studies have served to highlight both the similarities and differences between airway and nonairway smooth muscles.

Several current in-depth reviews have appeared that outline the molecular events that regulate airway smooth muscle contractile activity.[1-4] Consequently, this topic will be discussed only to orient the reader and will not be dwelled upon. Instead, emphasis will be placed on new and sometimes controversial areas of research, including: (1) the roles of phosphoinositides, diacylglycerol, and protein kinase C; (2) factors in addition to myosin phosphorylation and cytosolic Ca^{2+} content that may regulate contraction; and (3) processing and integration of simultaneous contractile and relaxant inputs.

This chapter is intended to provide a foundation for understanding the molecular processes that regulate airway smooth-muscle tone. It also is hoped that this review will underscore the fact that although our knowledge of this subject has increased substantially, it is far from complete.

II. CONTRACTION

A. REGULATION AND FUNCTION OF CONTRACTILE PROTEINS

Over the last decade, great strides have been made in understanding the biochemical basis for the regulation of smooth-muscle tone. Before 1975 a commonly held, but incorrect, concept was that smooth-muscle contraction was regulated in the same manner as striated muscle. The regulation of contraction in striated muscle is actin-based with Ca^{2+} playing a *permissive* role. At rest, the regulatory protein tropomyosin sterically inhibits the interaction of actin and myosin. The binding of Ca^{2+} to troponin, a tropomyosin-associated Ca^{2+} binding protein, induces a conformational change in tropomyosin. This conformational change eliminates steric hindrance such that actin can activate myosin ATPase, which, in turn, leads to muscle shortening.[5]

In contrast to the tropomyosin-based regulation of striated muscle, Ca^{2+} triggers contraction of smooth muscle by increasing myosin ATPase activity through activation of a phosphorylation cascade. Thus, Ca^{2+} has an *initiatory* role, rather than a permissive role, in smooth muscle.

1. Calcium

The molecular events that regulate airway smooth-muscle tone are depicted schematically in Figure 1. As in all muscle types, a rise in cytosolic Ca^{2+} content triggers contraction. As will be described in detail in Section II.B, contractile agonists interact with cell-surface receptors to stimulate the influx of extracellular Ca^{2+}, the release of intracellular Ca^{2+}, or both. Measurement of relative levels, if not precise molar concentrations, of cytosolic Ca^{2+} in smooth muscle has been made possible by employing techniques to detect the bioluminescence of aequorin or the fluorescence of fura-2 after treatment of cells or whole tissues with these Ca^{2+} indicators. Such studies have revealed a unique characteristic of the kinetics of agonist-induced changes in cytosolic Ca^{2+} levels in smooth muscle. Specifically, Ca^{2+} levels do not increase monotonically in response to contractile agonists, but rather reach a maximum within 1 min after agonist addition before declining to much lower levels over the next 5 min. This transient increase in Ca^{2+} content is observed in vascular,[7,8] gastrointestinal,[9] and airway smooth muscle.[10-12] An important observation emerging from these

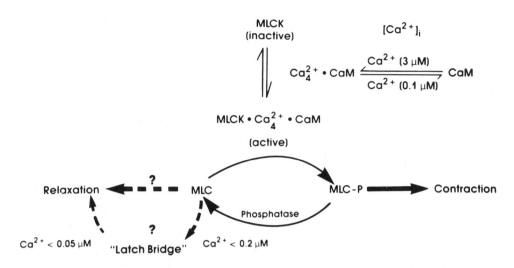

FIGURE 1. Activation of the contractile apparatus in smooth muscle. As the cytosolic concentration of Ca^{2+} $[Ca^{2+}]_i$) rises over a range of 0.1 to 3 μM, it binds to calmodulin (CaM). The active $Ca^{2+} \cdot$ CaM complex then binds to and activates myosin light chain kinase (MLCK). MLCK phosphorylates myosin light chain (MLC), which permits actin to activate myosin MgATPase. The resultant increase in cross-bridge turnover rate leads to muscle shortening and the establishment of tone. Even with the continued presence of the contractile agonist $[Ca^{2+}]_i$ rapidly falls, sometimes approaching the resting level (0.1 μM). Under these conditions, MLCK is inactivated and phosphatases dephosphorylate MLC. Tone is nonetheless maintained, perhaps by the formation of latch bridges. Latch bridges are dephosphorylated, slowly cycling cross bridges that maintain tension in the presence of low concentrations of cytosolic Ca^{2+} (approximately 0.05 to 0.2 μM). (From Torphy, T. J., *Rev. Clin. Basic Pharmacol.*, 6, 61, 1987. With permission.)

studies is that isometric force, unlike Ca^{2+} content, increases monotonically in response to contractile agonists and remains stable even as cytosolic Ca^{2+} content falls.

Although it is relatively safe to assume that cytosolic Ca^{2+} levels are low in resting cells and increase in contracting cells, precise measurement of cytosolic free Ca^{2+} concentrations is problematical. Nonetheless, reasonable estimates can be made. For example, data from skinned tracheal smooth muscle indicate that the threshold Ca^{2+} concentration is between 0.05 and 0.1 μM, whereas maximal contractile force is achieved with approximately 1 μM Ca^{2+}.[13] By analogy, the basal free Ca^{2+} content in intact smooth-muscle cells is 0.05 μM and increases to 1 μM during maximum agonist stimulation. Inferences from experiments with skinned smooth muscle are tenous, however, inasmuch as the precise amount of Ca^{2+} needed to activate the contractile apparatus varies with the concentration of intracellular Ca^{2+} binding proteins (e.g., calmodulin) present in the tissue,[13,14] and the concentration of these binding proteins is often changed by the skinning procedure. Nonetheless, estimates of Ca^{2+} content from studies with skinned airway smooth muscle are reasonably consistent with measurements made using fura-2.[11] Based upon results using this fluorescent Ca^{2+} indicator, the resting free Ca^{2+} concentration in cultured bovine tracheal smooth-muscle cells is 165 nM. Upon challenge with a maximal concentration (10 μM) of carbachol, the Ca^{2+} concentration increases to approximately 500 nM after 10 s before returning to an intermediate level (300 nM) by 60 s.[11]

2. Initiation of Contraction

The biochemical steps leading to force generation in smooth muscle have been reviewed in detail elsewhere.[1-4,6] Consequently, to serve as a foundation for subsequent discussions, only a brief description of these events will be provided here.

As the cytosolic Ca^{2+} concentration increases above baseline it binds to calmodulin, a ubiquitous intracellular receptor for Ca^{2+}. Calmodulin is a 16.7-kDa protein containing four

Ca^{2+} binding sites, each with a dissociation constant for Ca^{2+} in the micromolar range.[15,16] The binding of Ca^{2+} elicits a conformational change in calmodulin that exposes a hydrophobic binding region.[15,16] The hydrophobic region can then bind to and activate several different enzymes.[17] Thus, activation of calmodulin represents a key event by which Ca^{2+} regulates a variety of cellular processes.

One enzyme activated by Ca^{2+}/calmodulin is myosin light-chain kinase (MLCK). In mammalian airway smooth muscle, MLCK has a molecular weight of 160 kDa and is probably associated with both the thick (myosin) and thin (actin) filaments.[18,19] The endogenous substrate for MLCK is myosin light chain (MLC), a 20-kDa protein that resides on the myosin head. In both purified enzyme systems and intact tracheal smooth muscle, MLCK phosphorylates MLC at one serine and one threonine residue.[20-22] In intact smooth muscle, the amount of MLC monophosphorylated at the serine residue greatly exceeds the diphosphorylated form suggesting that phosphate incorporation into serine is more important physiologically.[22] Regardless, phosphorylation of MLC increases the maximum velocity of actin-activated myosin MgATPase activity several-fold and may also increase the ability of myosin to bind actin.[23,24] The net result is an increase in the cross-bridge turnover rate leading to muscle shortening (i.e., contraction) via the classic sliding filament model.[5,6]

At any instant the extent of MLC phosphorylation, and consequently myosin MgATPase activity, is determined by the relative rates of phosphorylation and dephosphorylation. A number of unique MLC phosphatases have been isolated from turkey gizzard and extensively characterized.[25,26] MLC phosphatase activity also has been isolated from airway smooth muscle, although it has not been characterized in depth.[27]

One question relating to the regulation of airway smooth-muscle contraction that has not yet been discussed concerns the quantitative relationship between the cytosolic free Ca^{2+} content and MLC phosphorylation. As discussed previously, free Ca^{2+} concentrations in airway smooth muscle range from 165 nM in resting tissue to 500 nM after stimulation with maximal concentrations of contractile agonists.[11] Is this range of Ca^{2+} concentrations adequate to regulate MLCK activity, MLC phosphorylation, and contraction in intact airway smooth muscle? This question has been addressed in an elegant study conducted by Taylor and Stull.[11] These investigators used fura-2 to determine cytosolic free Ca^{2+} concentrations in contracting bovine tracheal cells and correlated these values with the degree of MLC phosphorylation. In these studies, the relationship between Ca^{2+} content and MLC phosphorylation had a Hill coefficient of 2.7, indicating a marked degree of positive cooperativity. In fact, this positive cooperativity could be predicted by several intracellular biochemical parameters relating to: (1) the existence of multiple Ca^{2+} binding sites on calmodulin; (2) the absolute and relative cellular concentrations of calmodulin and MLCK; and (3) the increased affinity of Ca^{2+} for calmodulin produced as a result of the Ca^{2+}/calmodulin complex binding to MLCK.[14] Regardless, the net effect of this positive cooperativity is that small increases in free cytosolic Ca^{2+} can lead to a substantial increase in MLC phosphorylation.

3. Maintenance of Steady-State Tone: the "Latch Bridge"

In vitro studies indicating that MLC phosphorylation greatly enhances actin-activated myosin MgATPase activity led to the proposal of a simple, but intellectually satisfying model for the regulation of smooth-muscle contraction. This model held that an increase in cytosolic Ca^{2+} content leads to an activation of MLCK which, in turn, phosphorylates MLC. The muscle then contracts and tone is maintained until the cytosolic Ca^{2+} content decreases, thus reducing the activity of MLCK. Under these conditions, the activity of MLC phosphatases would lead to a net dephosphorylation of MLC, inactivation of myosin MgATPase, and relaxation.

The results of studies that carefully detailed the time course of agonist-induced MLC phosphorylation *in situ* in intact porcine carotid artery,[28-30] bovine trachealis,[31] and rabbit trachealis[32] were not consistent with the proposal outlined above. These experiments demonstrated that MLC undergoes rapid phosphorylation during the onset of contraction, but the phosphorylation is not sustained. Thus, steady-state tone is maintained in the face of falling levels of MLC phosphorylation. Steady-state tone nonetheless remains Ca^{2+} dependent, inasmuch as Ca^{2+} removal will result in relaxation.

In retrospect, it is easy to explain the transient nature of MLC phosphorylation following the exposure of smooth muscle to contractile agonists. This phenomenon is simply a reflection of transient increases in cytosolic free Ca^{2+} (see Section II.A.1). Not as readily apparent, however, is the mechanism by which smooth muscle maintains steady-state tension at the same time that MLC dephosphorylation is leading to "inactivation" of the contractile apparatus. To resolve this dilemma, Dillon and co-workers[29] suggested that force can be maintained by nonphosphorylated cross bridges called "latch bridges". Presumably, these latch bridges cycle at a very slow rate and are maintained as long as Ca^{2+} remains above some unspecified threshold concentration, a concentration below that necessary to activate calmodulin and MLCK.[33,34] Thus, MLC phosphorylation does not directly regulate steady-state force. Instead, MLC phosphorylation is thought to modulate muscle shortening velocity which, in turn, is a reflection of actomyosin ATPase activity.[29,30,34,35] According to this model, one population of rapidly cycling phosphorylated cross bridges is responsible for muscle shortening and the *establishment* of tone, whereas a second population of slowly cycling dephosphorylated cross bridges, or latch bridges, is responsible for the *maintenance* of steady-state tone. Note that this model implies that Ca^{2+} regulates contraction at two sites: (1) a low-affinity site (calmodulin) that modulates shortening velocity and is involved in the initiation of contraction and (2) a high-affinity site (latch bridge) that maintains tension as the cytosolic Ca^{2+} concentration declines. This paradigm is attractive teleologically inasmuch as reduced myosin MgATPase activity during tonic contraction would be reflected in a substantially reduced energy consumption. This is consistent with experimental results demonstrating the ability of smooth muscle to maintain active tension for prolonged periods at low metabolic cost.[36,37]

4. Mechanisms of Latch Bridge Formation

A major unresolved issue relating to the latch bridge hypothesis concerns the precise molecular mechanism by which latch bridges are formed. One attractive possibility involves caldesmon, an actin-associated protein with a molecular weight of approximately 140 kDa.[38,39] In its nonphosphorylated form, caldesmon both inhibits actin-activated myosin MgTPase activity and cross links actin and myosin filaments.[40,41] Phosphorylation by a Ca^{2+}/calmodulin-dependent enzyme, perhaps caldesmon itself, prevents caldesmon from binding to myosin.[42,43] Thus, in its unphosphorylated form, caldesmon may be responsible for latch bridge formation. However, as the concentration of Ca^{2+} rises and calmodulin is activated, caldesmon would be phosphorylated, thereby inactivating the latch state. This, of course, would occur simultaneously with MLC phosphorylation and the generation of phosphorylated, rapidly cycling cross bridges.

An alternative proposal holds that MLC phosphorylation is by itself necessary and sufficient to support the generation of latch bridges.[44] According to this hypothesis, the detachment rate of dephosphorylated cross bridges is substantially less than that of phosphorylated cross bridges. Thus, tension is maintained for a prolonged period even after MLC has been dephosphorylated.

Finally, an involvement of protein kinase C in latch bridge formation has been proposed based upon the activity of phorbol esters (activators of protein kinase C) in skinned vascular smooth muscle.[45] In these experiments, phorbol esters induced high stress in the presence of Ca^{2+} concentrations that alone could support neither the same degree of stress nor MLC phosphorylation. Potential physiologically relevant substrates for protein kinase C include MLC[46] and caldesmon.[47]

Whether one or more of the mechanisms discussed above contributes to latch bridge formation is not clear. It seems unlikely, however, that MLC phosphorylation is the primary mechanism regulating cross-bridge cycling and contraction. Hopefully, future studies will resolve this issue.

5. Inconsistencies in the Proposed Model

Very few areas of biological research are without controversies or inconsistencies. The regulation of smooth-muscle contraction is not among them. The results of several studies do not fit easily into the model proposed above. For example, contracting canine trachealis strips with muscarinic agonists produces a substantial and prolonged elevation of MLC phosphate content (i.e., the phosphorylation transient is subtle at best), even though short-ening velocity increases only transiently.[48-50] Indeed, studies with canine trachealis indicate that steady-state MLC phosphorylation is better correlated with isometric force than with shortening velocity.[48,51] Moreover, carbachol and serotonin increase MLC phosphorylation in Ca^{2+}-depleted canine trachealis without eliciting contraction, thus dissociating the phos-phorylation of MLC from both Ca^{2+} and force generation.[52] A lack of correlation between MLC phosphorylation and shortening velocity also is observed in K^+-depolarized swine carotid artery.[53] Finally, Siegman and co-workers[54] have reported that MLC phosphorylation remains elevated, while energy consumption and shortening velocity fall during electrically stimulated tetanic contractions of rabbit taenia coli.[54] In addition, increasing extracellular Ca^{2+} from 1.9 to 4.5 mM in preparations undergoing tetanic stimulation causes an increase in both shortening velocity and energy consumption without a concomitant increase in MLC phosphorylation.[54] This suggests that myosin MgATPase activity can be regulated by a direct action of Ca^{2+} on the contractile element as well as through a Ca^{2+}-dependent phosphory-lation mechanism.

Clearly, substantive issues regarding the roles of Ca^{2+} and MLC phosphorylation in regulating smooth-muscle function have yet to be resolved.

B. SIGNAL TRANSDUCTION

A variety of neurotransmitters and hormones influence the level of tone in airways following interaction with specific receptors located on the smooth-muscle cell membrane. The sequence of events and pathways responsible for the effects of contractile agents will be discussed in this section.

Interaction of an agonist with its membrane receptor initiates a complex sequence of events that ultimately leads to the functional response. Research indicates that in many systems, including smooth muscle, this signal-transduction process is initiated by the binding of the agonist-receptor complex to a guanine nucleotide-binding protein (G protein). The binding of the agonist-receptor complex activates the G protein, which then stimulates phospholipase C-mediated hydrolysis of phosphatidylinositol (PI), specifically PI bisphos-phate, which results in the formation of the intracellular second messengers, inositol 1,4,5-trisphosphate (IP_3) and 1,2-diacylglycerol (DAG). IP_3 mobilizes Ca^{2+} from intracellular stores, whereas DAG activates a Ca^{2+}-dependent, phospholipid-dependent protein kinase (protein kinase C[PKC]) which phosphorylates a variety of intracellular substrates.[55-57] Dis-cussion of this pathway will be separated into three sections: (1) receptor/G-protein coupling; (2) IP_3 formation and Ca^{2+} release; and (3) DAG production and PKC activation. Whenever possible, discussion will focus on findings in airway smooth muscle. It should be emphasized, however, that most of the information pertaining to these cellular signal transduction path-ways emanates from research conducted in nonsmooth-muscle systems. In addition, a sum-mary will be given of the research, largely using isolated smooth-muscle preparations, detailing the extracellular and intracellular sources of Ca^{2+} and the Ca^{2+} translocation processes that mediate contraction of airways.

1. Receptor/G-Protein Coupling

Research in recent years has provided evidence that membrane-associated G proteins play a critical role in membranal and transmembranal signal transduction mechanisms. These signal transduction mechanisms are responsible for a variety of cellular functions and effects, including regulation of ion channel activity, cell growth, vision, metabolic responses, intracellular second messenger formation, exocytosis, and phospholipase activity.[58-63] Several G proteins have been identified and characterized. They appear to be closely related heterotrimeric guanosine triphosphatases consisting of three subunits, designated α, β, and γ. In general, the β and γ subunits of different G proteins are quite similar. The unique nature of distinct G proteins is instead conferred by differences in the α subunits.

The following simplified sequence of events describes the mechanism of action of G proteins in modulating cellular function. The interaction of an agonist with its membrane receptor promotes the dissociation of GDP from the α subunit of the G protein, which increases the exchange of GDP for GTP. The binding of GTP to the G protein causes the dissociation of the $\beta\gamma$ subunits from the α subunit. This results in an activation of the α subunit, which can then interact with and modify the activity of the appropriate effector systems. G-protein activation is terminated through the hydrolysis of GTP by a GTPase present in the α subunit, which then reassociates with the $\beta\gamma$ subunits to form the inactive $\alpha\beta\gamma$ heterotrimer to complete the cycle.[58,59,61,63,64] This cycle of activation and inactivation will persist as long as the agonist is present.

The various G proteins have been studied and characterized experimentally with the use of (1) specific bacterial toxins, such as cholera and pertussis; (2) nonhydrolyzable analogs of GTP; (3) specific antisera against G proteins and individual subunits; and (4) oligonucleotide probes. The most widely researched G proteins are the stimulatory and inhibitory G proteins linked to the adenylate cyclase system, designated G_s (activated by cholera toxin) and G_i (inhibited by pertussis toxin), respectively,[65] and G_t (transducin), the G protein coupled to cyclic GMP-specific phosphodiesterase in retinal rod outer segments.[66] With regard to the present discussion, recent evidence suggests that a specific G protein is associated with phospholipase C, and thus is involved in the coupling between receptor activation, the formation of the intracellular second messengers IP_3 and DAG, and smooth-muscle contraction.[60,67,68] This G protein, designated G_p, has yet to be identified or purified, and direct activation of phospholipase C by a G protein remains to be demonstrated.[60,63,67,68] Nonetheless, GTP and nonhydrolyzable GTP analogs have been shown to stimulate the release of products of polyphosphoinositide breakdown in numerous systems including permeabilized platelets,[68] mast cells,[69] neutrophils,[70] smooth muscle,[71] and hepatocytes.[72] Furthermore, GTP analogs potentiate hormone-induced stimulation of phospholipase C.[71,73,74] Pertussis toxin has been used to attempt to identify the G protein controlling activation of PI turnover.[58,59,61] The results indicate that pertussis toxin inhibits receptor-mediated PI hydrolysis in some, but not all, cellular systems.[56,60,67,70,75] Differential susceptibility of receptor-mediated PI turnover to inhibition with cholera toxin has also been observed.[58,59,61] These data suggest that the G protein which couples receptor-mediated PI turnover is different from those that have been characterized to date.[69,75]

Although pertussis toxin markedly attenuates α_2-adrenoceptor-induced vasoconstriction in rats *in vivo*,[76] presumably by uncoupling α_2-adrenoceptor occupation with phospholipase C activation, there is no information on the effects of GTP or its analogues, or the bacterial toxins on agonist-induced PI turnover and contraction in airway smooth muscle. Nevertheless, the apparent integral role of the PI turnover pathway in this tissue (see Sections II.B.2. and II.B.3) suggests that G proteins play a vital role in signal transduction mechanisms in airways.

An important area of research will be the delineation of the G protein(s) responsible for regulating contraction of airway smooth muscle. It will be of interest to determine whether or not there are differences in the G proteins involved in receptor-phospholipase C activation in airway smooth muscle compared to inflammatory cells and vascular smooth muscle. Another fertile area for investigation is the role of G proteins (e.g., G_o) that are postulated to affect K^+ and Ca^{2+} membrane channel function in nonairway systems[77-79] in controlling the level of tone in airway smooth muscle.

2. Phosphatidylinositol Turnover: IP_3 Formation

The pioneering research of Hokin and Hokin[80] over 30 years ago demonstrated that acetylcholine stimulates ^{32}P incorporation into membrane phospholipids. Since this initial observation there has been a great deal of research investigating the stimulatory effects of agents on membrane phospholipid metabolism in numerous cellular systems. However, it is only within the last 15 years or so that the physiological importance and precise biochemical mechanisms underlying these experimental observations have been elucidated.[56,57,81] Thus, it is recognized now that stimulation of inositol lipid metabolism by hormones, neurotransmitters, and other stimuli plays a critical role in signal transduction mechanisms that control a range of cellular functions, including contraction, secretion, metabolism, phototransduction, and cell growth.[56,57,81]

The formation of the water-soluble IP_3 and the lipid-soluble DAG results from agonist-stimulated activation of phospholipase C and the consequent hydrolysis of PI 4,5-bisphosphate (PIP_2). The simultaneous formation of two intracellular second messengers which produce an array of effects results in a complex, yet flexible bifurcating system for the regulation of signal transduction processes and cellular functions following receptor activation.

It was initially hypothesized by Michell[82] that there is a link between agonist-induced increase in inositol lipid turnover and mobilization of intracellular calcium. Subsequent research supported this contention and provided convincing evidence that the trigger for intracellular release of calcium is IP_3, which, once formed from PIP_2, is released into the cytosol. Thus, it was first reported, using permeabilized rat pancreatic acinar cells, that submicromolar concentrations of IP_3 produce a rapid release, followed by slow reuptake, of Ca^{2+}.[83] Similar findings were observed in vascular[84-86] and airway[87] smooth muscles. Several experimental observations, including the use of metabolic inhibitors and cell fractionation techniques, indiate that the endoplasmic reticulum is the site of IP_3-induced Ca^{2+} release.[56,57,81] The mechanism whereby IP_3 produces Ca^{2+} release awaits clarification, although evidence suggests that IP_3 acts via a specific receptor to increase Ca^{2+} efflux from the endoplasmic reticulum, while having no effect on Ca^{2+} uptake into the organelle.[56,57,81,88,89] IP_3-induced Ca^{2+} release is temperature independent[90] and not inhibited by calcium channel inhibitors and other drugs affecting Ca^{2+} translocation.[91] There is some evidence for a G-protein coupling of IP_3-induced Ca^{2+} release from sarcoplasmic reticulum, although this has to be clarified.[56,92,93] Specific binding sites for IP_3 have been identified,[94,95] and the purification and characterization of an IP_3 receptor isolated from rat brain has been reported.[96]

Other than IP_3, there are numerous water-soluble inositol phosphates produced as a result of the hydrolysis of PIP_2, those of which have aroused the most interest being inositol 1,3,4,5-tetrakisphosphate (IP_4), the cyclic phosphates, and inositol 1,3,4-trisphosphate.[56,57,81,97] The physiological role of these products is unknown, although it can be envisaged that they act as additional second messengers contributing to the complex and versatile control of signal transduction and cellular functions associated with PIP_2 metabolism.

There have been a limited number of studies examining agonist-induced stimulation of the PI pathway in airway smooth muscle. In the first report, contraction of canine trachealis produced by carbachol was associated with an atropine-sensitive stimulation of PI turnover, as reflected by a decrease in the PI pool, an elevation in DAG and phosphatidic acid pools, and enhanced incorporation of $^{32}PO_4$ into PI.[98] No effect was observed with KCl, which induces a contraction that is primarily dependent on extracellular Ca^{2+} influx (see Section II.B.4). These data led to the proposal that pharmacomechanical coupling in airways, a process which involves intracellular Ca^{2+} mobilization, may be mediated by PI metabolism.[98] Similar findings were reported by Hashimoto and co-workers[87] using the same tissue, who observed that within 10 s 10μM acetylcholine markedly stimulated IP_3 formation, concomitant with a reduction in the amount of PIP_2 and stimulation of the levels of phosphatidic acid.[87] Serotonin (10 μM, but not histamine (10 μM) or prostaglandin $F_{2\alpha}$ ($PGF_{2\alpha}$) (0.1 μM) also stimulated PI metabolism.[87] Consistent with its proposed second messenger role, IP_3 causes a concentration-dependent (EC_{50} = 0.8 μM) release of Ca^{2+} from saponin-permeabilized tracheal smooth-muscle cells.[87] In a preliminary communication analyzing the temporal correlation between formation of inositol phosphates and contraction, it was reported that acetylcholine (10 μM) increases IP_3 levels in canine tracheal smooth muscle 1 s after addition, a time at which there is no significant contractile response.[99] Stimulation of PI metabolism has been reported for several agonists in bovine and guinea pig airways and also in cultured sheep airway smooth-muscle cells.[100-105]

It is noteworthy that cholinergic agonists and tachykinins induce contraction of bovine[101] and guinea pig[103] trachealis at concentrations 3 to 4 log units lower than those necessary to stimulate PI metabolism. One obvious interpretation of this finding is that contraction is not causally linked to IP_3 and DAG production. Alternatively, and perhaps more likely, this observation may reflect a large receptor reserve for these agonists, or a significant amplification step between PI hydrolysis and the eventual contraction.[103] In support of the receptor reserve postulate, the use of different concentrations of phenoxybenzamine to inactivate an increasing fraction of receptors, in addition to binding data, has revealed the presence of significant numbers of spare muscarinic receptors.[101] In contrast, these same procedures indicate that in bovine trachealis there are few or no spare receptors for histamine, which possesses a similar potency for eliciting contraction and stimulating PI turnover.[106]

Collectively, the above data provide relatively convincing evidence that the rapid agonist-induced degradation of phosphoinositides and formation of IP_3 are involved in the initiation of the contractile response to several bronchoconstrictor agents in mammalian airway smooth muscle. The role of IP_3 and other water-soluble inositol phosphates in the maintenance of contraction is uncertain. In addition, the importance of PI turnover in contraction of human airway smooth muscle, although likely, has not been reported.

3. Phosphatidylinositol Turnover: DAG Formation and PKC Activation

As indicated above, the other primary product of PIP_2 hydrolysis following receptor activation is DAG, a neutral lipid that is localized to the plasma membrane and whose main effect is the activation of a specific protein kinase, designated protein kinase C (PKC). PKC is a ubiquitous enzyme that has an absolute requirement for Ca^{2+} and a phospholipid, particularly phosphatidylserine, for activity.[56,57,107,108] PKC, which is a single polypeptide with two functionally distinct domains, has been shown to exist in several isozymic forms in different regions of the brain.[109,110] The molecular heterogeneity of this large family of proteins has recently been proposed to extend to seven subspecies of the kinase, some of which appear to possess differences in enzymological properties and expression, in addition to tissue distribution.[109-111] The physiological substrates, intracellular locations, and functional properties of the individual forms of PKC remain to be determined.

DAG markedly increases the affinity of PKC for Ca^{2+}, such that the enzyme becomes fully active without any net change in the intracellular Ca^{2+} concentration.[112] In most unstimulated cells, PKC is located in the cytosol.[56,108] Upon receptor stimulation the enzyme is translocated in a Ca^{2+}-dependent manner to the plasma membrane where it binds to phosphatidylserine.[56,108] Following activation, PKC phosphorylates intracellular proteins, and in this manner can alter cellular function. *In vitro* studies indicate that PKC phosphorylates a plethora of proteins, but it remains to be determined which of these serve as cellular substrates in intact cells and thus have physiological significance.[56,108]

Much of the information pertaining to the biological effects of the DAG/PKC pathway has been obtained from studies in a variety of systems utilizing phorbol esters, tumor-promoting agents that activate PKC.[108,111,113,114] However, although they are useful pharmacological tools to investigate the cellular effects of PKC activation, caution should be exercised in the interpretation of such data in view of the possibility that there may be other targets for these agents, especially when used in high concentrations.[56,108] In addition, a more fundamental consideration is that following receptor activation, DAG is normally produced only transiently before its degradation. Thus activation of PKC only occurs for a limited period. In contrast, phorbol esters intercalate into the membrane, are stable, degraded slowly, and cause prolonged activation of PKC[108,115] Accordingly, the observed experimental effects of phorbol esters may be, at least in part, a consequence of the sustained, rather nonphysiological stimulation of the enzyme.

Stimulation of canine[85,98] and bovine[100] trachealis with carbachol produces a rapid and, unlike in most other systems, sustained elevation in the levels of DAG or its degradation product, phosphatidic acid, concomitant with a reduction in contents of PIP_2 and an increase in the amount of water-soluble inositol phosphates, including IP_3. The changes in lipid mass are observed up to 60 min after stimulation, are Ca^{2+}-independent, and are not produced by exposure to elevated K^+.[98,100] The EC_{50} value for carbachol-induced alterations in PIP_2 hydrolysis and phosphatidic acid formation are similar (5 and 3 μM, respectively), but approximately 15- to 30-fold higher than the value for eliciting contraction. As indicated above, this may reflect the existence of a receptor reserve and significant amplification between generation of DAG and IP_3 and the ultimate physiological response.

Rasmussen and co-workers[116-118] proposed that activation of PKC in smooth muscle is responsible for the sustained phase of the contractile response, whereas IP_3 formation, intracellular Ca^{2+} release, and the resultant activation of Ca^{2+}/calmodulin-dependent enzymatic cascade are largely responsible for the initiation of the contraction. This hypothesis is based on the observation that administration of the Ca^{2+} ionophores, A23187 or ionomycin, alone produces a rapid but transient contraction, whereas the addition of a phorbol ester alone produces a sustained response that is slow to develop. The combination of calcium ionophore and phorbol ester produces a biphasic contraction which is similar in profile and magnitude to that elicited by carbachol.[117] In further support of this hypothesis, both carbachol and phorbol ester-induced contraction of bovine trachea are associated with phosphorylation of the same proteins.[119] However, the carbachol-induced elevation in the level of IP_3 in this tissue is sustained rather than transient.[100] which is not entirely consistent with its role being limited to the initiation of contraction. Furthermore, one study with rabbit aorta suggests that PKC plays only a minor role in maintaining smooth-muscle tone.[120] Rather surprisingly, phorbol ester-induced contractions of vascular tissues are associated with Ca^{2+} influx and are sensitive to inhibition by calcium channel inhibitors.[118,121] Furthermore, there is apparent synergy between phorbol esters and agents that activate voltage-dependent calcium channels.[56,118,121,123] Whether this represents a direct effect of phorbol esters on the membrane Ca^{2+} channel, is a consequence of activation of PKC, or is due to some other action remains to be determined.

It must be emphasized, however, that stimulation of the DAG/PKC pathway has been shown to inhibit PI turnover and agonist-induced elevation in intracellular Ca^{2+} in a variety of systems.[54] For example, in primary cultures of canine trachealis myocytes, phorbol 12-myristate 13-acetate abolishes histamine-induced release of intracellular Ca^{2+}.[124]

Although there is evidence for a role of the DAG/PKC pathway in the regulation of tone in several types of smooth muscles, the precise mechanism(s) and the relative importance of this system remain to be delineated. Furthermore, there is conflicting evidence as to whether the DAG/PKC system has a stimulatory or inhibitory influence. This may be related in part to the experimental limitations with phorbol esters. A major concern with the use of phorbol esters is that contraction elicited by these agents generally is observed only after a long latency period — up to 70 min[118]—whereas contraction produced by agonists known to induce PIP$_2$ hydrolysis occurs within seconds. It should be recognized, however, that the time to initiate contraction may depend markedly on the specific phorbol ester used.[123]

After being formed, DAG is rapidly metabolized via two different pathways to produce phosphatidic acid and arachidonic acid.[56,57,108] Phosphatidic acid has been postulated to act as a Ca^{2+}-ionophore[125] and products of arachidonic acid metabolism, including leukotrienes and prostanoids, produce a variety of effects in numerous tissues, including airway smooth muscle.[126]

A major objective of research delineating the importance of phospholipid metabolism in mediating contraction of airway smooth muscle will be the determination of the relative and temporal contributions of IP$_3$ and DAG, and the elucidation of the communication that exists between them. One issue to be resolved is whether or not the IP$_3$ and DAG/PKC pathways act in a complementary and synergistic manner to produce contraction of airway smooth muscle, with the former responsible for the initiation of contraction and the latter the maintenance of contraction.[56,57] In addition, the potential inhibitory effect of the DAG/PKC system on PI turnover and Ca^{2+} mobilization in airways needs to be clarified. The availability of potent and selective antagonists of IP$_3$, DAG, and PKC will assist greatly in these endeavors.

Although not addressed here, there is evidence that phospholipids other than PI/PIP$_2$ may be hydrolyzed following receptor activation to produce second messengers including DAG; the biological effects and physiological relevance of this are uncertain.[56,78,127]

4. Calcium Sources

The preceding discussion has dealt with the complex biochemical events and signal transduction mechanisms associated with the contraction of smooth muscle. Smooth-muscle contraction is dependent on the translocation of Ca^{2+} from extracellular and/or intracellular sources.[128] It has been postulated that the agonist-induced influx of Ca^{2+} from the extracellular compartment occurs through at least two different membrane channel types, voltage-dependent Ca^{2+} channels (VDCs) and receptor-operated Ca^{2+} channels (ROCs).[128,129] VDCs are activated by stimuli, most notably high K^+ solutions, that produce a reduction in the membrane potential, resulting in increased permeability to Ca^{2+}. Calcium influx through VDCs is attenuated by classical calcium channel inhibitors.[128] In many smooth muscles, activation of VDCs results in generation of action potentials, whereas in airway smooth muscle, stimulation of VDCs results in a graded depolarization of the membrane.[2,128,130] On the other hand, ROCs are stimulated by agonists that interact with specific membrane receptors. Activation of ROCs generally occurs with little or no change in membrane potential and is not affected appreciably by classical calcium channel inhibitors.[2,128,130] Activation of VDCs has been termed "electromechanical coupling", whereas activation of ROCs has been termed "pharmacomechanical coupling".[128,130,131]

In smooth muscle, the relative contribution of electromechanical and pharmacomechanical coupling and the relative importance of extracellular vs. intracellular Ca^{2+} sources to the contractile response depends on a variety of different factors, including species, the particular smooth muscle, the contractile stimulus and its concentration, and the specific phase of the contraction.[2,128,132,133] In airways there also may be regional differences.[133]

There are several potential intracellular sites for Ca^{2+} mobilization, although the predominant sources utilized under physiological conditions appear to be the endoplasmic reticulum and the inner surface of the plasma membrane.[128] A hitherto largely unrecognized source of Ca^{2+} involved in contraction of airways may be cartilage.[133,134]

In isolated smooth muscle a number of routine experimental procedures and standard agents can be utilized to delineate the excitation-contraction coupling mechanisms responsible for contraction produced by a given agonist. These include: (1) Ca^{2+}-deprivation studies; (2) ^{45}Ca flux measurements; (3) use of agents that affect extracellular or intracellular Ca^{2+} translocation; (4) fluorescent Ca^{2+}-sensitive dyes; and (5) electrophysiological analysis. Information from such experiments conducted in airway smooth muscle provide convincing evidence that, although differences do exist, contractile responses produced by agonists rely predominantly on the mobilization of Ca^{2+} released from intracellular stores, rather than the influx of Ca^{2+} from the extracellular environment.[2,130,133] Thus, in isolated airway smooth muscle from a variety of animals the contractile response produced by what can be termed "physiological" agonists, including acetylcholine, leukotrienes, and, to a lesser extent, histamine, are relatively resistant to the effects of classical calcium channel inhibitors and removal of Ca^{2+} from the external medium, and are not normally associated with stimulation of ^{45}Ca influx.[2,130,133] These findings suggest strongly that contractions produced by such agonists do not involve influx of appreciable amounts of extracellular Ca^{2+}, even though these agents produce membrane depolarization.[130] However, in view of the limitations of present-day techniques used for the measurement of Ca^{2+} influx, the possible involvement of transmembrane influx of a small amount of "trigger" Ca^{2+}, via ROCs insensitive to calcium channel inhibitors, cannot be dismissed.[130] These findings and conclusions are generally supported by the limited studies performed *in vivo* in experimental animals.[133] In contrast, contractions produced by "nonphysiological" agonists, such as KCl and tetra-ethylamine, are mediated largely by influx of significant amounts of Ca^{2+} via VDCs, as reflected by the associated increase in ^{45}Ca uptake and the attenuation of contraction by removal of extracellular Ca^{2+} and by calcium channel inhibitors.[2,130,133]

The above findings in animal airways appear to extend to human tissues. That is, there seems to be minor involvement of extracellular Ca^{2+} influx in eliciting contraction of human airways produced by agonists that interact with specific receptors.[133] For example, responses to cholinergic agonists, leukotrienes, and, to a lesser extent, histamine are less sensitive to inhibition by calcium channel inhibitors or Ca^{2+} deprivation than those elicited by KCl.[133,135-137] Furthermore, the VDC activator BAY k 8644 potentiates KCl-induced but not agonist-induced contraction of human bronchus.[138] These *in vitro* observations are supported by clinical studies which highlight the minimal efficacy of calcium channel inhibitors against bronchoconstriction elicited by a variety of stimuli.[133]

In summary, the data accumulated from *in vitro* and *in vivo* studies provide convincing evidence that agonist-induced contraction of mammalian airway smooth muscles is mediated predominantly by the mobilization of Ca^{2+} from intracellular stores, a generalization that is corroborated by findings that several agonists stimulate IP_3 production in airways. But differences between agonists exist in terms of the relative utilization of intracellular vs. extracellular Ca^{2+}. The development of specific inhibitors of ROCs as well as improved techniques for the detection of influx of small amounts of Ca^{2+} will greatly assist the elucidation of the importance of ROCs in excitation-contraction coupling mechanisms in airways.

III. CYCLIC NUCLEOTIDE-MEDIATED RELAXATION

The role of cyclic nucleotides in regulating smooth-muscle function has been the subject of scientific investigation for over 25 years. Although certain aspects of cyclic nucleotide function in smooth muscle remain unknown or even contentious (e.g., the identity of functionally relevant substrates for cyclic nucleotide-dependent protein kinases), one premise has gained virtually universal acceptance. That is, adenosine $3':5'$ cyclic monophosphate (cAMP) and guanosine $3':5'$ cyclic monophosphate (cGMP) act as second messengers to mediate smooth-muscle relaxation.[139-141] The evidence supporting a second messenger role for cyclic nucleotides specifically in airway smooth muscle has been reviewed extensively[4,6] and will not be presented here. Instead, this section will focus on the regulation of cyclic nucleotide content in airway smooth muscle and the biochemical mechanisms whereby cyclic nucleotides mediate their relaxant action.

A. CYCLIC AMP

1. Signal Transduction

Several endogenous (e.g., epinephrine, vasoactive intestinal polypeptide, prostaglandin E_2, prostacyclin) and exogenous (e.g., β_2-adrenoceptor agonists) bronchodilators are thought to act by a common mechanism. As depicted in Figure 2, these agents relax airway smooth muscle by interacting with cell-surface receptors to increase the generation of cAMP. In airway smooth muscle, as in other tissues, cAMP generation is under the dual regulatory control of both stimulatory (G_s) and inhibitory (G_i) G proteins. As described in Section II.B.1, receptor ligands that stimulate adenylate cyclase activity do so by promoting the binding of GTP to G_s. The G_s-GTP complex then activates adenylate cyclase, which converts MgATP into cAMP. Removal of the agonist inactivates G_s and adenylate cyclase activity returns to its basal state. Intracellular cAMP content then falls, primarily by phosphodiesterase-mediated metabolism of cAMP to $5'$-adenosine monophosphate (see Section III.C).

As mentioned above, adenylate cyclase activity in airway smooth muscle is also controlled by G_i. For example, muscarinic receptor stimulation inhibits adenylate cyclase activity in canine trachealis membrane preparations.[142] Muscarinic agonists also reduce agonist-stimulated cAMP content in intact canine trachealis strips[143,144] and cultured canine tracheal smooth-muscle cells.[145] Pertussis toxin eliminates the ability of muscarinic agonists to inhibit adenylate cyclase,[145] thus supporting a role for G_i in mediating the inhibitory effect. It would not be surprising to find that various other neurotransmitters, hormones, and autacoids also inhibit adenylate cyclase activity in airway smooth muscle, although this possibility has not been explored in a systematic manner.

2. Cyclic AMP-Dependent Protein Kinase

The intracellular target for cAMP in eukaryotic cells is cAMP-dependent protein kinase.[146-148] This tetrameric enzyme (R_2C_2) is composed of two identical catalytic subunits (C) along with two identical regulatory subunits (R) that each contain two high-affinity cAMP binding sites (see Figure 2). When the intracellular concentration of cAMP is low, the R subunits are tightly bound to the C subunits, thus inhibiting enzyme activity. As cellular cAMP content rises, it binds to the R subunits. Once all four binding sites on the R dimer are occupied by cAMP, a conformational change occurs that leads to the release and activation of the C subunits. In the intact cell, it is estimated that cAMP concentrations of approximately 1 μM must be reached to elicit half-maximal activation of cAMP-dependent protein kinase.[149] As will be discussed (Section III.A.3), cAMP-dependent protein kinase alters cellular activity by phosphorylating and consequently changing the activity of specific proteins (e.g., enzymes, receptors, ion channels).

As the intracellular concentrations of cAMP drops following the inactivation of adenylate cyclase, cAMP dissociates from the R subunit, which then rebinds to and inactivates the C subunit. The biologic response to cAMP is then terminated following the dephosphorylation of the relevant proteins by phosphoprotein phosphatases.[146,147]

cAMP-dependent protein kinase exists in two forms, designated type I and type II. The difference between these isozymes resides entirely in the structure and activity of the R subunits; the C subunits are identical.[148] The proportion of these isozymes can differ dra-

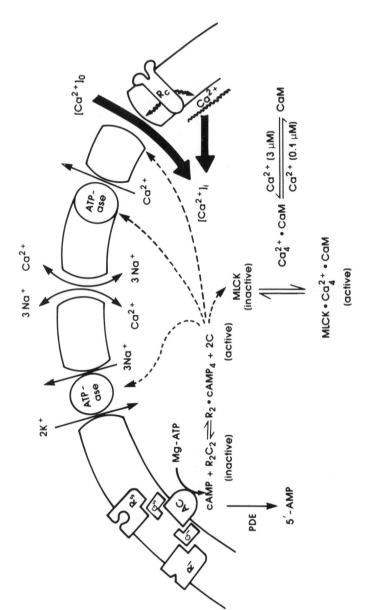

FIGURE 2. Biochemical mechanism of cAMP-mediated relaxation of smooth muscle. The interaction of relaxant agonists (e.g., epinephrine, prostaglandin E₂, vasoactive intestinal polypeptide) with specific cell-surface receptors (Rs) promotes the coupling of the stimulatory guanine nucleotide-binding protein (Gs) to adenylate cyclase (AC). The binding of Gs to AC increases the catalytic conversion of MgATP to cyclic AMP (cAMP). Cyclic AMP binds to and activates cAMP-dependent protein kinase (R₂C₂). The dashed lines represent hypothetical mechanisms by which the active catalytic subunit (C) of cAMP-dependent protein kinase can induce relaxation. These mechanisms include (1) a decrease in myosin light chain kinase (MLCK) activity; (2) a decrease in Ca²⁺ influx through voltage-dependent Ca²⁺ channels; (3) an increase in Ca²⁺ sequestration; and (4) an activation of Na⁺, K⁺-ATPase. An analogous pathway (not shown) exists for the guanylate cyclase/cGMP-dependent protein kinase cascade system. Other abbreviations: PDE, phosphodiesterase; Rᵢ, hormone receptor coupled to AC in an inhibitory manner; Gᵢ, inhibitory guanine nucleotide-binding protein; CaM, calmodulin; Rc, receptor for a contractile agonist. (From Torphy, T. J. and Gerthoffer, W. T., *Current Topics in Pulmonary Pharmacology and Toxicology*, Vol. I, Hollinger, M. A., Ed., Elsevier, Amsterdam, 1986, 2. With permission.)

matically among tissues and species. Canine trachealis, for example, contains equal amounts of each isozyme,[150] whereas bovine trachealis contains type II cAMP-dependent protein kinase almost exclusively.[151] Whether or not the differences in the R subunits are important physiologically is unknown. Krebs and Beavo[147] have suggested that relative affinities for cAMP and subcellular distribution — type I is primarily cytosolic, whereas type II is membrane bound — may represent functionally important differences between type I and type II isozymes. Autophosphorylation of type II holoenzyme, but not type I, also may represent an important distinction. Autophosphorylation of the R subunit of type II cAMP-dependent protein kinase decreases the affinity of the R subunit for the C subunit, thus favoring dissociation and activation of the holoenzyme.[148] That autophosphorylation may have a regulatory role *in vivo* is suggested by a study indicating that autophosphorylation of the type II isozyme in intact bovine trachealis is regulated by β-adrenoreceptor agonists and forskolin.[152]

3. Functional Effects

Relaxation of smooth muscle can occur via two general mechanisms: (1) reduction of cytosolic free Ca^{2+} concentration or (2) direct inhibition of contractile protein function. Evidence exists suggesting that cAMP can act through both of these mechanisms. The former mechanism is supported by data indicating that isoproterenol and forskolin can both prevent and reverse carbachol-induced rises in cytosolic Ca^{2+} (as measured by fura-2) in isolated bovine tracheal smooth-muscle cells.[153] This effect is observed, however, only if the relaxants are added shortly before (within 2 min) or after (within 10 s) the exposure of cells to carbachol.[153] If added alone for periods in excess of 2 min, isoproterenol causes a concentration-dependent *increase* in cytosolic Ca^{2+} in these cells.[153] Although difficult to explain, this unexpected finding may reflect a preferential accumulation of fura-2 in a subcellular compartment into which Ca^{2+} is being sequestered in response to β-adrenoreceptor stimulation.

Hypothetically, activation of the adenylate cyclase/cAMP/protein kinase cascade could reduce the cytosolic Ca^{2+} concentration by several mechanisms. Indeed, evidence supports the existence of at least three distinct pathways. In vascular[154,155] and uterine[156] smooth muscle, phosphorylation by cAMP-dependent protein kinase of one or more microsomal (M_r = 44 to 48 kDa) proteins is associated with an energy-dependent increase in vesicular Ca^{2+} uptake. However, a similar association has not been detected in microsomes prepared from airway smooth muscle,[157,158] perhaps because of differences in methodology.[140] Regardless, these results support the suggestion that increases in cAMP can induce smooth-muscle relaxation by promoting the export of Ca^{2+} across the sarcolemma or the uptake of Ca^{2+} into the sarcoplasmic reticulum. Activation of Na-K ATPase has been proposed as an additional mechanism of cAMP-induced relaxation of gastrointestinal,[159] vascular,[160] and airway smooth muscle.[161] An increase in Na-K ATPase activity could induce relaxation both by membrane hyperpolarization and by increasing Ca^{2+} extrusion across the sarcolemma through the Na^+-Ca^{2+} exchange.[159,161] Finally, using rabbit aortic smooth muscle, Meisheri and van Breemen[162] have proposed that cAMP inhibits Ca^{2+} influx through voltage-dependent Ca^{2+} channels.

Regulation of agonist-stimulated PI turnover represents another hypothetical mechanism by which cAMP could regulate cytosolic Ca^{2+} levels in airway smooth muscle. Thus far, conflicting results have been obtained in studies addressing this possibility. In bovine trachealis, isoproterenol does not reduce inositol monophosphate accumulation in response to several contractile agonists, including histamine, carbachol, and serotonin, when added 20 min before the spasmogens.[102] In contrast, simultaneous addition of a β-adrenoreceptor agonist (norepinephrine) and contractile agents to bovine trachealis reduces inositol phosphate accumulation in response to histamine, but not carbachol.[163] Although difficult to explain, the apparent inconsistency of these results may stem from the use of different β-adrenoreceptor agonist pretreatment times.[163]

Sparrow and co-workers[13] demonstrated that addition of the free catalytic subunit of cAMP-dependent protein kinase to skinned guinea pig trachealis both prevents and reverses Ca^{2+}-induced tension. Since removal of a functional cell membrane in these preparations prevents the tissue from regulating cytosolic Ca^{2+} content, this result strongly suggests that cAMP-dependent protein kinase can directly regulate the contractile element.

Investigations into the potential role of cAMP in mediating a direct inhibition of the contractile element have centered on the regulation of MLCK activity. Using immunoprecipitation techniques, de Lanerolle and co-workers[164] have demonstrated that forskolin-induced relaxation of methacholine-contracted canine trachealis strips is associated with phosphate incorporation into MLCK and a parallel dephosphorylation of MLC.[51] *In vitro* studies indicate that in the absence of Ca^{2+}/calmodulin, bovine tracheal MLCK can be phosphorylated by cAMP-dependent protein kinase at two sites.[18] Phosphorylation of both sites substantially reduces the affinity of MLCK for Ca^{2+}/calmodulin, which in effect reduces the Ca^{2+} sensitivity of MLCK.[18] In the presence of Ca^{2+}/calmodulin, cAMP-dependent protein kinase can phosphorylate only one site on MLCK, which is not sufficient to alter the affinity of MLCK for Ca^{2+}/calmodulin.[18] Presumably, then, this pathway would be activated most easily when cytosolic Ca^{2+} content is low. Keeping in mind that MLC phosphorylation is presumed to be important for the establishment, but not maintenance, of tone, inactivation of MLCK should be most effective at preventing rather than reversing contraction. In fact, the opposite is true in airway smooth muscle, since β-adrenoreceptor agonists reverse ongoing contractions much more effectively than they inhibit the establishment of contraction,[165] a phenomenon discussed in Section IV.B.3. Moreover, treatment of bovine tracheal smooth muscle with isoproterenol does not change the affinity of Ca^{2+}/calmodulin for MLCK, nor does it result in MLC dephosphorylation.[166] Thus, the role of MLCK phosphorylation in regulating airway smooth-muscle tone remains contentious.

Although it may be attractive to assume that a sole biochemical mechanism accounts for cAMP-mediated relaxation of airway smooth muscle, such an assumption is probably unfounded. Instead, it is likely several pathways act in concert to mediate the relaxant response to cAMP. Accordingly, attempts to identify a single, critical mechanism by which cAMP induces relaxation are likely to be fruitless.

B. CYCLIC GMP
1. Signal Transduction

The biochemical mechanism by which cGMP mediates smooth-muscle relaxation is analogous to the cascade system described for cAMP. The mechanism of guanylate cyclase activation, however, is different from adenylate cyclase activation. Two types of guanylate cyclase exist, a soluble form and a particulate form.[167,168] Nitric oxide, the common active product to which nitrovasodilators (e.g., sodium nitroprusside, hydroxylamine, nitroglycerin) are thought to be converted within the cell, chemically activates the soluble form of guanylate cyclase.[167,168] This activation may occur via a free-radical interaction with a heme moiety on the enzyme.[167,168] Recently, endothelium-derived relaxant factor (EDRF) has been identified as nitric oxide.[169]

Little is known about the regulation of the particulate guanylate cyclase. However, this enzyme is activated by atrial natriuretic factor,[170] an endogenous peptide hormone with vasodilator and diuretic properties. The receptor for atrial natriuretic factor co-purifies through several steps with particulate guanylate cyclase activity,[171] suggesting that both the receptor and enzyme exist on a single transmembrane protein. If this is indeed the case, then G proteins may not be involved with coupling the atrial natriuretic factor receptor with guanylate cyclase. Although not known to be an important endogenous physiologic regulator of airway smooth-muscle tone, exogenously added atrial natriuretic factor relaxes the guinea pig trachea with a potency equivalent to that of isoproterenol.[172]

2. Cyclic GMP-Dependent Protein Kinase

Cyclic GMP regulates cGMP-dependent protein kinase in much the same way as cAMP regulates cAMP-dependent protein kinase. However, there are two notable exceptions to this statement. First, unlike the effect of cAMP on cAMP-dependent protein kinase, cGMP does not promote dissociation of the cGMP-dependent protein kinase holoenzyme.[173] Accordingly, the activation state of cGMP-dependent protein kinase is determined solely by the amount of cyclic nucleotide bound to the enzyme, not by the dissociation-reassociation kinetics of catalytic and regulatory subunits. Second, low concentrations of cAMP (0.01 to 0.1 μM) activate cGMP-dependent protein kinase partially purified from canine airway and gastrointestinal smooth muscle, whereas high concentrations of cGMP ($>$10 μM) are required to activate cGMP-dependent protein kinase.[150,174] This raises the intriguing possibility that under certain conditions the physiologic responses to cAMP may be mediated by activation of both cGMP and cAMP-dependent protein kinases.

Information concerning the regulation of airway smooth-muscle cGMP-dependent protein kinase by relaxant agents is sketchy. It is known, however, that relaxation of bovine and canine tracheal smooth muscle induced by nitrovasodilators is associated with an increase in cGMP content and a concomitant activation of cGMP-dependent protein kinase.[175,176] That activation of cGMP-dependent protein kinase can indeed mediate airway smooth-muscle relaxation is supported by a recent study indicating that the potency of several analogues of cGMP in relaxing the guinea pig trachea is directly related to the potency of these compounds in activating purified cGMP-dependent protein kinase.[177]

3. Functional Effects

Functional studies support a role for both Ca^{2+} removal and direct interference with contractile protein activity in mediating the relaxant response to cGMP. The evidence for Ca^{2+} removal-sequestration is particularly strong. Nitroglycerin, an activator of the soluble guanylate cyclase, dampens the transient increase in cytosolic free Ca^{2+} observed after treating cultured vascular smooth-muscle cells with caffeine, an agent that induces Ca^{2+} release from sarcoplasmic reticulum.[178] In addition, atrial natriuretic factor and 8-bromo-cGMP reduce cytosolic free Ca^{2+} in primary cultures of rat aortic cells.[179] Interestingly, this affect is lost in parallel with a loss in cGMP-dependent protein kinase activity after these cells are passaged many times.[179] Reincorporating cGMP-dependent protein kinase using an osmolytic procedure reestablishes the responsiveness of these cells to atrial natriuretic factor and 8-bromo-cGMP, thus linking the decrease in cytosolic free Ca^{2+} with the presence of cGMP-dependent protein kinase activity.[179] Several studies with vascular smooth muscle suggest that phosphorylation of a microsomal protein(s), perhaps phospholamban, increases the activity of a membrane-associated Ca^{2+} pump.[180-183] Such an activation may account for the ability of cGMP to enhance Ca^{2+} removal from the cytosol.[180-183]

In addition to enhancing cytosolic Ca^{2+} removal, cGMP also may inhibit Ca^{2+} influx in vascular smooth muscle, perhaps by controlling the gating of ROCs.[184] On the other hand, one study with isolated bovine tracheal smooth-muscle cells suggests that cGMP inhibits Ca^{2+} influx through VDCs rather than ROCs.[153] Finally, cGMP may inhibit agonist-induced Ca^{2+} release in vascular smooth muscle by regulating receptor-linked phosphoinositide breakdown.[185]

Some evidence hints that in addition to regulating cytosolic Ca^{2+} content, cGMP also regulates contractile protein function. Addition of cGMP to skinned vascular smooth-muscle preparations reduces the sensitivity of these tissues to Ca^{2+}, presumably by altering contractile protein function.[186] In support of this suggestion, Karaki and co-workers[187] have

TABLE 1

**Characteristics of Canine Tracheal Cyclic Nucleotide
Phosphodiesterase Isozymes[192,193]**

Family[a]	Isozyme[b]	K_m (μM) cAMP	cGMP	Selective inhibitor[c]
Ic	Ca^{2+}/CaM-stimulated[d]	1	2	—
II	cGMP-stimulated	93[c]	80[c]	—
III	cGMP-inhibited	0.4	8	Milrinone, cilostamide, SK&F 94836
IV	cAMP-specific	4	38	Ro 20-1724, rolipram
V	cGMP-specific	135	4	Zaprinast, MY-5445

[a] Family designations are based upon kinetic characteristics along with primary protein and cDNA sequence.
[b] Isozyme nomenclature taken from Beavo.[189]
[c] Enzyme displays positive cooperativity.
[d] CaM, calmodulin.

reported that sodium nitroprusside relaxes intact vascular smooth muscle via four distinct cGMP-mediated mechanisms, one of which involves a decrease in the Ca^{2+} sensitivity of the contractile element. This suggestion was based on the observation that high concentrations of sodium nitroprusside inhibit norepinephrine-induced contraction while having very little effect on cytosolic Ca^{2+} levels, as assessed by fura-2 fluorescence. The mechanism by which activation of the cGMP/cGMP-dependent protein kinase cascade directly regulates the activity of the contractile proteins is unknown, but apparently does not involve phosphorylation of MLCK. Although MLCK is a substrate for cGMP-dependent protein kinase, phosphorylation does not inhibit the activity of MLCK, nor does it reduce the affinity of the enzyme for Ca^{2+}/calmodulin.[18]

C. CYCLIC NUCLEOTIDE PHOSPHODIESTERASES

The primary mechanism for terminating the actions of cyclic nucleotides in mammalian cells is hydrolysis of the 3'-phosphoester bond to form the inactive 5'-monophosphate product. This hydrolysis is catalyzed by a family of enzymes generically known as cyclic nucleotide phosphodiesterases (PDEs). Interest in PDEs, particularly as drug targets, has grown substantially over the last 5 years. This renaissance has been fueled by three factors: (1) the realization that several distinct PDE isozymes exist; (2) the demonstration that the role of these isozymes in regulating cyclic nucleotide content varies enormously among tissues; and (3) the synthesis of isozyme-selective PDE inhibitors.[188,189] Thus, with reference to the airway, targeting PDE inhibitors for specific isozymes may yield a new generation of bronchodilators that possess a marked degree of selectivity for bronchial smooth muscle.[190] General characteristics of PDE isozymes have been reviewed extensively elsewhere and will not be discussed in great detail here.[189] Instead, attention will be focused on the identity and role of PDE isozymes in airway smooth muscle.

PDE isozymes from both canine and human trachealis have been partially purified and characterized.[190-193] Using a combination of DEAE-Sepharose anion-exchange chromatography, calmodulin affinity chromatography, and isozyme-selective PDE inhibitors, five distinct PDE isozymes have been identified in canine trachealis.[192,193] A sixth distinct isozyme is present in human trachealis.[192] As shown in Table 1, isozymes in canine trachealis differ in their kinetic characteristics, endogenous activators (e.g., cGMP, Ca^{2+}/calmodulin) and inhibitors (e.g., cGMP), and susceptibility to isozyme-selective PDE inhibitors. Of the total PDE activity in canine trachealis homogenates, over 90% is present in the soluble fraction

(100,000 × g supernatant).[193] Differences exist in the subcellular distribution of the isozymes, with the cGMP-stimulated enzyme (PDE II) being present only in the soluble fraction and only very little of the cAMP-specific enzyme (PDE IV) being present in the particulate fraction.[193] The functional significance of this isozyme distribution is unknown.

Although valuable for the identification of PDE isozymes in various tissues, biochemical analyses of partially purified enzymes cannot accurately predict the importance of individual isozymes in regulating cyclic nucleotide content *in vivo*. That is, the mere presence of a particular isozyme in trachealis homogenates does not confirm its role in mediating cyclic nucleotide hydrolysis in intact tissues. Studies addressing this issue have been conducted with intact airway smooth muscle using isozyme-selective PDE inhibitors as probes for the functional role of the various PDE isozymes. Relaxation of canine trachealis following the administration of SK&F 94836, a selective inhibitor of the cGMP-inhibited PDE (PDE III; Table 1), is accompanied by an increase in cAMP content and activation of cAMP-dependent protein kinase.[194] Moreover, SK&F 94836 potentiates isoproterenol-induced relaxation and cAMP accumulation, but has no effect on the mechanical or biochemical responses to sodium nitroprusside,[194] an agent thought to relax airway smooth muscle by a cGMP-mediated mechanism.[175,176] These results suggest that the cGMP-inhibited PDE is important for the hydrolysis of cAMP, but not cGMP, in intact canine trachealis. A similar strategy has been used in an attempt to define the role of the cGMP-specific PDE (PDE V) and cAMP-specific PDE (PDE IV) in regulating cyclic nucleotide content in canine trachealis.[190,195] In these studies, zaprinast (a cGMP-specific PDE inhibitor) was shown to potentiate relaxation and cGMP accumulation in response to sodium nitroprusside, while having no effect on the responses to isoproterenol. In contrast, Ro 20-1724 (an inhibitor of the cAMP-specific PDE) potentiated the biochemical and mechanical effects of isoproterenol, but not the responses to sodium nitroprusside. These results suggest that the cGMP-specific PDE regulates cGMP content in the intact tissue, whereas the Ro 20-1724-inhibited PDE, like the cGMP-inhibited PDE, regulates cAMP content. Obviously, additional studies are required before the biologic function of the individual isozymes in airway smooth muscle can be defined with certainty.

IV. INTEGRATION OF CONTRACTILE AND RELAXANT PATHWAYS

A. BACKGROUND

To date, the vast majority of research aimed at discerning the physiological, pharmacological, and biochemical regulation of airway smooth-muscle tone has utilized isolated tissues removed from their normal environment and exposed only to selected inputs. Consequently, the findings from these studies represent a simplified version of events *in vivo* in which there are numerous simultaneous humoral, neuronal, and autacoid influences which are both excitatory and inhibitory in nature. The ultimate level of airway smooth-muscle tone in whole animals will reflect a balance of the concerted effects of these various contractile and relaxant inputs. An alteration in the contribution of one or more of the many factors influencing the absolute level of tone in airways may be responsible for the bronchospasm associated with asthma and other respiratory disorders.

B. FUNCTIONAL ANTAGONISM
1. Definition

A key issue when considering the net result of the effects of various excitatory and inhibitory inputs on the contractile state in airways is the phenomenon of "functional" or physiological" antagonism. Functional antagonism can be defined as, and results from, the interaction between two agonists which act via different mechanisms to produce directly opposing effects on a common effector system.[196] Accordingly, from a theoretical standpoint, a functional antagonist should attenuate the stimulatory influence of a variety of agonists regardless of the receptor type or biochemical mechanism(s) by which they produce their effects. This is in obvious contrast to the specific nature of receptor antagonism.

The nonselective nature of the inhibitory effects of a functional antagonist is advantageous in a disease such as asthma in which the etiology is likely to result from the concerted effects of several, rather than a single, mediators. This rationale forms the basis of present-day research efforts aimed at the development of bronchorelaxant agents that selectively target signal transduction pathways, for example, PDE inhibitors, ROC inhibitors, calmodulin antagonists, PKC inhibitors, and other modulators of the PI cycle.

2. Description

In airways, a classical example of the phenomenon of functional antagonism is the interaction between constrictor muscarinic agonists and the bronchorelaxant β-adrenoreceptor agonists, which have been investigated extensively in isolated tissues from several species.[143,197-201] It is observed that an inverse relationship exists between the initial level of tone produced by muscarinic agents and the ability of β-adrenoreceptor agonists to induce relaxation; this is reflected by an increase in the EC_{50} and a decrease in the maximum relaxation elicited by the bronchorelaxant agent as the muscarinic agonist concentration is increased.[143,197-201] In addition to being dependent upon the level of tone produced by an agonist, research indicates that the ability of β-adrenoreceptor agonist to relax airway smooth muscle is influenced markedly by the specific agonist producing contraction.[165,199-202] For example, the ability of β-adrenoreceptor agonists to reverse contraction produced by muscarinic agonists is less than when tissues are contracted to the same level of tone with LTD_4,[199,200] serotonin,[201] histamine,[201] or $PGF_{2\alpha}$.[202] These findings, which indicate that the potency and efficacy of bronchorelaxants depend on the initial degree of tone and also on the agent eliciting contraction, are supported by the limited number of *in vivo* studies performed in guinea pigs,[203] dogs,[204] and humans.[205] These data may explain, in part, the resistance of intense bronchospasm associated with a severe asthmatic attacks to treatment with bronchodilators, including β-adrenoreceptor agonists. Furthermore, the possibility exists that the relative sensitivity of individual asthmatics to bronchodilator therapy may depend on the predominant mediator that is responsible for the bronchoconstriction during an attack.

3. Order of Addition: Prevention vs. Reversal of Contraction

Another important experimental observation is that the ability of a bronchorelaxant functional antagonist to inhibit agonist-induced contraction of airways depends markedly on whether the inhibitory agent is given before or after initiation of contraction. In isolated guinea pig trachea, for example, salbutamol is much more effective at *reversing* rather than *preventing* contractions produced by carbachol and the peptidoleukotrienes.[165] Similar findings were obtained using cat trachea, in which isoproterenol was found to be a more effective inhibitor of acetylcholine-induced contraction when given following establishment of tone rather than when administered prior to initiation of contraction.[198]

The differential ability of β-adrenoreceptor agonists to antagonize contractions depending on whether they are given before or after addition of the contractile agonist also extends to other functional antagonists, including calcium channel inhibitors. Thus, several studies in isolated mammalian airway smooth muscle, including human, indicate that the calcium channel inhibitors are more effective at reversing agonist-induced contractions than in preventing their development.[133,135,206-208]

The consequences of these *in vitro* findings may extend to the clinical setting and suggest that certain functional antagonists, including β-adrenoreceptor agonists, may be less effective when given prophylactically than when given therapeutically to reverse an ongoing bronchospasm.

4. Underlying Mechanisms of Functional Antagonism

As indicated above, there are two characteristic features of functional antagonism in airways. First, the ability of bronchorelaxant agents such as β-adrenoreceptor agonists and calcium channel inhibitors to inhibit contraction is markedly affected by the nature of the agonist eliciting contraction. Second, the efficacy of bronchodilators is dependent on whether the relaxant agent is given prior to or following the initiation of contraction.

With regard to the former phenomenon, it has been proposed that this may be due to differences in the relative utilization of intracellular vs. extracellular Ca^{2+} sources, and to fundamental differences in the biochemical mechanisms responsible for contraction produced by the individual agonists.[165,198,199,201,202] For example, acetylcholine-induced contractions are less sensitive to the relaxant effects of isoproterenol than those produced by either serotonin or histamine, and are more reliant on the release of Ca^{2+} from intracellular sites.[139,198,201] In smooth muscle, β-adrenoreceptor activation and subsequent elevation in the intracellular levels of cAMP have been postulated to affect intracellular and extracellular Ca^{2+} translocation pathway at several loci and by a variety of mechanisms, including inhibition of extracellular Ca^{2+} influx, stimulation of Ca^{2+} sequestration, and promotion of Ca^{2+} efflux (see Section III.A.3). Accordingly, there may be a differential sensitivity of the many Ca^{2+} translocation pathways and Ca^{2+} release mechanisms to the effects of cAMP.[199,201] This could translate into differential potency and efficacy of a given concentration of β-adrenoreceptor agonist against contractions produced by agonists that utilize different Ca^{2+} sources.

Another factor to consider is the ability of certain contractile agonists to inhibit key biochemical processes involved in mediating the physiologic responses to selected bronchodilators. Methacholine inhibits activation of cAMP-dependent protein kinase produced by isoproterenol, PGE_2, or forskolin in canine trachealis, in parallel with its ability to antagonize functionally the relaxation produced by these agents.[143,144] In contrast, histamine does not inhibit the ability of β-adrenoreceptor agonists to induce relaxation, nor does it inhibit β-adrenoreceptor agonist-induced activation of cAMP-dependent protein kinase.[209]

One additional alternative proposal has been made. Specifically, Gunst and co-workers[210] have proposed that the differential sensitivity of contractile agents in airways to the relaxant effects of functional antagonists may be related to differences in the relative receptor reserves for the individual bronchoconstrictors.

Finally, the differences in the ability of functional antagonists to *prevent* and *reverse* bronchoconstriction in airways may be linked to a central theme of this chapter. Namely, evidence is accumulating which suggests that different fundamental biochemical processes are involved in the *development* vs. the *maintenance* of contraction (Section II.A.3). These different pathways may have corresponding differences in sensitivity to various inhibitory inputs. As an example, following receptor activation there is a marked but transient elevation in intracellular Ca^{2+} levels, which then return to, or come close to, baseline levels despite the persistence of the contractile response.[7-12] The secondary phase of agonist-induced contraction may thus be maintained by transmembrane influx of small amounts of Ca^{2+}, a hypothesis which is supported by Ca^{2+}-deprivation studies.[2,130,133] This may explain why calcium channel inhibitors are more effective when given subsequent to the development of contraction (low Ca^{2+} influx) than before its initiation (high Ca^{2+} influx and intracellular Ca^{2+} release).

Inhibition of MLCK activity can be used as another example to highlight the importance of timing in the actions of a functional antagonist. As discussed in Section II.A, MLCK activation may be more important for the establishment of tone than for its maintenance. Hypothetically, then, MLCK inhibitors (e.g., calmodulin antagonists) should be more effective in preventing contraction than reversing an ongoing contraction, a prediction borne out in studies conducted with bovine trachealis.[211]

In summary, functional antagonism is an important, physiologically relevant phenomenon which has been somewhat neglected and is inadequately understood. *In vivo* responses are regulated by complex interactions between excitatory and inhibitory inputs (functional antagonists), which have quite different and diverse basic mechanisms of action. The net affect of these many stimuli will determine the ultimate level of bronchomotor tone.

V. CONCLUSION

During the past few years, significant inroads have been made toward understanding the signal transduction pathways and biochemical events that are involved in regulating the level of airway smooth-muscle tone. Research, largely on isolated tissues, has emphasized the complexity of the many biochemical pathways that act in concert to produce the ultimate bronchomotor tone *in vivo*.

The substantial progress notwithstanding, several issues concerning the biochemical regulation of airway smooth-muscle tone remain unresolved. Some areas of particular interest include (1) unambiguous definition of the role of MLC phosphorylation in the regulation of contractility; (2) identification of important substrates for cyclic nucleotide-dependent protein kinases; (3) a delineation of the relative importance of the DAG/PKC and IP_3 pathways in the initiation and maintenance of the contractile response; (4) examination of the importance of other products of PIP_2 hydrolysis and the metabolites of the breakdown of other phospholipids in the contraction/relaxation cycle; and (5) determination of the identities and roles of various G proteins. Information relating to these and other important questions will be assisted by the identification of potent and selective inhibitors and activators of the numerous relevant cellular enzymes, receptors, and ion channels. These agents will also be crucial for determining the physiological relevance of the findings in isolated tissues to the regulation of airway smooth-muscle tone *in vivo*. Ultimately, a major issue to address is whether or not fundamental differences in key biochemical pathways exist between smooth muscle from normal vs. diseased airways, and whether or not any identified differences contribute to airway hyperreactivity in the asthmatic.

REFERENCES

1. **Kamm, K. E. and Stull, J. T.**, The function of myosin and myosin light chain kinase phosphorylation in smooth muscle, *Annu. Rev. Pharmacol. Toxicol.*, 25, 593, 1985.
2. **Rodger, I. W.**, Excitation-contraction coupling and uncoupling in airway smooth muscle, *Br. J. Clin. Pharmacol.*, 20, 255S, 1985.
3. **Stephens, N. L.**, Airway smooth muscle, *Am. Rev. Respir. Dis.*, 135, 960, 1987.
4. **Torphy, T. J. and Gerthoffer, W. T.**, Biochemical mechanisms of smooth muscle contraction and relaxation, in *Current Topics in Pulmonary Pharmacology and Toxicology*, Vol. 1, Hollinger, M. A., Ed., Elsevier Science Publishing, New York, 1986, 23.
5. **Ebashi, S.**, Regulatory mechanism of muscle contraction with special reference to the Ca-troponin-tropomyosin system, *Essays Biochem.*, 10, 1, 1974.
6. **Torphy, T. J.**, Biochemical regulation of airway smooth muscle tone: current knowledge and therapeutic implications, *Rev. Clin. Basic Pharmacol.*, 6, 61, 1987.
7. **Morgan, J. P. and Morgan, K. G.**, Stimulus-specific patterns of intracellular calcium levels in smooth muscle of ferret portal vein, *J. Physiol. (London)*, 351, 155, 1984.
8. **Rembold, C. M. and Murphy, R. A.**, Myoplasmic $[Ca^{2+}]$ determines myosin phosphorylation in agonist-stimulated swine arterial smooth muscle, *Circ. Res.*, 63, 593, 1988.
9. **Yagi, S., Becker, P. L., and Fay, F. S.**, Relationship between force and Ca^{2+} concentrations in smooth muscle as revealed by measurements on single cells, *Proc. Natl. Acad. Sci. U.S.A.*, 85, 4109, 1988.
10. **Takuwa, Y., Takuwa, N., and Rasmussen, H.**, Measurement of cytoplasmic free Ca^{2+} concentration in bovine tracheal smooth muscle using aequorin, *Am. J. Physiol.*, 253, C817, 1987.

11. **Taylor, D. A. and Stull, J. T.**, Calcium dependence of myosin light chain phosphorylation in smooth muscle cells, *J. Biol. Chem.*, 263, 14456, 1988.
12. **Gunst, S. J., Al-Hassani, M. H., and Gerthoffer, W. T.**, Receptor occupancy affects changes in intracellular free Ca^{2+} ($[Ca^{2+}]_i$) and myosin phosphorylation caused by muscarinic activation of canine tracheal smooth muscle, *Biophys. J.*, 55, 470a, 1989.
13. **Sparrow, M. P., Pfitzer, G., Gagelmann, M., and Rüegg, J. C.**, Effect of calmodulin, Ca^{2+}, and cAMP protein kinase on skinned tracheal smooth muscle, *Am. J. Physiol.*, 246, C308, 1984.
14. **Stull, J. T., Kamm, K. E., and Taylor, D. A.**, Calcium control of smooth muscle contractility, *Am. J. Med. Sci.*, 296, 241, 1988.
15. **Wolff, D. J. and Brostrom, C. P.**, Properties and functions of the calcium-dependent regulator protein, *Adv. Cyclic Nucleotide Res.*, 11, 27, 1979.
16. **Cheung, W. Y.**, Calmodulin plays a pivotal role in cellular regulation, *Science*, 207, 19, 1979.
17. **Klee, C. B. and Vanaman, T. C.**, Calmodulin, *Adv. Protein Chem.*, 35, 213, 1982.
18. **Nishikawa, M., de Lanerolle, P., Lincoln, T. M., and Adelstein, S.**, Phosphorylation of mammalian myosin light chain kinases by the catalytic subunit of cyclic AMP-dependent protein kinase and by cyclic GMP-dependent protein kinase, *J. Biol. Chem.*, 259, 8429, 1984.
19. **Sellers, J. R. and Pato, M. D.**, The binding of smooth muscle myosin light chain kinase and phosphatases to actin and myosin, *J. Biol. Chem.*, 259, 7740, 1984.
20. **Ikebe, M. and Hartshorne, D. J.**, Phosphorylation of smooth muscle myosin at two distinct sites by myosin light chain kinase, *J. Biol. Chem.*, 260, 10027, 1985.
21. **Ikebe, M., Hartshorne, D. J., and Elzinga, M.**, Identification, phosphorylation, and dephosphorylation of a second site for myosin light chain kinase on the 20,000-dalton light chain of smooth muscle myosin, *J. Biol. Chem.*, 261, 36, 1986.
22. **Colburn, J. C., Michnoff, C. H., Hsu, L.-C., Saughter, C. A., Kamm, K. E., and Stull, J. T.**, Sites phosphorylated in myosin light chain in contracting smooth muscle, *J. Biol. Chem.*, 263, 19166, 1988.
23. **Sellers, J. R.**, Mechanism of the phosphorylation-dependent regulation of smooth muscle heavy meromyosin, *J. Biol. Chem.*, 260, 15815, 1985.
24. **Wagner, P. D. and Vu, N.-D.**, Regulation of the actin-activated ATPase of aorta smooth muscle myosin, *J. Biol. Chem.*, 261, 7778, 1986.
25. **Pato, M. D. and Kerc, E.**, Purification and characterization of a smooth muscle phosphatase from turkey gizzards, *J. Biol. Chem.*, 260, 12359, 1985.
26. **Onishi, H., Umeda, J., Uchiwa, H., and Watanabe, S.**, Purification of gizzard myosin light-chain phosphatase, and reversible changes in ATPase and superprecipitation activities of actomyosin in the presence of purified preparations of myosin light-chain phosphatase and kinase, *J. Biol. Chem.*, 257, 265, 1982.
27. **Paietta, E. and Sands, H.**, Phosphoprotein phosphatase in bovine tracheal smooth muscle. Multiple fractions and multiple substrates, *Biochem. Biophys. Acta*, 523, 121, 1978.
28. **Driska, S. M., Askoy, M. D., and Murphy, R. A.**, Myosin light chain phosphorylation associated with contraction in arterial smooth muscle, *Am. J. Physiol.*, 240, C222, 1981.
29. **Dillon, P. F., Aksoy, M. O., Driska, S. P., and Murphy, R. A.**, Myosin phosphorylation and the cross-bridge cycle in smooth muscle, *Science*, 211, 495, 1981.
30. **Aksoy, M. O., Murphy, R. A., and Kamm, K. E.**, Role of Ca^{2+} and myosin light chain phosphorylation in regulation of smooth muscle, *Am. J. Physiol.* 242, C109, 1982.
31. **Silver, P. J. and Stull, J. T.**, Regulation of myosin light chain phosphorylation in tracheal smooth muscle, *J. Biol. Chem.*, 257, 6145, 1982.
32. **Gerthoffer, W. T. and Murphy, R. A.**, Myosin phosphorylation and regulation of the cross-bridge cycle in tracheal smooth muscle, *Am. J. Physiol.*, 244, C182, 1983.
33. **Chatterjee, M. and Murphy, R. A.**, Calcium-dependent stress maintenance without myosin phosphorylation in skinned smooth muscle, *Science*, 221, 464, 1983.
34. **Dillon, P. F., Murphy, R. A., and Claes, V.**, Tonic force maintenance with reduced shortening velocity in arterial smooth muscle, *Am. J. Physiol.*, 242, C102, 1982.
35. **Barany, M.**, ATPase activity of myosin correlated with the speed of muscle shortening, *J. Gen. Physiol.*, 50, 197, 1967.
36. **Gluck, E. and Paul, R. J.**, The aerobic metabolism of porcine carotid artery and its relationship to isometric force, *Pfluegers Arch.*, 370, 9, 1977.
37. **Paul, R. J.**, Chemical energetics of vascular smooth muscle, in *Handbook of Physiology*, Vol. 2, Sec. 2, Bohr, D. F., Somlyo, A. P., and Sparks, H. V., Eds., American Physiological Society, Bethesda, MD, 1980, 201.
38. **Clark, R., Ngai, P. K., Sutherland, C., Gröschel-Stewart, U., and Walsh, M. P.**, Vascular smooth muscle caldesmon, *J. Biol. Chem.*, 263, 8028, 1986.
39. **Marston, S. B. and Lehman, W.**, Caldesmon is a Ca^{2+}-regulatory component of native smooth muscle thin filaments, *Biochem. J.*, 231, 517, 1985.

40. **Ngai, P. K. and Walsh, M. P.**, Inhibition of smooth muscle actin-activated myosin Mg^{2+}-ATPase activity by caldesmon, *J. Biol. Chem.*, 259, 13656, 1984.

41. **Ikebe, M. and Reardon, S.**, Binding of caldesmon to smooth muscle myosin, *J. Biol. Chem.*, 263, 3055, 1988.

42. **Scott-Woo, G. C. and Walsh, M. P.**, Autophosphorylation of smooth muscle caldesmon, *Biochem. J.*, 252, 463, 1988.

43. **Sutherland, C. and Walsh, M. P.**, Phosphorylation of caldesmon prevents its interaction with smooth muscle myosin, *J. Biol. Chem.*, 264, 578, 1989.

44. **Hai, C.-H. and Murphy, R. A.**, Cross-bridge phosphorylation and regulation of latch state in smooth muscle, *Am. J. Physiol.*, 254, C99, 1988.

45. **Chatterjee, M. and Tejada, M.**, Phorbol ester-induced contraction in chemically skinned vascular smooth muscle, *Am. J. Physiol.*, 251, C356, 1986.

46. **Nishikawa, M., Hidaka, H., and Adelstein, R. S.**, Phosphorylation of smooth muscle heavy meromyosin by calcium-activated, phospholipid-dependent protein kinase, *J. Biol. Chem.*, 258, 14069, 1983.

47. **Umekawa, H. and Hidaka, H.**, Phosphorylation of caldesmon by protein kinase C, *Biochem. Biophys. Res. Commun.*, 132, 56, 1985.

48. **de Lanerolle, P. and Stull, J. T.**, Myosin phosphorylation during contraction and relaxation of tracheal smooth muscle, *J. Biol. Chem.*, 225, 9993, 1980.

49. **de Lanerolle, P., Condit, J. R., Jr., Tanenbaum, M., and Adelstein, R. S.**, Myosin phosphorylation, agonist concentration and contraction of smooth muscle, *Nature*, 298, 871, 1982.

50. **Gerthoffer, W. T.**, Calcium dependence of myosin phosphorylation and airway smooth muscle contraction and relaxation, *Am. J. Physiol.*, 250, C597, 1986.

51. **de Lanerolle, P.**, cAMP, myosin dephosphorylation, and isometric relaxation of airway smooth muscle, *J. Appl. Physiol.*, 64, 705, 1988.

52. **Gerthoffer, W. P.**, Dissociation of myosin phosphorylation and active tension during muscarinic stimulation of tracheal smooth muscle, *J. Pharmacol. Exp. Ther.*, 240, 8, 1987.

53. **Moreland, S., Moreland, R. S., and Singer, H. A.**, Apparent dissociation between myosin light chain phosphorylation and maximal velocity of shortening in KCl depolarized swine carotid artery: effect of temperature and KCl concentration, *Pfluegers Arch.*, 408, 139, 1986.

54. **Siegman, M. J., Butler, T. M., Mooers, S. U., and Michalek, A.**, Ca^{2+} can affect V_{max} without changes in myosin light chain phosphorylation in smooth muscle, *Pfluegers Arch.*, 401, 385, 1984.

55. **Majerus, P. W., Connolly, T. M., Deckmyn, H., Ross, T. S., Bross, T. E., Ishii, H., Bansal, V. S., and Wilson, D. B.**, The metabolism of phosphoinositide-derived messenger molecules, *Science*, 234, 1519, 1986.

56. **Abdel-Latif, A. A.**, Calcium-mobilizing receptors, polyphosphoinositides and the generation of second messengers, *Pharmacol. Rev.*, 38, 227, 1986.

57. **Berridge, M. J.**, Inositol trisphosphate and diacylglycerol: two interacting second messengers, *Annu. Rev. Biochem.*, 56, 159, 1987.

58. **Gilman, A. G.**, G Proteins: transducers of receptor-generated signals, *Annu. Rev. Biochem.*, 56, 615, 1987.

59. **Stryer, L. and Bourne, H. R.**, G Proteins: a family of signal transducers, *Annu. Rev. Cell Biol.*, 2, 391, 1986.

60. **Cockcroft, S.**, Polyphosphoinositide phosphodiesterase: regulation by a novel guanine nucleotide binding protein, G_p, *Trends Biochem. Sci.*, 12, 75, 1987.

61. **Iyengar, R. and Birnbaumer, L.**, Signal transduction by G-proteins, *ISI Atlas Sci. Pharmacol.*, 1, 213, 1987.

62. **Axelrod, J., Burch, R. M., and Jelsema, C. L.**, Receptor-mediated activation of phospholipase A_2 via GTP-binding proteins: arachidonic acid and its metabolites as second messengers, *Trends Neurosci.*, 11, 117, 1988.

63. **Casey, P. J. and Gilman, A. G.**, G Protein involvement in receptor-effector coupling, *J. Biol. Chem.*, 263, 2577, 1988.

64. **Weiss, E. R., Kelleher, D. J., Woon, C. W., Soparkar, S., Osowa, S., Heasley, L. E., and Johnson, G. L.**, Receptor activation of G proteins, *FASEB J.*, 2, 2841, 1988.

65. **Gilman, A. G.**, G Proteins and dual control of adenylate cyclase, *Cell*, 36, 577, 1984.

66. **Stryer, L.**, Cyclic GMP cascade of vision, *Annu. Rev. Neurosci.*, 9, 87, 1986.

67. **Fain, J. N., Wallace, M. A., and Wojcikiewicz, J. H.**, Evidence for involvement of guanine nucleotide-binding regulatory proteins in the activation of phospholipases by hormones, *FASEB J.*, 2, 2569, 1988.

68. **Haslam, R. J. and Davidson, M. M. L.**, Receptor-induced diacylglycerol formation in permeabilized platelets; possible role for a GTP-binding protein, *J. Recept. Res.*, 4, 605, 1984.

69. **Gomperts, B. D.**, Involvement of guanine nucleotide-binding protein in the gating of Ca^{2+} by receptors, *Nature*, 306, 64, 1983.

70. **Cockcroft, S. and Gomperts, B. D.,** Role of guanine nucleotide binding protein in the activation of polyphosphoinositide phosphodiesterase, *Nature,* 314, 534, 1985.
71. **Sasaguri, T., Hirata, M., and Kuriyama, H.,** Dependence on Ca^{2+} of the activities of phosphatidylinositol 4,5,-bisphosphate phosphodiesterase and inositol 1,4,5-trisphosphate in smooth muscle of the porcine coronary artery, *Biochem. J.,* 231, 497, 1985.
72. **Wallace, M. A. and Fain, J. N.,** Guanosine -5'-O-thiotriphosphate (GTP γs) stimulates phospholipase C activity in plasma membranes of rat hepatocytes, *J. Biol. Chem.,* 260, 9527, 1985.
73. **Litosch, I., Wallis, C., and Fain, J. N.,** 5-Hydroxytryptamine stimulated inositol phosphate production in a cell-free system from blowfly salivary glands: evidence for a role of GTP in coupling receptor activation to phosphoinositide breakdown, *J. Biol. Chem.,* 260, 5464, 1985.
74. **Litosch, I. and Fain, J. N.,** 5-Methyltryptamine stimulates phospholipase C-mediated breakdown of exogenous phosphoinositides by blowfly salivary gland membranes, *J. Biol. Chem.,* 260, 16052, 1985.
75. **Michell, B. and Kirk, C.,** G-Protein control of inositol phosphate hydrolysis, *Nature,* 323, 112, 1986.
76. **Nichols, A. J., Motley, E. D., and Ruffolo, R. R., Jr.,** Differential effect of pertussis toxin on pre- and postjunctional α_2-adrenoceptors in the cardiovascular system of the pithed rat, *Eur. J. Pharmacol.,* 145, 345, 1988.
77. **Brown, A. M. and Birnbaumer, L.,** Direct G protein gating of ion channels, *Am. J. Physiol.,* 254, 401, 1988.
78. **Exton, J. H.,** Mechanisms of calcium-mobilizing agonists: some variations on a young theme, *FASEB J.,* 2, 2670, 1988.
79. **Dunlap, K., Holz, G. G., and Rane, S. G.,** G Proteins as regulators of ion channel function, *Trends Neurosci.,* 10, 241, 1987.
80. **Hokin, M. R. and Hokin, L. E.,** Enzyme secretion and incorporation of P^{32} into phospholipids of pancreas slices, *J. Biol. Chem.,* 203, 967, 1953.
81. **Berridge, M. J. and Irvine, R. J.,** Inositol trisphosphate, a novel second messenger in cellular signal transduction, *Nature,* 312, 315, 1984.
82. **Michell, R. H.,** Inositol phospholipids and cell surface receptor function, *Biochem. Biophys. Acta,* 415, 81, 1975.
83. **Streb, H., Irvine, R. F., Berridge, M. J., and Schultz, I.,** Release of Ca^{2+} from a nonmitochondrial intracellular store in pancreatic acinar cells by inositol-1,4,5-trisphosphate, *Nature,* 360, 67, 1983.
84. **Suematsu, E., Hirata, M., Hashimoto, T., and Kuriyama, H.,** Inositol 1,4,5-trisphosphate releases Ca^{2+} from intracellular store sites in skinned single cells of porcine coronary artery, *Biochem. Biophys. Res. Commun.,* 120, 481, 1984.
85. **Somlyo, A. V., Bond, M., Somlyo, A. P., and Scarpa, A.,** Inositol trisphosphate-induced calcium release and contraction in vascular smooth muscle, *Proc. Natl. Acad. Sci., U.S.A.,* 82, 5231, 1987.
86. **Hashimoto, T., Hirata, M., Itoh, T., Kanmura, Y., and Kuriyama, H.,** Inositol 1,4,5-trisphosphate activates pharmacomechanical coupling in smooth muscle of the rabbit mesenteric artery, *J. Physiol.,* 370, 605, 1986.
87. **Hashimoto, T., Hirata, M., and Ito, Y.,** A role for inositol 1,4,5-trisphosphate in the initiation of agonist-induced contractions of dog tracheal smooth muscle, *Br. J. Pharmacol.,* 86, 191, 1985.
88. **Burgess, G. M., Irvine, R. F., Berridge, M. J., McKinney, J. S., and Putney, J. W., Jr.,** Actions of inositol phosphates on Ca^{2+} pools in guinea-pig hypatocytes, *Biochem. J.,* 224, 741, 1984.
89. **Irvine, R. F., Brown, K. D., and Berridge, M. J.,** Specificity of inositol trisphosphate-induced calcium release from permeabilized Swiss-mouse 3T3 cells, *Biochem. J.,* 222, 269, 1984.
90. **Smith, J. B., Smith, L., and Higgins, B. L.,** Temperature and nucleotide dependence of calcium release by myo-inositol 1,4,5-trisphosphate in cultured vascular smooth muscle cells, *J. Biol. Chem.,* 260, 14413, 1985.
91. **Biden, T. J., Prentki, M., Irvine, R. F., Berridge, M. J., and Wollheim, C. B.,** Inositol 1,4,5-trisphosphate mobilizes intracellular Ca^{2+} from permeabilized insulin-secreting cells, *Biochem. J.,* 223, 467, 1984.
92. **Ueda, T., Chueh, S.-H., Noel, M. W., and Gill, D. L.,** Influence of inositol 1,4,5-trisphosphate and guanine nucleotides on intracellular calcium release within N1E-115 neuronal cell line, *J. Biol. Chem.,* 251, 3184, 1986.
93. **Saida, K., Twort, C., and Van Breemen, C.,** The specific GTP requirement for inositol 1,4,5-trisphosphate-induced Ca^{2+} release from skinned vascular smooth muscle, *J. Cardiovasc. Pharmacol.,* 12, S47, 1988.
94. **Baukal, A. J., Guillemette, G., Rubin, R., Spät, A., and Catt, K. J.,** Binding sites for inositol trisphosphate in the bovine adrenal cortex, *Biochem. Biophys. Res. Commun.,* 133, 532, 1985.
95. **Spät, A., Fabiato, A., and Rubin, R. P.,** Binding of inositol trisphosphate by a liver microsomal fraction, *Biochem. J.,* 233, 929, 1986.
96. **Supattapone, S., Worley, P. F., Baraban, J. M., and Snyder, S. H.,** Solubilization, purification and characterization of an inositol trisphosphate receptor, *J. Biol. Chem.,* 263, 12132, 1988.

97. **Majerus, P. W., Connolly,T. M., Bansal, V. S., Inhorn, R. C., Ross, T. S., and Lips, D. L.,** Inositol phosphates: synthesis and degradation, *J. Biol. Chem.,* 263, 3051, 1988.

98. **Baron, C. B., Cunningham, M., Strauss, J. F., III, and Coburn, R. F.,** Pharmacomechanical coupling in smooth muscle may involve phosphatidylinositol metabolism, *Proc. Natl. Acad. Sci. U.S.A.,* 81, 6899, 1984.

99. **Duncan, R. A., Krzanowski, J. J., Jr., Davis, J. S., Polson, J. B., Coffey, R. G., Shimoda, T., and Szentivanyi, A.,** Polyphosphoinositide metabolism in canine tracheal smooth muscle (CTSM) in response to a cholinergic stimulus, *Biochem. Pharmacol.,* 36, 307, 1987.

100. **Takuwa, U., Takuwa, N., and Rasmussen, H.,** Carbachol induces a rapid and sustained hydrolysis of polyphosphoinositide in bovine tracheal smooth muscle measurements of the mass of polyphosphoinositides, 1,2-diacylglycerol, and phosphatidic acid, *J. Biol. Chem.,* 263, 14670, 1986.

101. **Grandordy, B. M., Cuss, F. M., Sampson, A. S., Palmer, J. B., and Barnes, P. J.,** Phosphatidylinositol response to cholinergic agonists in airway smooth muscle: relationship to contraction and muscarinic receptor occupancy, *J. Pharmacol. Exp. Ther.,* 238, 273, 1986.

102. **Grandordy, B. M., Cuss, F. M., and Barnes, P. J.,** Breakdown of phosphoinositides in airway smooth muscle: lack of influence of anti-asthmatic drugs, *Life Sci.,* 41, 1621, 1987.

103. **Grandordy, B. M., Frossard, N., Rhoden, K. J., and Barnes, P. J.,** Tachykinin-induced phospho-inositide breakdown in airway smooth muscle and epithelium: relationship to contraction, *Mol. Pharmacol.,* 33, 515, 1988.

104. **Mong, S., Hoffman, K., Wu, H.-L., and Crooke, S. T.,** Leukotriene-induced hydrolysis of inositol lipids in guinea pig lung: mechanism of signal transduction for leukotriene-D_4 receptors, *Mol. Pharmacol.,* 31, 35, 1987.

105. **Mong, S., Miller, J., Wu, H.-L., and Crooke, S. T.,** Leukotriene D_4 receptor-mediated hydrolysis of phosphatidylinositol and mobilization of calcium in sheep tracheal smooth muscle cells, *J. Pharmacol. Exp. Ther.,* 244, 508, 1988.

106. **Grandordy, B. M. and Barnes, P. J.,** Phosphoinositide turnover, *Am. Rev. Respir. Dis.,* 136, S17, 1987.

107. **Takai, Y., Kishimoto, A., Inoue, M., and Nishizuka, Y.,** Studies on a cyclic nucleotide-independent protein kinase and its proenzyme in mammalian tissues. I. Purification and characterization of an active enzyme from bovine cerebellum, *J. Biol. Chem.,* 252, 7603, 1977.

108. **Nishizuka, Y.,** Studies and perspectives of protein kinase C, *Science,* 233, 305, 1986.

109. **Huang, F. L., Yoshida, Y., Nakabayashi, H., and Huang, K.-P.,** Differential distribution of protein kinase C isozymes in the various regions of brain, *J. Biol. Chem.,* 262, 15714, 1987.

110. **Hidaka, J., Tanaka, T., Onoda, K., Hagiwara, M., Watanabe, M., Ohta, H., Ito, Y., Tsurudome, M., and Yoshida, T.,** Cell type-specific expression of protein kinase C isozymes in the rabbit cerebellum, *J. Biol. Chem.,* 263, 4523, 1988.

111. **Nishizuka, Y.,** The molecular heterogeneity of protein kinase C and its implications for cellular regulation, *Nature,* 334, 661, 1988.

112. **Kaibuchi, K., Takai, Y., and Nishizuka, Y.,** Cooperative roles of various membrane phospholipids in the activation of calcium-activated, phospholipid-dependent protein kinase, *J. Biol. Chem.,* 256, 7146, 1981.

113. **Castagna, M., Takai, Y., Kaibuchi, K., Sano, K., Kikkawa, U., and Nishizuka, Y.,** Direct activation of Ca^{2+}-activated, phospholipid-dependent protein kinase by tumor-promoting phorbol esters, *J. Biol. Chem.,* 257, 7847, 1982.

114. **Yamanishi, J., Takai, Y., Kaibuchi, K., Sano, K., Castagna, M., and Nishizuka, Y.,** Synergistic functions of phorbol ester and Ca^{2+} in serotonin release from human platelets, *Biochem. Biophys. Res. Commun.,* 112, 778, 1983.

115. **Nishizuka, Y.,** Phospholipid degradation and signal translation for protein phosphorylation, *Trends Biochem. Sci.,* 83, 13, 1983.

116. **Rasmussen, H., Forder, J., Kojima, I., and Scriabine, A.,** TPA-induced contraction of isolated rabbit vascular smooth muscle, *Biochem. Biophys. Res. Commun.,* 122, 776, 1984.

117. **Park, S. and Rasmussen, H.,** Activation of tracheal smooth muscle contraction: synergism between Ca^{2+} and activators of protein kinase C, *Proc. Natl. Acad. Sci. U.S.A.,* 82, 8835, 1985.

118. **Forder, J., Scriabine, A., and Rasmussen, H.,** Plasma membrane calcium flux, protein kinase C activation and smooth muscle contraction, *J. Pharmacol. Exp. Ther.,* 232, 267, 1985.

119. **Park, S. and Rasmussen, H.,** Carbachol-induced protein phosphorylation changes in bovine tracheal smooth muscle, *J. Biol. Chem.,* 261, 15734, 1986.

120. **Khalil, R. A. and Van Breemen, C.,** Sustained contraction of vascular smooth muscle: calcium influx or C-kinase activation?, *J. Pharmacol. Exp. Ther.,* 244, 537, 1988.

121. **Litten, R. Z., Suba, E. A., and Roth, B. L.,** Effects of a phorbol ester on rat aortic contraction and calcium influx in the presence and absence of BAY k 8644, *Eur. J. Pharmacol.,* 144, 185, 1987.

122. **Wakabayaski, I., Kakishita, E., Hatake, K., Hishida, S., and Nagai, K.,** Role of calcium in the potentiating effect of phorbol ester on KCl-induced vasocontraction, *Biochem. Biophys. Res. Commun.,* 156, 1195, 1988.

123. **Dale, M. M. and Obianime, A. W.**, 4β-PDBu contracts parenchymal strip and synergizes with raised cytoslic calcium, *Eur. J. Pharmacol.*, 141, 23, 1987.

124. **Kotlikoff, M. I., Murray, R. K., and Reynolds, E. E.**, Histamine-induced Ca^{2+} release and phorbol antagonism in cultured airway smooth muscle cells, *Am. J. Physiol.*, C561, 1987.

125. **Putney, J. W., Jr.**, Recent hypotheses regarding the phosphatidylinositol effect, *Life Sci.*, 29, 1183, 1981.

126. **Piper, P. J.**, Formation and actions of leukotrienes, *Physiol. Rev.*, 64, 744, 1984.

127. **Besterman, J. M., Duronio, V., and Cuatrecasas, R.**, Rapid formation of diacylglycerol from phosphatidylcholine: a pathway for generation of a second messenger, *Proc. Natl. Acad. Sci. U.S.A.*, 83, 6785, 1986.

128. **Bolton, T. B.**, Mechanism of action of transmitters and other substances on smooth muscle, *Physiol. Rev.*, 59, 606, 1979.

129. **Meisheri, K., Hwang, O., and Van Breemen, C.**, Evidence for two separate pathways in smooth muscle plasmalemma, *J. Membr. Biol.*, 59, 19, 1981.

130. **Rodger, I. W.**, Calcium channels, *Am. Rev. Respir. Dis.*, 136, S15, 1987.

131. **Somlyo, A. V. and Somlyo, A. P.**, Electromechanical and pharmacomechanical coupling in vascular smooth muscle, *J. Pharmacol. Exp. Ther.*, 159, 129, 1968.

132. **Farley, J. M. and Miles, P. R.**, Role of depolarization in acetylcholine-induced contractions of dog trachealis muscle, *J. Pharmacol. Exp. Ther.*, 201, 199, 1977.

133. **Fedan, J. S., Hay, D. W. P., and Raeburn, D.**, Ca^{2+} and respiratory smooth muscle function: is there a role for calcium entry blockers in asthma therapy?, in *Current Topics in Pulmonary Pharmacology and Toxicology*, Vol. 3, Hollinger, M. A., Ed., Elsevier, New York, 1988, 53.

134. **Raeburn, D., Rodger, I. W., Hay, D. W. P., and Fedan, J. S.**, The dependence of airway smooth muscle on extracellular Ca^{2+} for contraction is influenced by the presence of cartilage, *Life Sci.*, 38, 1499, 1986.

135. **Kohrogi, H., Horio, S., Ando, M., Sugiomoto, M., Honda, I., and Araki, S.**, Nifedipine inhibits human bronchial smooth muscle contractions induced by leukotrienes C_4 and D_4, prostaglandin $F_{2\alpha}$, and potassium, *Am. Rev. Respir. Dis.*, 132, 299, 1985.

136. **Raeburn, D., Roberts, J. A., Rodger, I. W., and Thomson, N. C.**, Agonist-induced contractile responses of human bronchial muscle *in vitro*: effects of Ca^{2+} removal, La^{3+} and PY 108068, *Eur. J. Pharmacol.*, 121, 251, 1986.

137. **Kannan, M. S. and Davis, C.**, Mode of action of calcium antagonists on responses to spasmogens and antigen challenge in human airway smooth muscle, *Respir. Physiol.*, 74, 15, 1988.

138. **Advenier, C., Naline, E., and Renier, A.**, Effects of Bay k 8644 on contraction of the human isolated bronchus and guinea-pig isolated trachea, *Br. J. Pharmacol.*, 88, 33, 1986.

139. **Kroeger, E. A.**, Role of cyclic nucleotides in modulating smooth muscle function, in *Biochemistry of Smooth Muscle Function*, Vol. 3, Stephens, N. L., Ed., CRC Press, Boca Raton, FL, 1985, 129.

140. **Hardman, J. G.**, Cyclic nucleotides and smooth muscle contraction: some conceptual and experimental considerations, in *Smooth Muscle: An Assessment of Current Knowledge*, Bülbring, E., Brading, A. F., Jones, A. W., and Tomita, T., Eds., Unviersity of Texas Press, Austin, 1981, 249.

141. **Kramer, G. L. and Hardman, J. G.**, Cyclic nucleotides and blood vessel contraction, in *Handbook of Physiology. The Cardiovascular System, Vol. 2, Vascular Smooth Muscle*, Bohr, D. F., Somlyo, A. P., and Sparks, H. S., Eds., American Physiologic Society, Bethesda, MD, 1980, 179.

142. **Jones, C. A., Madison, J. M., Tom-Moy, M., and Brown, J. K.**, Muscarinic cholinergic inhibition of adenylate cyclase in airway smooth muscle, *Am. J. Physiol.*, 253, C97, 1987.

143. **Torphy, T. J., Rinard, G. A., Rietow, M. G., and Mayer, S. E.**, Functional antagonism in canine tracheal smooth muscle: inhibition by methacholine of the mechanical and biochemical responses to isoproterenol, *J. Pharmacol. Exp. Ther.*, 227, 694, 1983.

144. **Torphy, T. J., Zheng, C., Peterson, S. H., Fiscus, R. R., Rinard, G. A., and Mayer, S. E.**, The inhibitory effect of methacholine on drug-induced relaxation, cyclic AMP accumulation and cAMP-dependent protein kinase activation in canine tracheal smooth muscle, *J. Pharmacol. Exp. Ther.*, 233, 409, 1985.

145. **Sankary, R. M., Jones, C. A., Madison, J. M., and Brown, J. K.**, Muscarinic cholinergic inhibition of cyclic AMP accumulation in airway smooth muscle: role of a pertussis toxin-sensitive protein, *Am. Rev. Respir. Dis.*, 138, 145, 1988.

146. **Greengard, P.**, Phosphorylated proteins as physiological effectors, *Science*, 199, 146, 1978.

147. **Krebs, E. G. and Beavo, J. A.**, Phosphorylation-dephosphorylation of enzymes, *Annu. Rev. Biochem.*, 48, 923, 1979.

148. **Flockhart, D. A. and Corbin, J. D.**, Regulatory mechanisms in the control of protein kinases, *CRC Crit. Rev. Biochem.*, 12, 133, 1982.

149. **Stull, J. T. and Mayer, S. E.**, Biochemical mechanism of adrenergic and cholinergic regulation of myocardial contractility, in *Handbook of Physiology, Vol. 2, The Cardiovascular System*, Berne, R. M., Speralakis, N., and Geiger, S. R., Eds., American Physiologic Society, Bethesda, MD, 1979, 741.

150. **Torphy, T. J., Freese, W. B., Rinard, G. A., Brunton, L. L., and Mayer, S. E.,** Cyclic nucleotide-dependent protein kinase in airway smooth muscle, *J. Biol. Chem.,* 257, 11609, 1982.

151. **Sands, H., Meyer, T. A., and Rickenberg, H. V.,** Adenosine 3′,5′-monophosphate-dependent protein kinase of bovine tracheal smooth muscle, *Biochim. Biophys. Acta,* 302, 267, 1973.

152. **Scott, C. W. and Mumby, M. C.,** Phosphorylation of type II regulatory subunit of cAMP-dependent protein kinase in intact smooth muscle, *J. Biol. Chem.,* 260, 2274, 1985.

153. **Felbel, J., Trockur, B., Ecker, T., Landgraf, W., and Hofmann, F.,** Regulation of cytosolic calcium by cAMP and cGMP in freshly isolated smooth muscle cells from bovine trachea, *J. Biol. Chem.,* 263, 16764, 1988.

154. **Brockbank, K. J. and England, P. J.,** A rapid method for the preparation of sarcolemmal vesicles from rat aorta, and the stimulation of Ca^{2+} uptake into the vesicles by cyclic AMP-dependent protein kinase, *FEBS Lett.,* 122, 67, 1980.

155. **Bhalla, R. C., Webb, R. C., Singh, D., and Brock, C.,** Role of cyclic AMP in rat aortic microsomal phosphorylation and calcium uptake, *Am. J. Physiol.,* 234, H508, 1978.

156. **Nishikori, K. and Maeno, H.,** Close relationship between adenosine 3′,5′-monophosphate dependent endogenous phosphorylation of a specific protein and stimulation of calcium uptake in rat uterine microsomes, *J. Biol. Chem.,* 254, 6099, 1979.

157. **Sands, H., Mascali, J., and Paietta, E.,** Determination of calcium transport and phosphoprotein phosphatase activity in microsomes from respiratory and vascular smooth muscle, *Biochim. Biophys. Acta,* 500, 223, 1977.

158. **Sands, H. and Mascali, J.,** Effects of cAMP and of protein kinase on the calcium uptake of various smooth muscle organelles, *Arch. Int. Pharmacodyn. Ther.,* 236, 180, 1978.

159. **Scheid, C. R., Honeyman, T. W., and Fay, F. S.,** Mechanism of β-adrenergic relaxation of smooth muscle, *Nature (London),* 277, 32, 1979.

160. **Webb, R. C. and Bohr, D. F.,** Relaxation of vascular smooth muscle by isoproterenol, dibutyryl-cyclic AMP and theophylline, *J. Pharmacol. Exp. Ther.,* 217, 26, 1981.

161. **Gunst, S. J. and Stropp, J. Q.,** Effect of Na-K adenosine triphosphatase activity on relaxation of canine tracheal smooth muscle, *J. Appl. Physiol.,* 64, 635, 1988.

162. **Meisheri, K. D. and van Breemen, C.,** Effects of β-adrenergic stimulation on calcium movements in rabbit aortic smooth muscle: relationship with cyclic AMP, *J. Physiol.,* 331, 429, 1982.

163. **Hall, I. P. and Hill, S. J.,** β-Adrenoceptor stimulation inhibits histamine-stimulated inositol phospholipid hydrolysis in bovine tracheal smooth muscle, *Br. J. Pharmacol.,* 95, 1204, 1988.

164. **de Lanerolle, P., Nishikawa, M., Yost, D. A., and Adelstein, R. S.,** Increased phosphorylation of myosin light chain kinase after an increase in cyclic AMP in intact smooth muscle, *Science,* 223, 1415, 1983.

165. **Hay, D. W. P., Muccitelli, R. M., Wilson, K. A., Wasserman, M. A., and Torphy, T. J.,** Functional antagonism by salbutamol suggests differences in the relative efficacies and dissociation constants of the peptidoleukotrienes in guinea-pig trachea, *J. Pharmacol. Exp. Ther.,* 244, 71, 1988.

166. **Miller, J. R., Silver, P. J., and Stull, S. T.,** The role of myosin light chain kinase phosphorylation in beta-adrenergic relaxation of tracheal smooth muscle, *Mol. Pharmacol.,* 24, 235, 1983.

167. **Rapoport, R. M. and Murad, F.,** Endothelium-dependent and nitrovasodilator-induced relaxation of vascular smooth muscle: role of cGMP, *J. Cyclic Nucleotide Res.,* 9, 281, 1983.

168. **Waldman, S. A. and Murad, F.,** Cyclic GMP synthesis and function, *Pharmacol. Rev.,* 39, 163, 1987.

169. **Moncada, S., Radomski, M. W., and Palmer, R. M. J.,** Endothelium-derived relaxing factor: identification as nitric oxide and role in the control of vascular tone and platelet function, *Biochem. Pharmacol.,* 37, 2495, 1988.

170. **Waldman, S. A., Rapoport, R., and Murad, F.,** Atrial natriuretic factor selectively activates particulate guanylate cyclase and elevates cGMP in rat tissues, *J. Biol. Chem.,* 259, 14332, 1984.

171. **Kuno, T., Andersen, J. W., Kamisaki, Y., Waldman, S. A., Chang, L. T., Saheki, S., Leitman, D. C., Nakane, M., and Murad, F.,** Co-purification of an atrial natriuretic factor receptor and particulate guanylate cyclase from rat lung, *J. Biol. Chem.,* 261, 5817, 1986.

172. **Hamel, R. and Ford-Hutchinson, A. W.,** Relaxant profile of synthetic atrial natriuretic factor on guinea-pig pulmonary tissues, *Eur. J. Pharmacol.,* 121, 151, 1986.

173. **Lincoln, T. M., Dills, W. L., and Corbin, J. D.,** Purification and subunit composition of guanosine 3′:5′-monophosphate-dependent protein kinase from bovine lung, *J. Biol. Chem.,* 252, 4269, 1977.

174. **Miller, C. A., Barnette, M. S., Ormsbee, H. S., III, and Torphy, T. J.,** Cyclic nucleotide-dependent protein kinases in the lower esophageal sphincter, *Am. J. Physiol.,* 251, G794, 1986.

175. **Katsuki, S. and Murad, F.,** Regulation of adenosine cyclic 3′,5′-monophosphate and guanosine cyclic 3′,5′-monophosphate levels and contractility in bovine tracheal smooth muscle, *Mol. Pharmacol.,* 13, 330, 1977.

176. **Fiscus, R. R., Torphy, T. J., and Mayer, S. E.,** Cyclic GMP-dependent protein kinase activation in canine tracheal smooth muscle by methacholine and sodium nitroprusside, *Biochem. Biophys. Acta,* 805, 382, 1984.

177. **Francis, S. H., Noblett, B. D., Todd, B. W., Wells, J. N., and Corbin, J. D.,** Relaxation of vascular and tracheal smooth muscle by cyclic nucleotide analogs that preferentially activate purified cGMP-dependent protein kinase, *Mol. Pharmacol.,* 34, 506, 1988.

178. **Kobayashi, S., Kanaide, H., and Nakamura, M.,** Cytosolic-free calcium transients in cultured vascular smooth muscle cells: microfluorometric measurements, *Science,* 229, 553, 1985.

179. **Cornwell, T. L. and Lincoln, T. M.,** Regulation of intracellular Ca^{2+} levels in cultured vascular smooth muscle cells: reduction of Ca^{2+} by atriopeptin and 8-bromo-cyclic GMP is mediated by cyclic GMP-dependent protein kinase, *J. Biol. Chem.,* 264, 1146, 1989.

180. **Popescu, L. M., Panoiu, C., Hinescu, M., and Nutu, O.,** The mechanism of cGMP-induced relaxation in vascular smooth muscle, *Eur. J. Pharmacol.,* 107, 393, 1985.

181. **Furukawa, K.-I., Tawada, Y., and Shigekawa, M.,** Regulation of the plasma membrane Ca^{2+} pump by cyclic nucleotides in cultured vascular smooth muscle cells, *J. Biol. Chem.,* 263, 8058, 1988.

182. **Rashatwar, S. S., Cornwell, T. L., and Lincoln, T. M.,** Effects of 8-bromo-cGMP on Ca^{2+} levels in vascular smooth muscle cells: possible regulation of Ca^{2+}-ATPase by cGMP-dependent protein kinase, *Proc. Natl. Acad. Sci. U.S.A.,* 84, 5685, 1987.

183. **Raeymaekers, L., Hofmann, F., and Casteels, R.,** Cyclic GMP-dependent protein kinase phosphorylates phospholamban in isolated sarcoplasmic reticulum from cardiac and smooth muscle, *Biochem. J.,* 252, 269, 1988.

184. **Godfraind, T.,** EDRF and cyclic GMP control gating of receptor-operated calcium channels in vascular smooth muscle, *Eur. J. Pharmacol.,* 126, 341, 1986.

185. **Rapoport, R. M.,** Cyclic guanosine monophosphate inhibition of contraction may be mediated through inhibition of phosphatidylinositol hydrolysis in rat aorta, *Circ. Res.,* 58, 407, 1986.

186. **Pfitzer, G., Hofmann, F., DiSalvo, J., and Rüegg, J. C.,** cGMP and cAMP inhibit tension development in skinned coronary arteries, *Pfluegers Arch.,* 401, 277, 1984.

187. **Karaki, H., Sato, K., Ozakai, H., and Murakami, K.,** Effects of sodium nitroprusside on cytosolic Ca^{2+} level in vascular smooth muscle, *Eur. J. Pharmacol.,* 156, 259, 1988.

188. **Weishaar, R. E., Cain, M. H., and Bristol, J. A.,** A new generation of phosphodiesterase inhibitors: multiple molecular forms of phosphodiesterase and the potential for drug selectivity, *J. Med. Chem.,* 28, 537, 1985.

189. **Beavo, J. A.,** Multiple isozymes of cyclic nucleotide phosphodiesterase, *Adv. Second Messenger Phosphoprotein Res.,* 22, 1, 1988.

190. **Torphy, T. J.,** Action of mediators on airway smooth muscle: functional antagonism as a mechanism for bronchodilator drugs, *Agents Actions Suppl.,* 23, 37, 1988.

191. **Silver, P. J., Hamel, L. T., Perrone, M. H., Bentley, R. C., Bushover, C. R., and Evans, D. B.,** Differential pharmacologic sensitivity of cyclic nucleotide phosphodiesterase isozymes isolated from cardiac muscle, arterial and airway smooth muscle, *Eur. J. Pharmacol.,* 150, 85, 1988.

192. **Cieslinski, L. B., Reeves, M. L., and Torphy, T. J.,** Cyclic nucleotide phosphodiesterases (PDEs) in canine and human tracheal smooth muscle, *FASEB J.,* 2, A1065, 1988.

193. **Torphy, T. J. and Cieslinski, L. B.,** Characterization and selective inhibition of cyclic nucleotide phosphodiesterase isozymes in canine tracheal smooth muscle, *Mol. Pharmacol.,* 37, 206, 1990.

194. **Torphy, T. J., Burman, M., Huang, L. B. F., and Tucker, S. S.,** Inhibition of the low k_m cyclic AMP phosphodiesterase in intact canine trachealis by SK&F 94836: mechanical and biochemical effects, *J. Pharmacol. Exp. Ther.,* 246, 843, 1988.

195. **Torphy, T. J., Burman, M., and Huang, L. B. F.,** Role of phosphodiesterase (PDE) isozymes in regulating cyclic nucleotide content in canine trachealis, *FASEB J.,* 2, A1066, 1988.

196. **Van den Brink, F. G.,** The model of functional interaction. II. Experimental verification of a new model: the antagonism of β-adrenoceptor stimulants and other agonists, *Eur. J. Pharmacol.,* 22, 279, 1973.

197. **Buckner, C. K. and Saini, R. K.,** On the use of functional antagonism to estimate dissociation constants for *beta* adrenergic receptor agonists in isolated guinea-pig trachea, *J. Pharmacol. Exp. Ther.,* 194, 565, 1975.

198. **Mitchell, H. W. and Denborough, M. A.,** Drug interactions in cat isolated tracheal smooth muscle, *Clin. Exp. Pharmacol. Physiol.,* 6, 249, 1979.

199. **Torphy, T. J., Burman, M., Schwartz, L. W., and Wasserman, M. A.,** Differential effects of methacholine and leukotriene D_4 on cyclic nucleotide content and isoproterenol-induced relaxation in the opossum trachea, *J. Pharmacol. Exp. Ther.,* 237, 332, 1986.

200. **Torphy, T. J.,** Differential relaxant effects of isoproterenol on methacholine- versus leukotriene D_4-induced contraction in the guinea-pig trachea, *Eur. J. Pharmacol.,* 102, 549, 1984.

201. **Russell, J. A.,** Differential inhibitory effect of isoproterenol on contractions of canine airways, *J. Appl. Physiol.,* 57, 801, 1984.

202. **Heaslip, R. J., Giesa, F. R., Rimele, T. J., and Grimes, D.,** Sensitivity of the PGF$_{2\alpha}$-versus carbachol-contracted trachea to relaxation by salbutamol, forskolin and prenalterol, *Eur. J. Pharmacol.*, 128, 73, 1986.
203. **Farmer, J. B. and Lehrer, D. N.,** The effect of isoprenaline on the contraction of smooth muscle produced by histamine, acetylcholine or other agents, *J. Pharm. Pharmacol.*, 18, 649, 1966.
204. **Jenne, J. W., Shaughnessy, T. K., Druz, W. S., Manfredi, C. J., and Vestal, R. E.,** In vivo functional antagonism between isoproterenol and bronchoconstrictants in the dog, *J. Appl. Physiol.*, 63, 812, 1987.
205. **Barnes, P. J. and Pride, N. B.,** Dose-response curves to inhaled β-adrenoceptor agonists in normal and asthmatic subjects, *Br. J. Clin. Pharmacol.*, 15, 677, 1983.
206. **Cheng, J. B. and Townley, R. G.,** Pharmacological characterization of effects of nifedipine on isolated guinea-pig and rat tracheal smooth muscle, *Arch. Int. Pharmacodyn. Ther.*, 263, 228, 1983.
207. **Ahmed, F., Foster, R. W., and Small, R. C.,** Some effects of nifedipine in guinea-pig isolated trachealis, *Br. J. Pharmacol.*, 84, 861, 1985.
208. **Horio, S., Kohrogi, H., Ando, M., Sugimoto, M., and Araki, S.,** Preventive and reverse effects of nifedipine on human bronchoconstriction "in vitro", *Arch. Int. Pharmacodyn. Ther.*, 267, 80, 1984.
209. **Rinard, G. A., Puckett, A. M., and Torphy, T. J.,** unpublished observations, 1985.
210. **Gunst, S. J., Stropp, J. Q., and Flavahan, N. A.,** Analysis of receptor reserves in canine tracheal smooth muscle, *J. App. Physiol.*, 62, 1755, 1987.
211. **Silver, P. J. and Stull, J. T.,** Effects of the calmodulin antagonist, fluphenazine, on phosphorylation of myosin and phosphorylase in intact smooth muscle, *Mol. Pharmacol.*, 23, 665, 1983.
212. **Beavo, J. A. and Reifsnyder, D. H.,** Primary sequence of cyclic nucleotide phosphodiesterase isozymes and the design of selective inhibitors, *Trends Pharmac. Sci.*, 11, 150, 1990.

Chapter 3

AIRWAY SMOOTH MUSCLE: ELECTROPHYSIOLOGICAL PROPERTIES AND BEHAVIOR

R. C. Small, J. P. Boyle, R. W. Foster, and D. M. Good

TABLE OF CONTENTS

I. Introduction 70

II. General Electrophysiological Properties of Airway Smooth Muscle 70
    A. Resting Membrane Potential 70
    B. Passive Electrical Properties of Airway Smooth Muscle 70
    C. Rectification in Airway Smooth Muscle 72
    D. Spontaneous Activity 72
    E. Action Potentials in Airway Smooth Muscle after K^+ Channel
       Blockade 74

III. Ion Channels in Airway Smooth Muscle 75
    A. K^+ Channels 76
    B. Ca^{2+} Channels 79
    C. Chloride Channels 79

IV. Modulation of the Electrical Activity of Airway Smooth Muscle by
Epithelium-Derived Relaxant Factor and by Neurotransmitters 80
    A. Epithelium-Derived Relaxant Factor 80
    B. Neuroeffector Transmission in Airway Smooth Muscle 80
    C. Cholinergic Nerves 80
    D. Noradrenergic Nerves 81
    E. Nonadrenergic, Noncholinergic Nerves 81

V. Electrophysiological Effects of Exogenous Spasmogens 82
    A. Potassium Chloride (KCl) and Tetraethylammonium (TEA) 82
    B. Agonists at Muscarinic Cholinoreceptors and Histamine H_1
       Receptors 83
    C. Leukotrienes 85

VI. Electrophysiological Effects of Exogenous Relaxant Agents 85
    A. Agonists at β-Adrenoreceptors 85
    B. Methylxanthines 88
    C. K^+ Channel-Opening Drugs 88
    D. Ca^{2+} Antagonists and Ca^{2+} Agonists 90

Acknowledgments 90

References 90

I. INTRODUCTION

To our knowledge, the earliest review of the electrophysiological properties of airway smooth muscle is that of Kirkpatrick,[1] published in 1981. Most of the literature cited in that review involved recordings of membrane potential changes made either by means of the sucrose-gap technique or by means of conventional intracellular glass microelectrodes. Furthermore, such recordings were made solely from the trachealis muscle of a very limited number of mammalian species.

Since 1981 an increasing number of laboratories have studied the electrophysiological properties of airway smooth muscle. Tissue has been obtained from a greater variety of species, including the human. A few studies have now been made of smooth muscle taken from airways of smaller caliber than the trachea. In addition, the techniques of preparing isolated cells and patch-clamp recording have enabled studies of membrane potential to be supplemented by analysis of current flow through individual ion channels in the plasmalemma.

In common with many other fields of biological science, study of the electrophysiology of airway smooth muscle has entered a phase of rapid growth. Accordingly, our understanding of the workings of this tissue in health and disease seems set for marked improvement.

II. GENERAL ELECTROPHYSIOLOGICAL PROPERTIES OF AIRWAY SMOOTH MUSCLE

A. RESTING MEMBRANE POTENTIAL

For most species examined, the resting membrane potential of trachealis cells lies in the range -45 to -60 mV (Table 1). Smooth-muscle cells from bronchi or bronchioles have not been extensively investigated, but, in the dog, there is some evidence for higher resting membrane potential in the smaller caliber airways.[18,21]

B. PASSIVE ELECTRICAL PROPERTIES OF AIRWAY SMOOTH MUSCLE

The passive electrical, or cable, properties of any cell are defined by the spatial and temporal changes which are observed when membrane potential is displaced by the passage of current through some part of the cell membrane. The space constant (λ) and the time constant (τ) characterize the passive electrical properties of the cell membrane. These two constants depend on the resistance (R_m) and capacitance (C_m) of the cell membrane, λ being proportional to R_m/C_m and τ being proportional to $R_m \cdot C_m$. These constants are commonly measured for a single excitable cell, but, since smooth-muscle cells often exhibit electrical coupling through low-resistance gap junctions, a more useful measure of these parameters can be made in strips of smooth muscle containing a number of cells.

The space constant defines the distance that a voltage change will spread passively along the cell (or cells) under test. If a constant current is passed into the test preparation for an effectively infinite time, to establish a transmembrane potential change V_o at that point and a transmembrane potential change V_x at a distance x from the point of current injection, then the expression:

$$V_x = V_o \cdot e^{-x/\lambda} \qquad (1)$$

describes the relationship between these voltage changes and the space constant. If the special case where $x = \lambda$ is considered, then

$$V_x = V_o \cdot e^{-1} \qquad (2)$$

TABLE 1
Electrical Properties of Airway Smooth Muscle

Tissue	Species	Resting transmembrane potential (mV)	Spontaneous activity (slow waves)	Space constant (mm)	Time constant (ms)	Ref.
	Human	−20 to −50	Zero	—	—	2
Trachealis		−45	High incidence	—	—	3
	Ox	−47	Low incidence	—	—	4
		−47		2.6	306	5
	Cat	−68	Zero	—	—	6
	Guinea pig	−40	High incidence	—	—	7
		−40		—	—	8
		−61		—	—	9
		−50		—	—	10
		−51		—	—	11
		−42		—	—	12
	Dog	−54	Zero	—	—	13
		−47	Zero	1.6	—	14
		−59	Zero	3.2	449	15
		−60	Zero	2.1	306	16
		−55	Zero	2.2	282	17
		−60	Low incidence in lower trachea	—	—	18
		−61	Zero	—	—	19
	Ferret	−58	Zero	—	—	20
2nd Generation bronchus	Dog	−63	Zero	—	—	18
1 mm Bronchiole	Dog	−70	Zero	—	—	21

and can thus be defined as the distance at which the voltage change across the membrane falls to 1/e (0.3701) of its original value.

The space constants for canine and bovine trachealis (determined by using the partition stimulation technique of Abe and Tomita)[22] are in the range 1.5 to 3.5 mm (Table 1). It should be noted that individual cells in canine trachealis rarely exceed 1 mm in length, suggesting that these smooth-muscle cells are electrically coupled through gap junctions.

Results obtained using microelectrodes to inject current into cells of the ferret trachealis did not suggest the existence of such coupling.[20] However, it should be noted that the use of intracellular current injection allows the voltage to decay in three dimensions. This complicates subsequent analysis.[23] Electrotonic potentials induced by large, extracellular, current-passing electrodes spread along the longitudinal axis of the muscle bundles, thereby avoiding the problems of three-dimensional decay.[22] Accordingly, the partition stimulation technique of Abe and Tomita[22] remains the preferred method of assessing the value of λ in smooth muscle.

The time constant defines the time required for a voltage change to occur in response to an injection of constant current. If such constant current is applied to the cell/tissue strip beginning when the time (t) is equal to zero, then the relationship between the charge (Q) on the membrane and the time constant is given by:

$$Q_t = Q_o \cdot e^{-t/\tau} \qquad (3)$$

Where Q_t is the charge at time t and Q_o is the membrane charge at t = 0. Since $Q = C_m V$, and assuming that C_m is a constant, this equation transforms to:

$$V_t = V_o \cdot e^{-t/\tau} \tag{4}$$

When the case where $t = \tau$ is considered, τ can be shown to be the time taken for the transmembrane potential to reach $1/e$ of its steady-state value.

The time constants for bovine and canine trachealis are in the range 280 to 450 ms (Table 1). These figures are very large in comparison to those found in spontaneously active tissue such as intestinal or uterine smooth muscle,[22,24] but are similar to the constants for quiescent smooth muscle such as vas deferens and anococcygeus.[25,26]

In airway smooth muscle, λ and τ are both increased by the application of the K^+ channel blocking agent tetraethylammonium (TEA),[14,17] presumably because TEA increases membrane resistance. It is likely, therefore, that the membrane resistance of airway smooth-muscle cells is governed, at least in part, by the K^+ permeability of the plasmalemma.

C. RECTIFICATION IN AIRWAY SMOOTH MUSCLE

When the resistance of a conductor is dependent on the voltage across it, then the conductor acts as a rectifier. Rectification may be seen in response to current flow in either direction across the conductor. The plasmalemma of trachealis cells exhibits rectifying behavior. Anodal current passed into trachealis cells evokes hyperpolarization, while cathodal current evokes depolarization. Although the amplitude of these electronic potentials is dependent on the current passed into or out of the cell, the membrane potential change evoked by the passage of cathodal current is much smaller than that evoked by an equivalent anodal current due to membrane rectification.[4,14,15,17] Under normal conditions the rectifying behavior of the trachealis cells acts to prevent the discharge of regenerative action potentials in response to cathodal current injection.

Since rectification by the cell membrane is by definition associated with changes in R_m, it may be related to changes in the activity of plasmalemmal ion channels. A number of different, voltage-dependent K^+ channels have been shown to exist in smooth-muscle cell membranes (see Section III), some of which open in response to depolarization. The resultant outward current flow will tend to limit any depolarizing shift in membrane potential. In airway smooth muscle, spontaneous action potentials are not observed and it is difficult to elicit action potentials by cathodal current injection. Hence, outward current carried by K^+ channels may be sufficient to prevent regenerative action potential discharge.

The proposal that membrane rectification is K^+ channel dependent is supported by the finding that the K^+ channel blocker, TEA, causes an increase in membrane resistance[15,17] and a decrease in rectification.[4,14,15,17] 4-Aminopyridine (4-AP), another K^+ channel blocker, appears to act in a manner different from TEA, since it decreases membrane resistance and fails to modify rectification in canine tracheal smooth muscle.[17]

D. SPONTANEOUS ACTIVITY

Under *in vitro* conditions, airway smooth muscle is often electrically quiescent. However, trachealis isolated from a number of species may exhibit spontaneous rhythmic fluctuations in membrane potential. These oscillations, or slow waves, are commonly seen when recording from human or guinea pig trachealis (Figure 1) and are occasionally seen in records obtained from bovine trachealis or from the thoracic end of canine trachealis. The smooth-muscle cells of the bronchi and bronchioles from the dog and the trachealis of the cat and ferret lack any spontaneous electrical activity (Table 1).

Slow-wave activity recorded from a cell may be relatively constant in frequency and amplitude or may exhibit complex patterns where the amplitude or, more rarely, the frequency varies.[3] The maximum amplitude of slow waves only rarely exceeds 20 mV[1,3,18,27] and, while slow-wave frequency in bovine, canine, and human trachealis is approximately 0.3 Hz,[1,3,18] in guinea pig tracheal cells it varies from 0.5 to 1.6 Hz.[3,8,11,28,29]

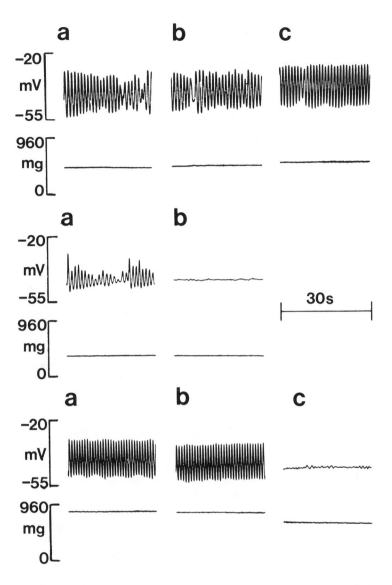

FIGURE 1. Effects of Bay K8644 and nifedipine on the electrical and mechanical properties of guinea pig isolated trachealis. In each row of records the upper trace represents membrane potential and the lower trace the mechanical activity of a contiguous segment of trachea. In each row all electrical records were taken from the same cell. Upper row: activity recorded before (a) and 1.5 min (b) or 9 min (c) after Bay K8644 1 μM. Middle row: activity recorded before (a) and 1.5 min (b) after nifedipine 1 μM. Lower row: activity recorded in a tissue pretreated with Bay K8644 1 μM (a) and 1.5 min (b) or 9 min (c) following addition of nifedipine 1 μM. Note in (c) that the slow waves were at the point of being abolished 9 min after the addition of nifedipine. Bay K8644 clearly delays slow-wave suppression induced by nifedipine. (From Allen, S. L., Foster, R. W., Small, R. C., and Towart, R., *Br. J. Pharmacol.*, 86, 171, 1985. With permission.)

Slow-wave activity seems to be dependent on the extracellular Ca^{2+} concentration and is abolished by Ca^{2+}-free media[12,30] or by organic inhibitors of Ca^{2+} influx such as nifedipine and verapamil (Figure 1).[10,27,28,31] The depolarizing phase of each slow wave is therefore likely to be due to an increase in membrane Ca^{2+} conductance. However, such Ca^{2+} conductance changes have yet to be demonstrated in airway smooth muscle.[1] Nevertheless, slow-wave activity provides evidence for a membrane Ca^{2+} oscillator[32] in airway smooth muscle.

If the depolarizing phase of each slow wave represents Ca^{2+} influx into the cell, the cytosolic concentration of free Ca^{2+} $[Ca^{2+}]_i$ might be expected to oscillate in synchrony with the pattern of slow-wave discharge. Measurement of $[Ca^{2+}]_i$ can be made in excitable cells using fluorescent Ca^{2+} indicators such as fura-2 or the Ca^{2+}-sensitive photoprotein, aequorin.[19,35,36] Measurements of this kind have been made in isolated airway smooth muscle,[19,33-36] but no reports of $[Ca^{2+}]_i$ fluctuations which could be associated with slow-wave activity have yet appeared. Presently reported experiments, however, fall short of the ideal kind in which both electrical activity and $[Ca^{2+}]_i$ are simultaneously measured. Despite the fact that direct evidence for Ca^{2+} influx during the depolarizing phase of slow waves is not available, it is our conviction that such Ca^{2+} influx occurs and that slow waves therefore act as nascent action potentials. This conviction is stengthened by the observation that bursts of slow-wave activity are often associated with tension development by the muscle.[1,11,18,28]

There is good evidence that slow-wave discharge is of myogenic rather than neurogenic origin (Figure 2).[11,12,37] Honda and Tomita[3] have reported that indomethacin suppresses both mechanical tone and slow-wave discharge in guinea pig trachealis. Accordingly, these authors suggested that the synthesis of prostaglandins is responsible for initiating slow-wave discharge and hence tone production. However, other laboratories have shown that flurbiprofen and indomethacin, at concentrations which abolish the prostaglandin-dependent tone of guinea pig trachealis, do not abolish slow-wave activity.[38,39] In all probability, slow-wave discharge is an intrinsic behavior pattern for the plasmalemma of the airway smooth-muscle cell. The basal discharge process may well be stimulated by the actions of prostaglandins or other endogenous or exogenous spasmogens.

Cooling[9,12,28] or the addition of ouabain[18] inhibits slow-wave activity, but it is not clear if this indicates slow-wave dependence on the supply of metabolic energy or is the result of nonspecific depression of muscle activity. However, it is clear that slow-wave discharge is potential dependent, as shifts in membrane potential in the depolarizing or hyperpolarizing directions result in abolition of slow-wave activity.[1]

Low-resistance gap junctions between trachealis cells may provide a route by which slow-wave activity could be transmitted through the tissue. Synchronization of slow-wave discharge has been suggested by extracellular recording of compound electrical activity[28] and by intracellular recording of activity from a number of cells in a small area of tissue.[8] The simplest explanation of the synchrony of slow-wave discharge is that the cells are electrically coupled. However, many cells, even in tissue from species which do exhibit slow waves, are electrically quiescent and, in spite of electrical coupling, the trachealis does not behave as a true syncytium. Different patterns of activity can be recorded even from adjacent muscle bundles in the same tracheal segment.[40]

E. ACTION POTENTIALS IN AIRWAY SMOOTH MUSCLE AFTER K^+ CHANNEL BLOCKADE

Although the rectifying properties of airway smooth muscle usually prevent the discharge of regenerative action potentials, the addition of the K^+ channel blocking agent, TEA, to the bathing medium allows action potentials to be generated in response to cathodal current injection.[14,15,17,41] TEA itself causes concentration-dependent depolarization, and this may be sufficient to initiate action potential discharge.[4,10,14,17,28,30,42]

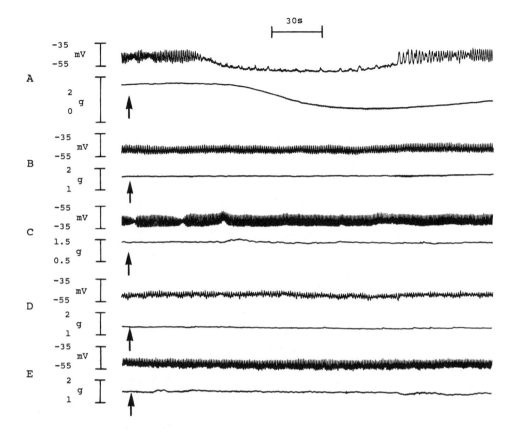

FIGURE 2. Effects of tetrodotoxin, hexamethonium, guanethidine, and propranolol on the electrical and mechanical responses of hyoscine-treated guinea pig isolated trachealis to nicotine (100 μM). Each pair of traces represents results from a different preparation. In each case hyoscine (1 μM) was present throughout. The upper trace represents membrane potential changes, while the lower trace represents the mechanical activity of a contiguous segment of trachea. Nicotine (100 μM) was introduced at the arrow and was allowed to superfuse the tissues for 4 min. (A) Control; (B) tetrodotoxin (0.3 μM) present throughout; (C) hexamethonium (500 μM) present throughout; (D) guanethidine (50 μM) present throughout; (E) propranolol (1 μM) present throughout. Note that tetrodotoxin, hexamethonium, guanethidine, and propranolol were each able to suppress the electrical and mechanical responses to nicotine, but did not suppress the electrical slow-wave discharge. (From Boyle, J. P., Davies, J. M., Foster, R. W., Morgan, G. P., and Small, R. C., *Br. J. Pharmacol.*, 90, 733, 1987. With permission.)

Action potential generation in bovine, canine, feline, and guinea pig trachealis is associated with an increase in tension.[4,10,14,17,29,40-42] Both the action potentials and the mechanical effects are resistant to Na^+-free media[41] and tetrodotoxin,[31] but are sensitive to procedures which will reduce Ca^{2+} influx. These include tissue exposure to a Ca^{2+}-free medium containing EGTA[41] or to a Ca^{2+} influx inhibitor such as gallopamil (D600), verapamil, or nifedipine.[10,17,31] The rising (depolarizing) phase of the action potential in trachealis is therefore likely to be associated with an increase in membrane permeability to Ca^{2+}, probably due to the opening of voltage-operated calcium channels (VOCs) (see Section III). Action potentials in trachealis therefore resemble those observed in other smooth muscles.

III. ION CHANNELS IN AIRWAY SMOOTH MUSCLE

Until recently, very little information about currents due to the movement of specific ions across smooth-muscle cell membranes in general, and airway smooth-muscle membranes in particular, has been obtained by direct measurement. Difficulties associated with attempting to voltage clamp smooth muscle have included the geometry of the cells, the syncytial nature of the tissue, and the often large values of λ and τ.[43] These factors have cast doubt on the adequacy of any clamp of tissue potential or current and, as a result, about the validity of data thus obtained.

Two developments have refined our ability to measure the activity of ion channels in the plasmalemma and the flow of current through such channels. Firstly, single, viable smooth-muscle cells can now be isolated from tissues using a mixture of digestive enzymes (typically collagenase and elastase) and mechanical agitation. Secondly, the patch clamp technique[44] allows adequate voltage or current clamping of cells exhibiting the spindle-shaped profile of smooth muscle. The patch clamp recording pipette establishes such a very high resistance glass-membrane seal that the serial resistance (membrane resistance + pipette resistance) is small in comparison. If voltage clamp of the cell is to be performed, the serial resistance is normally further reduced by disrupting the membrane under the pipette tip. This has the additional effect of dialyzing the cell with the pipette solution. It is also possible, using a variant of this technique, to record current flowing through single-ion channels in patches of membrane.

A. K⁺ CHANNELS

In most tissues, including smooth muscle, the easiest channels to identify due to their relatively high conductances and high density, are K^+ channels (Figure 3). In consequence, these channels have been studied more than any other and have been classified in most detail. K^+ channels have been classified according to their dependence on voltage for activation, their dependence on Ca^{2+} for activation, their unitary conductance, and their sensitivity to a variety of blockers or toxins.

Up to nine different K^+-selective channels have been identified in smooth muscle using the above criteria.[45,46] In addition, two channels have been described that will permit the passage of K^+, but which are not selective for this ion.[45] Some of these channels have only been identified from recordings of whole-cell currents, while others have been identified on the basis of records of current flow through single channels in isolated membrane patches. Indirect evidence also exists for a further type of K^+ channel in smooth muscle. Such evidence is based on data obtained using drugs which are known to act by increasing the K^+ permeability of the cell membrane (see Section VI.C).

Several laboratories have studied K^+ channels in isolated trachealis cells using both whole cell and isolated patch recording configurations. Cells dispersed from canine trachealis by treatment with collagenase and elastase have been identified as smooth muscle using antismooth-muscle actin[47] or myosin[48] and retained the morphological[48] and physiological[47] properties seen in intact tissue. When studied in both the cell-attached[47] and the inside-out patch configuration,[47,49] the principal channel detected in both porcine and canine airway smooth muscle was highly selective for K^+ over other cations, and had a reversal potential that was close to Ek (the K^+ equilibrium potential).[47,49] The channel was voltage activated (i.e., depolarization increased both the frequency of opening and the time spent in the open state) and Ca^{2+} activated (i.e., increases in $[Ca^{2+}]_i$ increased both the opening frequency and the duration of the open state). The conductance of this channel in symmetrical K^+ solutions was approximately 270 pS and ion movement through it was blocked by external TEA or reduced by TEA or Cs^{+}[47] applied to the cytoplasmic side of the membrane.

On the basis of these observations this channel can be identified as the "maxi" or big K^+ channel which has been described in many tissues. The high density of this channel, its Ca^{2+} and voltage dependence and its susceptibility to blockade by TEA all suggest that it may play an important role in the rectifying behavior of the airway smooth-muscle cell membrane.[47] Depolarization accompanied by a small increase in $[Ca^{2+}]_i$ would cause an increase in the open probability (P_o) of the channel. The membrane potential will therefore

77

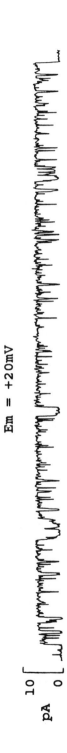

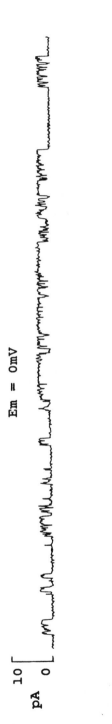

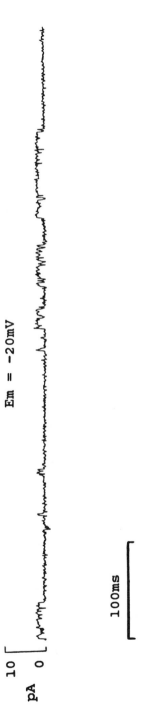

Em = +20mV

Em = 0mV

Em = -20mV

100ms

FIGURE 3.   Currents associated with the opening of single K$^+$ channels in an inside-out plasmalemmal patch from a smooth-muscle cell isolated from guinea pig trachealis. Each trace represents activity recorded after the patch had been clamped at the indicated potential for at least 10 s. The media bathing the external and internal surfaces of the membrane patch contained Na$^+$ and K$^+$ equivalent to that normally found in extracellular fluid and cytosol, respectively. The high (100 pS) unitary conductance of the illustrated K$^+$ channels suggests that they are the "maxi" K$^+$ channels responsible for the rectifying behavior of the plasmalemma. Note how depolarization increases the probability of channel opening, the duration of channel opening, and the unitary current amplitude. Experiment conducted at 22°C. (From Boyle, J. P., Foster, R. W., and Small, R. C., unpublished observations.)

be driven in the direction of Ek, so limiting the depolarization evoked by the excitatory stimulus.

As mentioned above, TEA-induced blockade of K^+ channels abolishes plasmalemmal rectification and allows regenerative action potentials to be discharged in response to cathodal current injection into trachealis cells. Evidence that similar K^+ channels may limit the depolarization induced by structurally specific spasmogenic agents has been obtained using guinea pig trachealis and canine bronchus. In these tissues, cholinesters or histamine evoke depolarization on which may be superimposed rapid, hyperpolarizing transients.[29,38,39,50] These transients probably represent the synchronous opening of groups of Ca^{2+}- and voltage-dependent K^+ channels, the required Ca^{2+} being provided from intracellular stores.[39] Addition of TEA to acetylcholine- (ACh) or histamine-treated tissue not only induced further depolarization, but also abolished the hyperpolarizing transients. However, TEA did not augment ACh- or histamine-induced tension development.[39] In feline trachealis, application of TEA clearly increased the mechanical response to cathodal current injection.[41] The differing effects of TEA on mechanical responses to structurally specific spasmogens and cathodal current injection may reflect differing underlying processes of excitation-contraction coupling.

Two further Ca^{2+}-activated K^+ channels have been described in cells from bovine trachealis.[51,52] In cell-attached patches they could not be discriminated from each other, but recording from isolated inside/out or outside/out patches revealed two channels on the basis of their different unitary conductances (120 and 50 pS).[51] Whole-cell voltage clamp recordings revealed two K^+ currents in response to a depolarizing step, an early current (peak within 100 ms) and a late current (peak within 300 to 1000 ms).[52] Both currents were Ca^{2+} dependent and were abolished by removal of Ca^{2+} from the extracellular fluid or by treatment with Ca^{2+} influx blockers such as Ni^{2+}. When Ca^{2+} release from intracellular stores was inhibited by pretreatment of cells with caffeine or ryanodine, the late current was inhibited, but the early current persisted. In Ca^{2+}-free media containing EGTA, the late current could be evoked by treatment of the cell with caffeine, histamine, 5-hydroxytryptamine (5HT), ACh, or phenylephrine. A similar response could be obtained by including inositol 1,4,5-trisphosphate (IP_3) in the patch pipette.[52] Unfortunately, the protocols for the whole-cell and isolated patch experiments were different and it is not possible to determine the role of each of the two K^+ channels observed in the membrane patches in contributing to the two recorded K^+ currents.

More recently, whole-cell voltage clamp experiments have identified two K^+ currents in canine trachealis cells.[53,54] One of these currents is calcium dependent and resembles current carried by the "maxi" K^+ channel described above. The other current is Ca^{2+} independent and is classified as a delayed rectifier current. This delayed rectifier current is voltage dependent and is blocked by internal Cs^+ and external TEA. The delayed rectifier current reverses when membrane potential is raised above the K^+ equilibrium potential. It is unaffected by the "maxi" K^+ channel blocker charybdotoxin or substitution of Mn^{2+} for Ca^{2+}. Similar outward currents have been identified in other smooth muscles[55-57] and may be responsible for the downstroke (return of membrane potential towards its resting value) of action potentials or slow waves.[45]

Evidence from other types of smooth muscle suggests that further K^+ channels may be revealed in trachealis, e.g., a channel showing inward (anomalous) rectification and probably one or more cation-selective channels. One intriguing possibility is that the K^+ channel which opens in response to drugs such as cromakalim (BRL 34915) or pinacidil will be identified. On the basis of observations made in tissues other than smooth muscle,[58,59] the channel opened by these compounds may be an ATP-sensitive K^+ channel. However, although these drugs are very active in causing hyperpolarization in airway smooth muscle (see Section VI.C), no ATP-sensitive K^+ channel has yet been observed in this tissue.

B. Ca²⁺ CHANNELS

Although K^+ channels form the bulk of the channel activity seen in smooth-muscle cell membranes, inward current through Ca^{2+} channels can be easily identified and therefore analyzed. Technically, the problems of recording from Ca^{2+} channels are very similar to those when recording from K^+ channels. However, since K^+ channel activation will produce currents that interfere with the recorded Ca^{2+} current, in whole-cell recording TEA is usually included in the external solution and K^+ is often replaced by Cs^+ in the internal solution to reduce such interference.

Voltage-gated Ca^{2+} channels have been divided into three types on the basis of channel kinetics, unitary conductance, sensitivity to blockers and toxins, and characteristics of their activation and inactivation processes. These channels are known as T, N, or L types.[60,61] However, this classification is based on studies of the Ca^{2+} channels of neuronal cell membranes. Only two types of voltage-gated Ca^{2+} channels have been reported in smooth muscle. These correspond to the T-type (transient) and L-type (long-lasting) channels.[62-64]

Recent whole-cell voltage clamp experiments on canine airway smooth muscle have revealed the existence of a calcium current that activates at potentials positive to -45 mV and is maximal at $+15$ mV.[62] This current was blocked by Mn^{2+}, Cd^{2+}, and Co^{2+}, but was relatively insensitive to blockade by the dihydropyridine, nifedipine. However, the dihydropyridine Ca^{2+} agonist Bay K8644 increased the current. These findings, plus the rapid inactivation of the current and its current-voltage characteristics, suggest that it is carried by channels showing T-type characteristics.[62] L-type channel behavior was not seen in these experiments, although the presence of this channel was not discounted.

A voltage-dependent calcium current can be evoked in cells isolated from the smooth muscle of human bronchi.[65] This current activates at -26 mV, is maximal at $+18$ mV, reverses at $+52.5$ mV, and is blocked by Co^{2+} or the dihydropyridine PN 200-110 (isradipine). Bay K8644 enhances this inward current. This Ca^{2+} current therefore resembles that described in cells from canine trachealis and it may be that a very similar channel is responsible for the currents measured in the two tissues.

The Ca^{2+} currents from these two species did apparently differ in one important way; the current recorded in human bronchial cells did not show the rapid inactivation reported in cells from the dog. However, this difference may only be one of interpretation, since a second phase of calcium current was noted in the records obtained in the dog and, although this was not analyzed, it can be seen in the published records that it does not inactivate over the period of the voltage step (150 ms).

The existence of voltage-independent, receptor-operated calcium channels has not yet been demonstrated in airway smooth muscle.

C. CHLORIDE CHANNELS

Cl^- channels may also play an important role in the control of trachealis cell function. Although current measurement has indicated the presence of Cl^- channels in other smooth-muscle cells,[66,67] their existence in airway smooth muscle has yet to be directly demonstrated. However, there is good indirect evidence to suggest their existence.

In porcine trachealis, phorbol 12,13-dibutyrate causes a depolarization which is inhibited by substitution of Na^+ and/or Cl^- by an impermeant anion.[68] In canine trachealis,[69] substitution of Cl^- by an impermeant anion lowers membrane resistance, causes depolarization, reduces the amplitude of cholinergic excitatory postjunctional potentials (EJPs) and decreases ACh-induced depolarization. EJPs exhibit a reversal potential close to E_{cl}. Accordingly, it has been suggested that a Cl^- conductance change (activated by Ca^{2+}) may underlie the decrease in membrane resistance which accompanies ACh-induced depolarization.[69]

IV. MODULATION OF THE ELECTRICAL ACTIVITY OF AIRWAY SMOOTH MUSCLE BY EPITHELIUM-DERIVED RELAXANT FACTOR AND BY NEUROTRANSMITTERS

A. EPITHELIUM-DERIVED RELAXANT FACTOR

Fedan et al.[70] have recently reviewed the substantial literature which suggests that the airway epithelium generates a substance (epithelium-derived relaxant factor; EpDRF) which can modulate the excitability of the airway smooth muscle. Many authors have observed that epithelial removal results in the potentiation of spasmogens such as ACh and histamine. Accordingly, the belief has grown that EpDRF can reduce the sensitivity of the airway smooth muscle to spasmogenic substances.

If EpDRF is tonically released from epithelial cells, even in the absence of exogenous spasmogens, then it might be expected that the electrical properties of the airway smooth muscle in epithelium-denuded tissue should differ from those of the smooth muscle in epithelium-intact tissue. This possibility has been examined in canine bronchus, where removal of the epithelium caused no change in resting membrane potential, but increased the depolarization evoked by ACh.[50] In guinea pig trachea, too, removal of the epithelium did not affect the resting membrane potential of trachealis cells.[118a] In epithelium-intact tissue, the resting membrane potential (mean $\pm$ SE mean) was -51 ± 2 mV, while in epithelium-denuded tissue the equivalent value was -52 ± 1 mV. These findings suggest that if EpDRF is released tonically from epithelial cells, it fails to modulate the resting membrane potential of the underlying smooth-muscle cells. However, when airway smooth muscle is exposed to ACh in the absence of epithelium, the absence of EpDRF allows ACh to become more potent regarding both evoking contraction and evoking depolarization.[50]

B. NEUROEFFECTOR TRANSMISSION IN AIRWAY SMOOTH MUSCLE

Electrical field stimulation of intrinsic nerves in airway smooth muscle, exhibiting either spontaneous or spasmogen-induced tone, yields a triphasic mechanical response.[1,6,21,71] The initial phase of this response is a contraction which is atropine sensitive. This is followed by a relaxation which is only partially inhibited by β-adrenoreceptor antagonists.[1,6,21,37,71] All of these responses are abolished by treatment with tetrodotoxin (TTX). It is therefore evident that airway smooth muscle is innervated by cholinergic excitatory and adrenergic and noncholinergic, nonadrenergic inhibitory nerves.

C. CHOLINERGIC NERVES

An atropine- and TTX-sensitive wave of depolarization accompanied by a mechanical twitch is seen in the trachealis of cat, dog, and ox and in bronchiolar muscle from the dog when these tissues are subjected to electrical field stimulation.[6,16,21,72] This transient depolarization is referred to as an excitatory junctional or postjunctional potential (EJP) and represents the electrical response to acetylcholine release from parasympathetic nerve terminals. Stimulation of extrinsic parasympathetic nerves in isolated preparations of ferret and guinea pig trachealis also results in EJPs that are blocked by atropine.[12,20]

The latency of EJPs evoked either by field stimulation or by extrinsic nerve stimulation is in the range 100 to 400 ms[1,12,16,20,72] and EJP amplitude falls as distance from the stimulating electrodes increases.[21] About 50% of muscle cells in canine bronchioles discharge an action potential if the amplitude of the EJP exceeds 35 mV.[21] In guinea pig trachealis, repetitive stimulation may lead to increased depolarization and subsequent damped oscillations in membrane potential, but does not cause the firing of action potentials[12] (see Section II.C).

EJPs evoked in reponse to single stimuli delivered every few minutes decline in amplitude. The addition of indomethacin at the start of such experiments prevents this from occurring. Since the response to exogenous ACh is unaltered by the addition of indomethacin, it is likely that one of the actions of endogenous eicosanoids is to inhibit the release of ACh from nerve terminals.[16,21,73,74] There is also evidence that, in the cat, noradrenaline released from sympathetic nerves may act prejunctionally to limit the release of ACh evoked by repetitive stimulation.[75]

D. NORADRENERGIC NERVES

In the presence of muscarinic blockade, field stimulation of trachealis from guinea pig, cat, and ox and bronchiolar smooth muscle from the dog results in a relaxation whose amplitude is reduced by antagonists at β-adrenoreceptors such as propranolol.[1,6,21,37] No electrical or mechanical response can be elicited to single stimuli applied either to the extrinsic sympathetic nerves supplying guinea pig trachealis[12] or (in the presence of a muscarinic antagonist) by field stimulation in guinea pig, cat, and ox trachealis or canine bronchioles.[1,6,21,37]

Repetitive stimulation of extrinsic sympathetic nerves or repetitive field stimulation in the presence of muscarinic blockade results in relaxation and suppression of slow-wave activity.[12,37] At high frequencies of stimulation hyperpolarization usually accompanies slow-wave suppression.[12,37] Repetitive field stimulation of feline trachealis or canine bronchioles under the same conditions evokes a similar response.[6,21] Since the hyperpolarization is abolished by propranolol, it represents the inhibitory postjunctional effect of noradrenaline on airway smooth muscle. The hyperpolarization in feline trachealis is accompanied by a reduction in membrane resistance (electrotonic potentials are reduced in amplitude during the hyperpolarization).[6] This reduction in membrane resistance is also seen in the presence of β-agonists (see below) and is probably due to the opening of membrane K^+ channels.

Agents known to block α-adrenoreceptors have no effect on the electrical or mechanical consequences of stimulation of extrinsic sympathetic nerves.[12]

E. NONADRENERGIC, NONCHOLINERGIC NERVES

Although the major response to electrical field stimulation of the trachealis in the presence of muscarinic cholinoreceptor and β-adrenoreceptor blockade is relaxation, there are reports in guinea pig and human airways of an excitatory response.[76,77] However, the electrophysiological consequences of nonadrenergic, noncholinergic (NANC) excitatory neurotransmission are unknown.

Feline trachealis, subjected to field stimulation in the presence of atropine, propranolol, and 5HT, relaxes without change in either membrane resistance or membrane potential.[6] In guinea pig trachealis treated with hyoscine and propranolol, electrical field stimulation causes relaxation which is not accompanied by slow-wave suppression or any change in membrane potential.[37] These findings suggest that the NANC inhibitory neurotransmitter in guinea pig and feline airway smooth muscle acts to produce relaxation by a mechanism that does not involve changes in membrane potential. Since hyperpolarization is not observed, the action of the inhibitory transmitter probably does not involve K^+ channel opening. The NANC inhibitory transmitter in bovine trachealis may have a similar mechanism of action, since field stimulation in the presence of atropine produces relaxation without hyperpolarization.[1] However, the results obtained using this tissue are difficult to assess, since the published records were obtained from experiments where a β-adrenoreceptor antagonist and (in some cases) an antagonist at muscarinic cholinoreceptors were not included in the bathing medium.[1,71]

The identity of the NANC inhibitory neurotransmitter in airways is still the subject of some controversy. Evidence obtained in other smooth muscles suggests that the transmitter is likely to be either a purine (adenosine or adenosine 5′-triphosphate [ATP]) or a peptide (vasoactive intestinal polypeptide [VIP]).

Do purines mimic the mechanical and electrical effects of the NANC inhibitory neurotransmitter? Adenosine causes relaxation of guinea pig tracheal smooth muscle at high concentrations, but this is accompanied by an increase in slow-wave amplitude and a decrease in slow-wave frequency.[78] ATP causes a concentration-dependent relaxation of guinea pig trachealis. No associated electrical changes occur until very high concentrations are applied when slow waves are suppressed and a small, transient hyperpolarization is seen.[78] However, this suppression of slow-wave activity may be a feature of the NANC inhibitory transmitter action in this tissue if the transmitter is present in high concentration. Evidence for this includes the observation that, in the presence of hyoscine and propranolol, stimulation of intramural nerves with high concentrations of nicotine causes slow-wave suppression without changes in membrane potential.[37] The K^+ channel inhibitors TEA, 4-AP, and procaine have little effect on relaxant responses to purines in guinea pig trachealis, suggesting that K^+ channel opening is not an important feature of their action.[78] In feline trachealis, ATP induces relaxation at concentrations which have no effect on the electrical properties of the membrane. However, in this tissue, repeated application of ATP caused desensitization (as assessed by a reduction in the size of the mechanical response) to ATP, but had no effect on the response to field stimulation.[6] In bovine trachealis ATP either had no effect on membrane potential, or at high concentrations produced hyperpolarization.[1,71]

Does VIP mimic the mechanical and electrical effects of the NANC inhibitory transmitter? The actions of VIP on guinea pig, feline, and bovine trachealis are accompanied by an increase in membrane potential (hyperpolarization)[6,71,79] and a reduction in amplitude in bovine,[71] or loss in guinea pig,[79] of slow waves. The K^+ channel inhibitors TEA and 4-AP cause a large reduction in the relaxant potency of VIP in guinea pig trachealis, suggesting that K^+ channel opening may play an important role in the actions of VIP.[79]

The identity of the NANC inhibitory transmitter is therefore still a matter of conjecture, and although there is a large body of evidence favoring VIP, electrophysiological findings indicate that acceptance of this peptide as the transmitter is premature. Identification of the transmitter as ATP, VIP, or some other substance must therefore await the development of either specific antagonists or improved assay techniques.

V. ELECTROPHYSIOLOGICAL EFFECTS OF EXOGENOUS SPASMOGENS

A. POTASSIUM CHLORIDE (KCl) AND TETRAETHYLAMMONIUM (TEA)

In feline and canine airways smooth muscle, increasing the external potassium concentration ($[K^+]_o$) evokes a concentration-dependent spasm which is accompanied by graded depolarization, but not by action potential discharge.[41,50,80-82] Similar mechanical and electrical changes are seen in guinea pig trachealis, although it should be noted that low concentrations of KCl may transiently increase slow-wave activity. Higher concentrations of KCl evoke depolarization sufficient to abolish slow waves.[38,83]

TEA-induced spasm of trachealis in dog, ox, or guinea pig is associated with depolarization, initiation, or promotion of slow waves and the discharge of action potentials.[4,14,17,28,40,42,84,85] In human tracheal muscle, TEA induces depolarization and the promotion of slow waves.[3] The single concentration of TEA tested in the study of human tissue would have been subthreshold for the initiation of action potentials in airway smooth muscle from all other species that have been tested. Accordingly, it is likely that higher concentrations of TEA would have evoked action potentials in human trachealis. As discussed above, these effects are attributable to the K^+ channel blocking activity of TEA and the consequent reduction in membrane K^+ conductance. TEA is a relatively nonspecific blocker of K^+ channels,[45] and so may inhibit not only K^+ channels that contribute to the maintenance of resting membrane potential, leading to depolarization, but also those K^+ channels that open in response to depolarization. Therefore, the overall effect of this blockade will not only be a decrease in resting membrane potential, but also reduced membrane rectification and an increased probability of action potential discharge.

The mechanism by which TEA and KCl exert their spasmogenic effects seems to involve the opening of VOCs in the plasmalemma, leading to influx of extracellular Ca^{2+}. Since these channels are highly dependent on membrane potential for their activation, the depolarizing actions of KCl and TEA are important for their ability to produce spasm. This has been demonstrated in canine trachealis[80] where, in double sucrose gap experiments, reversal of K^+-induced depolarization by long anodal current pulses almost completely suppressed the accompanying spasm.

$^{45}Ca^{2+}$ influx promoted by KCl[83,86,87] or TEA[30] has been demonstrated in guinea pig trachealis and the KCl-induced influx can be inhibited by verapamil or D600, which block Ca^{2+} flux through VOCs.[86,87] Verapamil and other organic inhibitors of Ca^{2+} influx also block or reverse KCl- or TEA-evoked changes in slow-wave activity, action potential production, and spasm.[10,17,31] In contrast, the spasmogenic actions of KCl or TEA on trachealis[88] or KCl on bronchial smooth muscle[89] are potentiated by Bay K8644, an agent which promotes the cellular influx of Ca^{2+} through VOCs. Further evidence of the dependence of KCl and TEA on an extracellular source of Ca^{2+} to activate the contractile proteins of the smooth-muscle cells is the suppression of KCl- and TEA-induced mechanical changes which occur when cells are exposed to Ca^{2+}-free, EGTA-containing media.[4,30,41,83,85] Since slow-wave activity and action potentials in this tissue are also dependent on extracellular calcium (see this chapter), treatment with Ca^{2+}-free solutions also prevents slow-wave induction by TEA and KCl. However, the magnitude of KCl- and TEA-induced depolarizations seems to be independent of VOC status (open or closed). This is shown by the observation that Ca^{2+} influx inhibitors have little effect on the changes in resting membrane potential induced by these agents.[17,42,82]

B. AGONISTS AT MUSCARINIC CHOLINORECEPTORS AND HISTAMINE H₁ RECEPTORS

Agonists at muscarinic cholinoreceptors (ACh and carbachol) induce depolarization of bovine, human, and canine trachealis[3,4,15,17,18,81,82] which may be associated with the initiation or promotion of slow-wave activity[1,3,17,90] and decreased membrane resistance.[15,17] ACh also causes concentration-dependent depolarization of guinea pig trachealis that may, at low concentrations, be associated with an increase in slow-wave frequency.[29] Higher concentrations of ACh abolish slow-wave activity due to the large depolarization.[28,29,39] In guinea pig trachealis and canine bronchus the marked depolarization induced by ACh or methacholine is often accompanied by the appearance of an increased level of "noise" and rapid, hyperpolarizing transients in the membrane potential record.[29,38,39,50] This "noise" and the associated voltage transients are abolished by treatment with TEA or procaine and may represent the opening of plasmalemmal K^+ channels triggered by the release of Ca^{2+} from intracellular stores (Figure 4).[39]

The effects of histamine on the electrical behavior of airway smooth muscle are similar to the effects of ACh. In canine, porcine, bovine, and guinea pig trachealis and in canine bronchus, histamine evokes a depolarization[4,8,9,15,18,29,90] which in canine trachealis is accompanied by a fall in membrane resistance.[15] Histamine-induced slow-wave activity occurs in bovine and porcine trachealis[1,4,71,90] and, at low concentrations, in guinea pig trachealis.[29] At high concentrations histamine induces depolarization which suppresses slow-wave activity in guinea pig trachealis and often leads to increased membrane "noise" and rapid, hyperpolarizing transients in the membrane potential record.[29,39] The addition of TEA or procaine abolishes both "noise" and transients.[39]

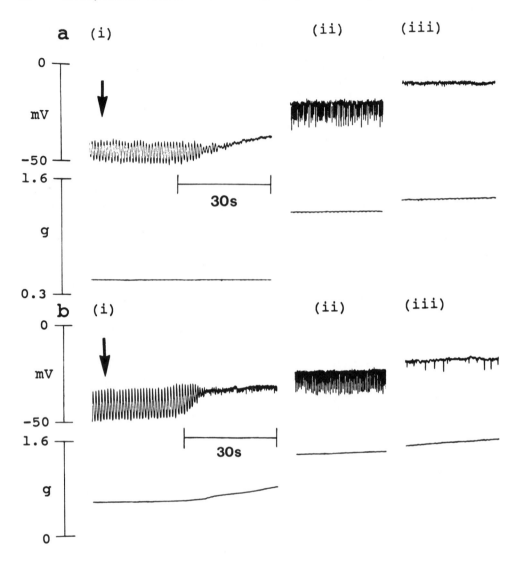

FIGURE 4.   The effects of acetylcholine (1 m*M*) on the electrical and mechanical activity of guinea pig isolated trachealis and their modification by 10 m*M* tetraethylammonium (a) and 5 m*M* procaine (b). Indomethacin (2.8 μ*M*) was present throughout. In each panel the upper trace represents membrane potential and the lower trace the mechanical activity of a contiguous segment of trachea. In both (a) and (b) all electrical recordings are taken from the same cell. (i) Onset of action of acetylcholine added at arrow; note depolarization and abolition of spontaneous slow waves. (ii) 4 min after acetylcholine addition; note spasm, membrane noise, and rapid, hyperpolarizing transients. (iii) 4 min after addition of 10 m*M* TEA (a) or 5 m*M* procaine (b); note reduced membrane noise and suppression of rapid, hyperpolarizing transients in each case. (From Boyle, J. P., Davies, J. M., Foster, R. W., Good, D. M., Kennedy, I., and Small, R. C., *Br. J. Pharmacol.*, 93, 319, 1988. With permission.)

The spasmogenic actions of ACh and histamine on airway smooth muscle are, in contrast to the actions of TEA and KCl, largely independent of the opening of VOCs. Double sucrose gap experiments have shown that ACh-induced spasm of canine trachealis is not potential-dependent and that anodal current not only failed to abolish such spasm, but actually augmented it.[82] Confirmation that the actions of ACh and histamine are independent of the opening of VOCs comes from experiments involving inhibitors of calcium influx. Nicardipine, nifedipine, or verapamil, at concentrations known to inhibit the actions of Ca^{2+} (tested in Ca^{2+}-free, K^+-rich physiological salt solution), KCl, or TEA on guinea pig trachealis, failed to have any significant effect on the actions of ACh or histamine.[10,31,91,92] Additionally, the dihydropyridine Ca^{2+}-agonist Bay K8644 failed to potentiate ACh or histamine in guinea pig trachea[88] and failed to potentiate carbachol in human bronchus.[89]

Since the actions of ACh and histamine are independent of VOC opening, it might be argued that Ca^{2+} influx must occur through receptor-operated calcium channels.[93] However, measurements of $^{45}Ca^{2+}$ influx in guinea pig tracheal smooth muscle have failed to detect any significant influx induced by ACh or histamine.[29] However, under the same conditions a KCl- or TEA-induced increase in $^{45}Ca^{2+}$ influx could be detected.[30,83] The ability of ACh and histamine to promote slow-wave activity probably represents some stimulation of Ca^{2+} influx through VOCs, though this may be of negligible importance for initiating tension development.

ACh- and histamine-induced tension development in tracheal smooth muscle therefore seems to depend on an intracellular source of activator Ca^{2+}.[29] The fact that ACh- and histamine-induced responses are relatively resistant to Ca^{2+}-free, EGTA-containing physiological salt solutions[4,30,41,91] supports this idea. Therefore, it is likely that agonists at muscarinic cholinoreceptors and histamine H_1 receptors initiate tension development in airway smooth muscle by causing the release of Ca^{2+} from intracellular stores.[27] The increase in $[Ca^{2+}]_i$ may then be sufficient to cause some Ca^{2+}-activated K^+ channels to open, thereby offsetting the spasmogen-induced depolarization.[38,39]

The second messenger involved in mobilizing Ca^{2+} from intracellular stores in response to muscarinic and histamine H_1 agonists is probably inositol-1,4,5-triphosphate (IP_3). In airway smooth muscle, histamine and carbachol induce an increase in inositol phospholipid hydrolysis, leading to the production of IP_3 and diacylglycerol (DAG).[94-98] Furthermore, IP_3 can evoke spasm of saponin-skinned trachealis[97] and, following intracellular injection in bovine trachealis, can induce a Ca^{2+}-activated outward K^+ current (probably through release of Ca^{2+} from an intracellular store).[52]

DAG causes activation of protein kinase C, an effect that is mimicked by phorbol esters. In porcine trachealis, phorbol 12,13-dibutyrate (PDB) causes a small depolarization and contraction which are inhibited by Na^+ and/or Cl^- substitution or by amiloride, but which are not affected by verapamil or ouabain.[68] PDB is without effect on the depolarization induced by high $[K^+]_o$, but causes 80% suppression of the carbachol-induced depolarization and a rightward shift of the carbachol concentration-effect curve.[99] In the presence of PDB, carbachol-evoked contraction becomes as sensitive to the effects of verapamil or Ca^{2+}-free bathing media as responses to high $[K^+]_o$. This effect seems to represent the conversion of carbachol-evoked contraction from pharmacomechanical to electromechanical coupling. Such a mechanistic change would lead to an increased dependence of the carbachol response on extracellular sources of activator Ca^{2+}.[99]

C. LEUKOTRIENES

The electrophysiological effects of leukotrienes in airway smooth muscle have been little studied. However, in guinea pig trachealis, concentrations of leukotriene D_4 causing near-maximal spasm evoke depolarization and an increase in slow-wave frequency. Ultimately, the slow waves are abolished by the developing depolarization.[38]

VI. ELECTROPHYSIOLOGICAL EFFECTS OF EXOGENOUS RELAXANT AGENTS

A. AGONISTS AT β-ADRENORECEPTORS

β-adrenoreceptor agonists, such as adrenaline, isoprenaline, and procaterol, suppress spasmogen-induced tone in bovine and canine trachealis. This effect is associated with hyperpolarization of the muscle cells.[1,15,19,71,75] Isoprenaline tested in human trachealis[3] and isoprenaline, terbutaline, and adrenaline tested in guinea pig trachealis[11,28,100] suppress spontaneous tone, suppress slow waves, and cause hyperpolarization. Since the slow-wave inhibition and hyperpolarization are inhibited by propranolol (Figure 5),[1,11,75,100] but not by phentolamine,[11] it seems certain that these electrophysiological changes are mediated by β-adrenoreceptor activation.

Electrotonic potentials induced by current pulses of alternating polarity are reduced in size during β-agonist-induced hyperpolarization,[19,71,75] showing that this increase in membrane potential represents an increase in membrane conductance. Since isoprenaline-induced hyperpolarization approaches the predicted value of the K^+ equilibrium potential of trachealis muscle,[1,100] it is likely that this conductance change involves the opening of membrane K^+ channels. However, if isoprenaline opens K^+ channels, such channels are not permeable to $^{86}Rb^+$ or sensitive to apamin.[100,101]

The membrane potential changes that accompany β-agonist-induced relaxation do not seem to be essential for the mechanical effects of these compounds. Although it has been suggested that slow waves may be involved in the generation and maintenance of tone in some airway smooth muscles,[3,11,28] their abolition by inhibitors of Ca^{2+} influx does not lead to suppression of spontaneous tone.[29,31] In view of this, and since other airway smooth muscle does not exhibit slow-wave activity, it is extremely unlikely that suppression of slow waves plays a major role in β-adrenoreceptor agonist-induced relaxation. Slow-wave suppression is probably secondary to the β-agonist-induced hyperpolarization and reflects the potential-dependence of slow-wave discharge.

The hyperpolarization itself does not seem to be essential for the relaxation evoked by β-agonists. K^+ channel blockade with TEA or procaine inhibits, in guinea pig trachealis, the hyperpolarization induced by isoprenaline without affecting the relaxant action.[100] If the K^+ equilibrium potential is moved closer to 0 mV by performing experiments in an isosmotic medium containing 120 mM K^+, the opening of K^+ channels will only cause a very small current flow and hence little or no hyperpolarization. Isoprenaline tested in guinea pig trachealis under these conditions retains its relaxant action.[100,102]

A similar hyperpolarization of airway smooth muscle is observed during relaxation induced by the adenylate cyclase activator, forskolin, or by the membrane-permeable cyclic nucleotide, dibutyryl-cyclic AMP.[11] Since β-agonists are known to act via activation of adenylate cyclase and subsequent intracellular accumulation of cAMP, it seems likely that the hyperpolarization induced by agonists at β-adrenoreceptors is caused by this cyclic nucleotide.

The fundamental process by which β-adrenoreceptor activation leads to relaxation probably involves a decrease in $[Ca^{2+}]_i$, reduced sensitivity of the intracellular contractile machinery to Ca^{2+}, or a combination of these factors. Experiments with trachealis skinned of its plasma membrane suggest that isoprenaline does not directly reduce the responsiveness of the contractile machinery to Ca^{2+}.[41,103] However, in the intact cell the activation of β-adrenoreceptors could reduce the Ca^{2+} sensitivity of the contractile proteins by mechanisms involving cyclic nucleotide accumulation and protein kinase activation.

Recent evidence obtained using the fluorescent Ca^{2+} indicator fura-2 in canine trachealis indicates that the β-agonist, procaterol, causes a fall in $[Ca^{2+}]_i$ under resting conditions and can reduce the size of Ca^{2+} transients induced by ACh, histamine, or 5HT.[19] In contrast, experiments using the Ca^{2+} fluorophor aequorin have suggested that isoprenaline increases $[Ca^{2+}]_i$.[36] This single report of the ability of isoprenaline to increase $[Ca^{2+}]_i$ in airway smooth muscle needs confirmation by other laboratories and is difficult to reconcile with data obtained for procaterol.

If reduction in $[Ca^{2+}]_i$ is the mechanism by which β-agonists induce relaxation, then this could result from inhibition of IP_3 formation, inhibition of Ca^{2+} influx, increased Ca^{2+} efflux, or increased uptake into intracellular stores. In bovine trachealis, β-agonists reduce

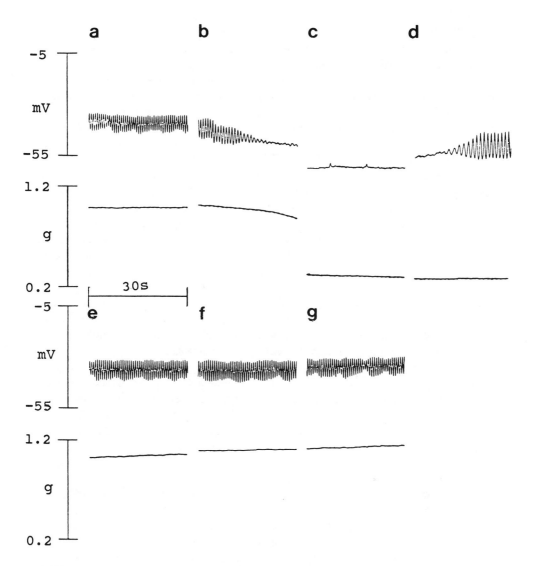

FIGURE 5. The effects of propranolol (1 μ*M*) on the electrical and mechanical responses of guinea pig isolated trachealis to isoprenaline (0.1 μ*M*). In all records the upper trace represents membrane potential and the lower trace the mechanical activity of a contiguous segment of trachea. All electrical records are taken from the same cell. Activity was recorded (a) before, (b) 1 min, and (c) 4 min after the initial challenge with isoprenaline (0.1 μ*M*), (d) 2 min and (e) 10 min after washout of isoprenaline using Krebs solution containing propranolol 1 μ*M*. Activity was also recorded (f) 1 min and (g) 4 min after a second challenge with isoprenaline (0.1 μ*M*) in the presence of propranolol. Note the ability of propranolol to abolish both the electrical and mechanical responses to isoprenaline. (From Allen, S. L., Beech, D. J., Foster, R. W., Morgan, G. P., and Small, R. C., *Br. J. Pharmacol.*, 86, 843, 1985. With permission.)

inositol-phospholipid turnover by a cAMP-dependent process.[104] It may be that this provides part of the mechanism by which β-agonist relaxation is achieved. Evidence for isoprenaline-induced stimulation of Ca^{2+} uptake into intracellular stores has been obtained in feline trachealis,[41] but inhibition of Ca^{2+} influx or stimulation of Ca^{2+} efflux by β-agonists has not yet been directly demonstrated in airway smooth muscle.

B. METHYLXANTHINES

The electrophysiological effects of methylxanthines in airway smooth muscle have been little studied. However, in guinea pig trachealis, aminophylline and theophyline evoke relaxation accompanied by slow-wave supression and hyperpolarization.[11,103] Although the evidence is somewhat indirect, it seems likely that the effects of the methylxanthines on membrane potential changes are mediated by the opening of K^+ channels that are impermeable to ^{86}Rb. Aminophylline-induced hyperpolarization approaches the K^+ equilibrium potential, can be reduced by K^+ channel blockers such as TEA and procaine, and is abolished in a medium containing 120 mM K^+.[103]

The methylxanthine-induced hyperpolarization seems similar to that induced by β-agonists and is not crucial for relaxation. Low concentrations of aminophylline can cause relaxation without causing electrical changes, and treatment that reduces or abolishes hyperpolarization (TEA, procaine, 120 mM K^+_o media) does not prevent aminophylline-induced relaxation.[103] Methylxanthines inhibit cyclic nucleotide phosphodiesterases and so will increase cytosolic cAMP and cGMP concentrations. This may well explain some of the similarities between the electrophysiological effects of methylxanthines and those of agonists at β-adrenoreceptors.

Aminophylline does not directly reduce the responsiveness of the intracellular contractile machinery to Ca^{2+}, but is very effective in counteracting contractile responses to KCl, ACh, or histamine.[103] Like the agonists at β-adrenoreceptors, alkylxanthines can inhibit histamine-stimulated inositol phosphate accumulation in bovine trachealis.[104,105]

In addition to their relaxant actions, the xanthines also possess the ability to produce spasm of airway smooth muscle, probably by releasing Ca^{2+} from intracellular sites of sequestration. This process does not seem to depend on raised intracellular concentrations of cAMP, since neither forskolin nor the phosphodiesterase inhibitor AH 21-132 share this action.[106] However, the mechanism by which this occurs has not been studied electrophysiologically.

C. K^+ CHANNEL-OPENING DRUGS

In guinea pig trachealis, K^+ channel-opening drugs such as cromakalim (BRL 34915) suppress slow-wave activity and mechanical tone and evoke hyperpolarization (Figure 6).[107] These effects seem to be attributable to the opening of ^{86}Rb-permeable, but apamin-insensitive, K^+ channels in the plasma membrane. Other drugs identified as K^+ channel openers, e.g., pinacidil, are also relaxant on airway smooth muscle[108] and may share a mechanism of action similar to that of cromakalim.

The relaxant action of cromakalim (and probably other K^+ channel openers) seems to be unique in that it depends on membrane hyperpolarization caused by an increase in the K^+ conductance of the membrane.[109] That this is the mechanism by which these compounds cause relaxation in airway smooth muscle is suggested by several observations. In guinea pig trachealis, the log concentration-relaxation and log concentration-hyperpolarization curves of cromakalim are virtually coincident. TEA and procaine reduce both the hyperpolarization and the relaxation induced by cromakalim, and, in the presence of K^+-rich (120 mM) physiological salt solutions, neither cromakalim nor pinacidil evoke relaxation.[107,108,110]

The specific type of K^+ channel that is opened by these drugs in smooth muscle is still unknown, but evidence from vascular smooth muscle and cardiac muscle has led to the suggestion that it is either the Ca^{2+}-dependent, high-conductance K^+ channel[111,112] or an ATP-modulated K^+ channel.[58] The sulfonylurea compounds tolbutamide and glibenclamide are specific blockers of ATP-modulated K^+ channels in cardiac muscle, neurones, and pancreatic β-cells.[58,113,114] Recent observations made in a variety of smooth muscles suggest that these agents can antagonize K^+ channel-opening drugs.[115-117] It may therefore be that cromakalim and other K^+ channel openers relax trachealis muscle by opening K^+ channels which resemble the ATP-regulated channel detected in other tissues.

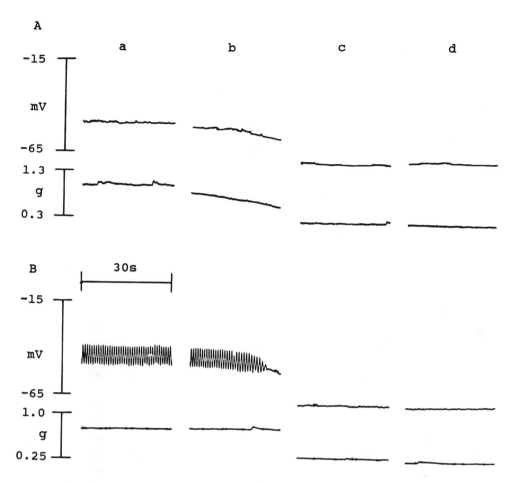

FIGURE 6. Effects of cromakalim (10 μM) on the electrical and mechanical properties of guinea pig isolated trachealis. The upper (A) and lower (B) rows of records indicate results obtained from a quiescent and a spontaneously active cell, respectively. In each row of records the upper trace represents membrane potential and the lower trace the mechanical activity of a contiguous segment of trachea. In (A) activity was recorded (a) before, (b) 2 min, (c) 4 min, and (d) 8 min after addition of cromakalim 10 μM. In (B) activity was recorded (a) before, (b) 1 min, (c) 4 min, and (d) 8 min after addition of cromakalim 10 μM. (From Allen, S. L., Boyle, J. P., Cortijo, J., Foster, R. W., Morgan, G. P., and Small, R. C., *Br. J. Pharmacol.*, 89, 395, 1986. With permission.)

It is possible that the bronchial hyperresponsiveness characteristic of asthma might partly be explained by hyperresponsiveness of airway smooth muscle. The latter type of hyperresponsiveness could be caused by altered gating properties of plasmalemmal K^+ channels. If the threshold at which such channels are opened is shifted towards 0 mV, then membrane rectification would be reduced. This would allow VOCs to open in response to less intense stimuli and might augment, or even trigger, contraction.[107] K^+ channel-opening drugs could act to prevent depolarization reaching critical thresholds for VOC opening and thus reduce hyperresponsiveness. However, when K^+ channel blockers such as TEA are used to reduce rectification, structurally specific spasmogens are not potentiated.[39] Accordingly, any relationship between dysfunction of the K^+ channels responsible for rectification and airway hyperresponsiveness is unlikely to be a simple one.

The nitro compound, nicorandil, shares many of the properties of the K^+ channel openers. In guinea pig trachealis, nicorandil causes inhibition or abolition of slow waves and hyperpolarization.[101] Hyperpolarization is also seen in canine trachealis.[118] The hyperpolarization induced by nicorandil is independent of $[Cl]_o$ in the range 18 to 134 mM, but is abolished when $[K^+]_o$ is raised to, or above, 20 mM. Furthermore, nicorandil-induced hyperpolarization is accompanied by an increase in membrane conductance.[118] The hyperpolarization is reduced by procaine and TEA,[101,118] but not by apamin.[101] It is associated with an increase in ^{86}Rb efflux.[101] However, nicorandil differs from the K^+ channel openers such as cromakalim inasmuch as low concentrations of nicorandil cause a relaxation that is apparently not accompanied by electrical changes. Procaine can reduce nicorandil-induced hyperpolarization without affecting its relaxant action, and nicorandil retains some relaxant activity even in conditions of high $[K^+]_o$.[101] It is likely, therefore, that the relaxant effects of nicorandil depend not only on hyperpolarization, but also on the activity of this agent as an activator of guanylate cyclase.[101,118]

D. Ca²⁺ ANTAGONISTS AND Ca²⁺ AGONISTS

In guinea pig trachealis not exposed to spasmogens, organic inhibitors of Ca^{2+} influx such as gallopamil (D600), verapamil, and nifedipine, abolish slow waves without greatly altering the resting membrane potential or mechanical tone.[10,27,28,88]

The failure of these agents to relax spontaneous tone probably reflects the source of activator Ca^{2+} utilized by prostaglandins in maintaining tone. It is likely that prostaglandin-induced tone depends on Ca^{2+} release from intracellular stores. Inhibitors of Ca^{2+} influx therefore have very little effect on spontaneous tone.

The dihydropyridine Bay K8644 acts to promote the influx of Ca^{2+} through VOCs. In guinea pig trachealis, Bay K8644 promotes Ca^{2+} influx, but causes little or no change in the resting membrane potential of the cells. Bay K8644 causes no change in slow-wave activity, but delays the slow-wave supression induced by nifedipine (Figure 1).[88]

ACKNOWLEDGMENTS

The authors' work has been sponsored by the Asthma Research Council, the British Lung Foundation, the Mason Medical Research Foundation, the North Western Regional Health Authority, the Wellcome Trust, Sandoz AG, and various companies within the U.K. pharmaceutical industry. The collaboration of Dr. S. L. Allen, Dr. J. Cortijo, Dr. J. Davies, Dr. J. S. Dixon, Dr. G. P. Morgan, Dr. A. H. Weston, F. Ahmed, and B. I. Okpalugo is gratefully acknowledged.

REFERENCES

1. **Kirkpatrick, C. T.,** Tracheobronchial smooth muscle, in *Smooth Muscle: an Assessment of Current Knowledge,* Bülbring, E., Brading, A. F., Jones, A. W., and Tomita, T., Eds., Edward Arnold, London, 1981, 385.
2. **Zorychta, E. and Richardson, J. B.,** Control of smooth muscle in human airways, *Bull. Eur. Physiopathol. Respir.,* 16, 581, 1980.
3. **Honda, K. and Tomita, T.,** Electrical activity in isolated human tracheal muscle, *Jpn. J. Physiol.,* 37, 333, 1987.
4. **Kirkpatrick, C. T.,** Excitation and contraction in bovine tracheal smooth muscle, *J. Physiol.,* 244, 263, 1975.
5. **Kirkpatrick, C. T. and Tomita, T.,** The spread of neural excitation compared with passive current spread in tracheal smooth muscle, *Ir. J. Med. Sci.,* 147, 80, 1978.
6. **Ito, Y. and Takeda, K.,** Non-adrenergic inhibitory nerves and putative transmitters in the smooth muscle of cat trachea, *J. Physiol.,* 330, 497, 1982.
7. **Clark, L. A. and Small, R. C.,** Simultaneous recording of electrical and mechanical activity from smooth muscle of the guinea-pig isolated trachealis, *J. Physiol.,* 300, 5P, 1979.
8. **McCaig, D. J. and Souhrada, J. F.,** Alteration of electrophysiological properties of airway smooth muscle from sensitised guinea-pigs, *Respir. Physiol.,* 41, 49, 1980.

9. **Souhrada, M. and Souhrada, J. F.,** Re-assessment of electrophysiological and contractile characteristics of sensitised airway smooth muscle, *Respir. Physiol.,* 46, 17, 1981.

10. **Ahmed, F., Foster, R. W., and Small, R. C.,** Some effects of nifedipine in guinea-pig isolated trachealis, *Br. J. Pharmacol.,* 84, 861, 1985.

11. **Honda, K., Satake, T., Takagi, K., and Tomita, T.,** Effects of relaxants on electrical and mechanical activities in the guinea-pig tracheal muscle, *Br. J. Pharmacol.,* 87, 665, 1986.

12. **McCaig, D. J.,** Electrophysiology of neuroeffector transmission in the isolated, innervated trachea of the guinea-pig, *Br. J. Pharmacol.,* 89, 793, 1986.

13. **Stephens, N. L. and Kroeger, E. A.,** Effects of hypoxia on airway smooth muscle mechanics and electrophysiology, *J. Appl. Physiol.,* 28, 630, 1970.

14. **Kroeger, E. A. and Stephens, N. L.,** Effect of tetraethylammonium on tonic airway smooth muscle: initiation of phasic electrical activity, *Am. J. Physiol.,* 228, 633, 1975.

15. **Suzuki, H., Morita, K., and Kuriyama, H.,** Innervation and properties of the smooth muscle of the dog trachea, *Jpn. J. Physiol.,* 26, 303, 1976.

16. **Ito, Y. and Tajima, K.,** Actions of indomethacin and prostaglandins on neuroeffector transmission in the dog trachea, *J. Physiol.,* 319, 379, 1981.

17. **Kannan, M. S., Jager, L. P., Daniel, E. E., and Garfield, R. E.,** Effects of 4-aminopyridine and tetraethylammonium chloride on the electrical activity and cable properties of canine tracheal smooth muscle, *J. Pharmacol., Exp. Ther.,* 227, 706, 1983.

18. **Souhrada, M., Klein, J. J., Berend, N., and Souhrada, J. F.,** Topographical differences in the physiological responses of canine airway smooth muscle, *Respir. Physiol.,* 52, 245, 1983.

19. **Fujiwara, T., Sumimoto, K., Itoh, T., and Kuriyama, H.,** Relaxing actions of procaterol, a beta$_2$-adrenoceptor stimulant, on smooth muscle cells of the dog trachea, *Br. J. Pharmacol.,* 93, 199, 1988.

20. **Coburn, R. F.,** Neural co-ordination of excitation of ferret trachealis muscle, *Am. J. Physiol.,* 246, C459, 1984.

21. **Inoue, T. and Ito, Y.,** Characteristics of neuro-effector transmission in the smooth muscle layer of the dog bronchiole and modification by autacoids, *J. Physiol.,* 370, 551, 1986.

22. **Abe, Y. and Tomita, T.,** Cable properties of smooth muscle, *J. Physiol.,* 96, 87, 1968.

23. **Tomita, T.,** Electrical properties of mammalian smooth muscle, in *Smooth Muscle,* Bulbring, E., Brading, A. F., Jones, A. W., and Tomita, T., Eds., Edward Arnold, London, 1970, 197.

24. **Abe, Y.,** The hormonal control and the effects of drugs and ions on the electrical and mechanical activity of the uterus, in *Smooth Muscle,* Bulbring, E., Brading, A. F., Jones, A. W., and Tomita, T., Eds., Edward Arnold, London, 1970, 396.

25. **Bywater, R. A. R. and Taylor, G. S.,** The passive membrane properties and excitatory junction potentials of the guinea-pig vas deferens, *J. Physiol.,* 300, 303, 1980.

26. **Creed, K. E.,** Membrane properties of the smooth muscle cells of the rat anococcygeus muscle, *J. Physiol.,* 245, 49, 1975.

27. **Small, R. C. and Foster, R. W.,** Airways smooth muscle: an overview of morphology, electrophysiology and aspects of the pharmacology of contraction and relaxation, in *Asthma: Clinical Pharmacology and Therapeutic Progress,* Kay, A. B., Ed., Blackwell Scientific, London, 1986, 101.

28. **Small, R. C.,** Electrical slow waves and tone of guinea-pig isolated trachealis muscle: effects of drugs and temperature changes, *Br. J. Pharmacol.,* 77, 45, 1982.

29. **Ahmed, F., Foster, R. W., Small, R. C., and Weston, A. H.,** Some features of the spasmogenic actions of acetylcholine and histamine in guinea-pig isolated trachealis, *Br. J. Pharmacol.,* 83, 227, 1984.

30. **Foster, R. W., Small, R. C., and Weston, A. W.,** Evidence that the spasmogenic action of tetraethylammonium in guinea-pig trachealis is both direct and dependent on the cellular influx of calcium ion, *Br. J. Pharmacol.,* 79, 255, 1983.

31. **Foster, R. W., Okpalugo, B. I., and Small, R. C.,** Antagonism of Ca^{2+} and other actions of verapamil in guinea-pig isolated trachealis, *Br. J. Pharmacol.,* 81, 499, 1984.

32. **Berridge, M. J. and Galione, A.,** Cytosolic calcium oscillators, *FASEB J.,* 2, 3074, 1988.

33. **Himpens, B. and Somlyo, A. P.,** Free-calcium and force transients during depolarization and pharmacomechanical coupling in guinea-pig smooth muscle, *J. Physiol.,* 395, 507, 1988.

34. **DeFeo, T. T., Briggs, G. M., and Morgan, K. G.,** Ca^{2+} signals obtained with multiple indicators in mammalian vascular muscle cells, *Am. J. Physiol.,* 253, H1456, 1987.

35. **Takuwa, Y., Takuwa, N., and Rasmussen, H.,** Measurement of cytoplasmic free Ca^{2+} concentration in bovine tracheal smooth muscle using aequorin, *Am. J. Physiol.,* 253, C817, 1987.

36. **Takuwa, Y., Takuwa, N., and Rasmussen, H.,** The effects of isoproterenol on intracellular calcium concentration, *J. Biol. Chem.,* 263, 762, 1988.

37. **Boyle, J. P., Davies, J. M., Foster, R. W., Morgan, G. P., and Small, R. C.,** Inhibitory responses to nicotine and transmural stimulation in hyoscine-treated guinea-pig isolated trachealis: an electrical and mechanical study, *Br. J. Pharmacol.,* 90, 733, 1987.

38. **McCaig, D. J. and Rodger, I. W.**, Effects of leukotriene D_4 on the mechanical and electrical properties of guinea-pig isolated trachealis, *Br. J. Pharmacol.*, 94, 729, 1988.

39. **Boyle, J. P., Davies, J. M., Foster, R. W., Good, D. M., Kennedy, I., and Small, R. C.**, Spasmogen action in guinea-pig isolated trachealis: involvement of membrane K^+-channels and the consequences of K^+-channel blockade, *Br. J. Pharmacol.*, 93, 319, 1988.

40. **Dixon, J. S. and Small, R. C.**, Evidence of poor conduction of muscle excitation in the longitudinal axis of guinea-pig isolated trachea, *Br. J. Pharmacol.*, 79, 75, 1983.

41. **Ito, Y. and Itoh, T.**, The roles of stored calcium in contraction of cat tracheal smooth muscle produced by electrical stimulation, acetylcholine and high K^+, *Br. J. Pharmacol.*, 83, 667, 1984.

42. **Imaizumi, Y. and Watanabe, M.**, The effect of tetraethylammonium chloride on potassium permeability in the smooth muscle cell membrane of canine trachea, *J. Physiol.*, 316, 33, 1981.

43. **Bolton, T. B., Tomita, T., and Vassort, G.**, Voltage-clamp and the measurement of ionic conductances in smooth muscle, in *Smooth Muscle: an Assessment of Current Knowledge*, Bülbring, E., Brading, A. F., Jones, A. W., and Tomita, T., Eds., Edward Arnold, London, 1981, 47.

44. **Hamill, O. P., Marty, A., Neher, E., Sakmann, B., and Sigworth, F. J.**, Improved patch-clamp techniques for high-resolution current recording from cells and cell-free membrane patches, *Pfluegers Arch.*, 391, 85, 1981.

45. **Cook, N. S.**, The pharmacology of potassium channels and their therapeutic potential, *TIPS*, 9, 21, 1988.

46. **Dubas, F., Stein, P. G., and Anderson, P. A. V.**, Ionic currents of smooth muscle cells isolated from the ctenophore Mnemiopsis, *Proc. R. Soc. London Ser. B.*, 233, 99, 1988.

47. **McCann, J. D. and Welsh, M. J.**, Calcium-activated potassium channels in canine airway smooth muscle, *J. Physiol.*, 372, 113, 1986.

48. **Tom-Moy, M., Madison, J. M., Jones, C. A., De Lanerolle, P., and Brown, J. K.**, Morphologic characterisation of cultured smooth muscle cells isolated from the tracheas of adult dogs, *Anat. Rec.*, 218, 313, 1987.

49. **Huang, H. M., Dwyer, T. M., and Farley, J. M.**, Patch clamp recording of single calcium-activated K-channels in tracheal smooth muscle from swine, *Biophys. J.*, 51, 50a, 1987.

50. **Gao, Y. and Vanhoutte, P. M.**, Removal of the epithelium potentiates acetycholine in depolarising canine bronchial smooth muscle, *J. Appl. Physiol.*, 65, 2400, 1988.

51. **Isenberg, G. and Klöckner, U.**, Elementary currents through single Ca-activated potassium channels (smooth muscle cells isolated from trachea or urinary bladder), *Pfluegers Arch.*, 405, R62, 1987.

52. **Klöckner, U. and Isenberg, G.**, Calcium-activated potassium currents as an indicator for intracellular (i.c.) Ca-transients. (Single smooth muscle cells from trachea and urinary bladder, *Pfluegers Arch.*, 405, R61, 1987.

53. **Kotlikoff, M. I.**, Potassium currents in isolated airway smooth muscle cells, *Am. Rev. Respir. Dis.*, 135, A273, 1987.

54. **Kotlikoff, M. I.**, Ion channels in airway smooth muscle, in *Airway Smooth Muscle in Health and Disease*, Coburn, R. F., Ed., Plenum Press, New York, 1989, 169.

55. **Walsh, J. V. and Singer, J. J.**, Identification and characterization of major ionic currents in isolated smooth muscle cells using the voltage-clamp technique, *Pfluegers Arch.*, 408, 83, 1987.

56. **Singer, J. J. and Walsh, J. V.**, Passive properties of the membrane of single freshly isolated smooth muscle cells, *Am. J. Physiol.*, 239, C154, 1980.

57. **Benham, C. D. and Bolton, T. B.**, Patch-clamp studies of slow potential-sensitive potassium channels in longitudinal smooth muscle cells of rabbit jejunum, *J. Physiol.*, 340, 469, 1983.

58. **Escande, D., Thuringer, D., Lequern, S., and Cavero, I.**, The potassium channel opener cromakalim (BRL 34915) activates ATP-dependent K^+-channels in isolated cardiac myocytes, *Biochem. Biophys. Res. Commun.*, 154, 620, 1988.

59. **Mondot, S., Mestre, M., Caillard, C. G., and Cavero, I.**, RP 49356: A vasorelaxant agent with potassium channel activating properties, *Br. J. Pharmacol.*, 96, 813P, 1989.

60. **McCleskey, E. W., Fox, A. P., Feldman, D., and Tsien, R. W.**, Different types of calcium channels, *J. Exp. Biol.*, 124, 177, 1986.

61. **Tsien, R. W., Benham, C. D., Fox, A. P., Hess, P., Lipscombe, D., McCleskey, E. W., Madison, D. V., and Rosenberg, R. L.**, Calcium channels: functional insights and structural implications, *Biophys. J.*, 51, 2a, 1987.

62. **Kotlikoff, M. I.**, Calcium currents in isolated canine airway smooth muscle cells, *Am. J. Physiol.*, 254, C793, 1988.

63. **Mironneau, J.**, Calcium currents gated by potential in smooth muscle cells, *J. Muscle Res. Cell Motil.*, 9, 456, 1988.

64. **Bolton, T. B., MacKenzie, I., Aaronson, P. I., and Lim, S. P.**, Calcium channels in smooth muscle cells, *Biochem. Soc. Trans.*, 16, 492, 1988.

65. **Marthan, R., Martin, C., Amédée, T., and Mironneau, J.,** Calcium channel currents in isolated smooth muscle cells from human bronchus, *J. Appl. Physiol.,* 66, 157, 1988.

66. **Byrne, N. G. and Large, W. A.,** Membrane mechanism associated with muscarinic receptor activation in single cells freshly dispersed from the rat anococcygeus muscle, *Br. J. Pharmacol.,* 92, 371, 1987.

67. **Byrne, N. G. and Large, W. A.,** Mechanism of action of alpha-adrenoceptor activation in single cells freshly dissociated from the rabbit portal vein, *Br. J. Pharmacol.,* 94, 475, 1988.

68. **Baba, K. and Coburn, R. F.,** Effect of phorbol ester on the membrane potential and tension in swine tracheal smooth muscle, *FASEB J.,* 2, A331.203, 1988.

69. **Daniel, E. E., Serio, R., Jury, J., Pashley, M., and O'Byrne, P.,** Effects of inflammatory mediators on neuromuscular transmission in canine trachea in vitro, in *Mechanisms in Asthma: Pharmacology, Physiology and Management,* Armour, C. L. and Black, J. L., Eds., Alan R. Liss, New York, 1988.

70. **Fedan, J. S., Hay, D. W. P., Farmer, S. G., and Raeburn, D.,** Epithelial cells: modulation of airway smooth muscle reactivity, in *Asthma: Basic Mechanisms and Clinical Management,* Barnes, P. J., Rodger, I. W., and Thomspon, N. C., Eds., Academic Press, London, 1988, 143.

71. **Cameron, A. R., Johnston, C. F., Kirkpatrick, C. T., and Kirkpatrick, M. C. A.,** The quest for the inhibitory neurotransmitter in bovine tracheal smooth muscle, *Q. J. Exp. Physiol.,* 68, 413, 1983.

72. **Cameron, A. R. and Kirkpatrick, C. T.,** A study of excitatory neuromuscular transmission in the bovine trachea, *J. Physiol.,* 270, 733, 1977.

73. **Inoue, T., Ito, Y., and Takeda, K.,** Prostaglandin-induced inhibition of acetylcholine release from neuronal elements of dog tracheal tissue, *J. Physiol.,* 349, 553, 1984.

74. **Inoue, T. and Ito, Y.,** Pre- and post-junctional actions of prostaglandin I_2, carbocyclic thromboxane A_2 and leukotriene C_4 in dog tracheal muscle, *Br. J. Pharmacol.,* 84, 289, 1985.

75. **Ito, Y. and Tajima, K.,** Dual effects of catecholamines on pre- and post-junctional membranes in the dog trachea, *Br. J. Pharmacol.,* 75, 433, 1982.

76. **Andersson, R. G. G. and Grunsstrom, N.,** The excitatory non-cholinergic non-adrenergic nervous system of the guinea-pig airways, *Eur. J. Respir. Dis.,* 64, 141, 1983.

77. **Barnes, P. J.,** Neuropeptides in human airways, in *Mechanisms in Asthma: Pharmacology, Physiology, and Management,* Armour, C. L. and Black, J. L., Eds., Alan R. Liss, New York, 1988.

78. **Boyle, J. P., Davies, J. M., Foster, R. W., Morgan, G. P., and Small, R. C.,** Electrical and mechanical effects of adenosine and ATP in guinea-pig isolated trachealis, *Br. J. Pharmacol.,* 91, 491P, 1987.

79. **Boyle, J. P., Davies, J. M., Gosling, J. A., and Small, R. C.,** Pharmacological, electrophysiological and immunocytochemical studies of VIP in guinea-pig isolated trachealis, *Pfluegers Arch.,* 411, R201, 1988.

80. **Coburn, R. F. and Yamaguchi, T.,** Membrane potential-dependent and -independent tension in the canine tracheal muscle, *J. Pharmacol. Exp. Ther.,* 201, 276, 1977.

81. **Farley, J. M. and Miles, P. R.,** Role of depolarisation in acetylcholine-induced contractions of dog trachealis muscle, *J. Pharmacol. Exp. Ther.,* 201, 199, 1977.

82. **Coburn, R. F.,** Electromechanical coupling in canine trachealis muscle, *Am. J. Physiol.,* 236, C177, 1979.

83. **Foster, R. W., Small, R. C., and Weston, A. H.,** The spasmogenic action of potassium chloride in guinea-pig trachealis, *Br. J. Pharmacol.,* 80, 553, 1983.

84. **Richards, I. S., Murlas, C. G., Ousterhout, J. M., and Sperelakis, N.,** 8-Bromo-cyclic GMP abolishes TEA-induced slow action potentials in canine trachealis muscle, *Eur. J. Pharmacol.,* 218, 299, 1986.

85. **Richards, I. S., Ousterhout, J. M., Sperelakis, N., and Murlas, C. G.,** cAMP suppresses Ca^{2+}-dependent electrical activity of airway smooth muscle induced by TEA, *J. Appl. Physiol.,* 62, 175, 1987.

86. **Raeburn, D. and Rodger, I. W.,** Lack of effect of leukotriene D_4 on Ca^{2+} uptake in airway smooth muscle, *Br. J. Pharmacol.,* 83, 499, 1984.

87. **Weiss, G. B., Pang, I. H., and Goodman, F. R.,** Relationship between ^{45}Ca movements, different calcium components and responses to acetylcholine and potassium in tracheal smooth muscle, *J. Pharmacol. Exp. Ther.,* 233, 389, 1985.

88. **Allen, S. L., Foster, R. W., Small, R. C., and Towart, R.,** The effects of the dihydropyridine BAY K8644 in guinea-pig isolated trachealis, *Br. J. Pharmacol.,* 86, 171, 1985.

89. **Advenier, C., Naline, E., and Renier, A.,** Effects of Bay K8644 on contraction of the human isolated bronchus and guinea-pig isolated trachea, *Br. J. Pharmacol.,* 88, 33, 1986.

90. **Mitchell, H. W.,** Electromechanical effects of tetraethylammonium and K^+ on histamine-induced contraction in pig isolated tracheal smooth muscle, *Lung,* 165, 129, 1987.

91. **Cerrina, J., Advenier, C., Renier, A., Floch, A., and Duroux, P.,** Effects of diltiazem and other Ca^{2+} antagonists on guinea-pig tracheal muscle, *Eur. J. Pharmacol.,* 94, 241, 1983.

92. **Advenier, C., Cerrina, J., Duroux, P., Floch, A., and Renier, A.,** Effects of five different organic calcium antagonists on guinea-pig isolated trachea, *Br. J. Pharmacol.,* 82, 727, 1984.

93. **Bolton, T. B.,** Mechanism of action of transmitters and other substances on smooth muscle, *Physiol. Rev.,* 59, 606, 1979.

94. **Barnes, P. J., Cuss, F. M., and Grandordy, B. M.,** Spasmogens and phosphatidylinositol breakdown in bovine trachealis smooth muscle, *Br. J. Pharmacol.,* 87, 65P, 1986.

95. **Grandordy, B. M., Cuss, F. M., Sampson, A. S., Palmer, J. B., and Barnes, P. J.,** Phosphatidylinositol response to cholinergic agonists in airway smooth muscle: relationships to contraction and muscarinic receptor occupancy, *J. Pharmacol. Exp. Ther.,* 238, 273, 1986.

96. **Hall, I. P. and Hill, S. J.,** β_2-Adrenoceptor stimulation inhibits histamine-stimulated inositolphospholipid hydrolysis in bovine tracheal smooth muscle, *Br. J. Pharmacol.,* 95, 1204, 1989.

97. **Hashimoto, T., Hirata, M., and Ito, Y.,** A role for inositol 1,3,5-triphosphate in the initiation of agonist-induced contractions of dog tracheal muscle, *Br. J. Pharmacol.,* 86, 191, 1985.

98. **Baron, C. B., Cunningham, M., Strauss, J. F., and Coburn, R. F.,** Pharmacomechanical coupling in smooth muscle may involve phosphatidyl-inositol metabolism, *Proc. Natl. Acad. Sci. U.S.A.,* 81, 6899, 1984.

99. **Coburn, R. F. and Baba, K.,** Phorbol ester-induced conversion of pharmacomechanical coupling to electromechanical coupling in the response of swine tracheal smooth muscle to carbachol, *FASEB J.,* 2, A331.204, 1988.

100. **Allen, S. L., Beech, D. J., Foster, R. W., Morgan, G. P., and Small, R. C.,** Electrophysiological and other aspects of the relaxant action of isoprenaline in guinea-pig isolated trachealis, *Br. J. Pharmacol.,* 86, 843, 1985.

101. **Allen, S. L., Foster, R. W., Morgan, G. P., and Small, R. C.,** The relaxant action of nicorandil in guinea-pig isolated trachealis, *Br. J. Pharmacol.,* 87, 117, 1986.

102. **Kumar, M. A.,** The basis of beta adrenergic bronchodilation, *J. Pharmacol. Exp. Ther.,* 206, 528, 1978.

103. **Allen, S. L., Cortijo, J., Foster, R. W., Morgan, G. P., Small, R. C., and Weston, A. H.,** Mechanical and electrical aspects of the relaxant action of aminophylline in guinea-pig isolated trachealis, *Br. J. Pharmacol.,* 88, 473, 1986.

104. **Hall, I. P., Donaldson, J., and Hill, S. J.,** Cyclic AMP-mediated inhibition of histamine-induced inositol phospholipid hydrolysis in bovine tracheal smooth muscle, *Br. J. Pharmacol.,* 96, 748P, 1989.

105. **Murray, R. K., Fluharty, S. J., and Kotlikoff, M. I.,** Phorbol ester blocks histamine-induced inositol triphosphate (IP3) production in cultured airway smooth muscle, *Am. Rev. Respir. Dis.,* 137, A309, 1988.

106. **Small, R. C., Boyle, J. P., Cortijo, J., Curtis-Prior, P. B., Davies, J. M., Foster, R. W., and Hofer, P.,** The relaxant and spasmogenic effects of some xanthine derivatives acting on guinea-pig isolated trachealis muscle, *Br. J. Pharmacol.,* 94, 1091, 1988.

107. **Allen, S. L., Boyle, J. P., Cortijo, J., Foster, R. W., Morgan, G. P., and Small, R. C.,** Electrical and mechanical effects of BRL34915 in guinea-pig isolated trachealis, *Br. J. Pharmacol.,* 89, 395, 1986.

108. **Bray, K. M., Newgreen, D. T., Small, R. C., Southerton, J. S., Taylor, S. G., Weir, S. W., and Weston, A. H.,** Evidence that the mechanism of the inhibitory action of pinacidil in rat and guinea-pig smooth muscle differs from that of glyceryl trinitrate, *Br. J. Pharmacol.,* 91, 421, 1987.

109. **Nakao, K., Okabe, K., Kitamura, K., Kuriyama, H., and Weston, A. H.,** Characteristics of cromakalim-induced relaxations in the smooth muscle cells of guinea-pig mesenteric artery and vein, *Br. J. Pharmacol.,* 95, 795, 1988.

110. **Arch, J. R. S., Buckle, D. R., Bumstead, J., Clarke, G. D., Taylor, J. F., and Taylor, S. G.,** Evaluation of the potassium channel activator cromakalim (BRL 34915) in the guinea pig: comparison with nifedipine, *Br. J. Pharmacol.,* 95, 763, 1988.

111. **Trieschmann, U., Pichlmaier, M., Klockner, U., and Isenberg, G.,** Vasorelaxation due to K-agonists: single channel recording from isolated human vascular myocytes, *Pfluegers Arch.,* 411, R199, 1988.

112. **Gelband, C. H., Lodge, N. J., Talvenheimo, J. A., and van Breeman, C.,** BRL 34915 increases P_{open} of the large conductance Ca^{2+} activated K^+ channel isolated from rabbit aorta in planer lipid bilayers, *Biophys. J.,* 53, 149a, 1988.

113. **Bernadi, H., Fosset, M., and Lazdunski, M.,** Characterization, purification and affinity labelling of the brain [3H] glibenclamide-binding protein, a putative neuronal ATP-regulated K^+ channel, *Proc. Natl. Acad. Sci. U.S.A.,* 85, 9816, 1988.

114. **Zunkler, B. J., Lenzen, S., Manner, K., Panten, U., and Trube, G.,** Concentration-dependent effects of tolbutamide, meglitinide, glipizide, glibenclamide and diazoxide on ATP-regulated K^+ currents in pancreatic β-cells, *Naunyn-Schmiedeberg's Arch. Pharmacol.,* 337, 225, 1988.

115. **Quast, U. and Cook, N. S.,** Potent inhibitors of the effects of the K^+ channel opener BRL 34915 in vascular smooth muscle, *Br. J. Pharmacol.,* 93, (Suppl.), 204P, 1988.

116. **Wilson, C., Buckingham, R. E., Mootoo, S., Parrott, L. S., Hamilton, T. C., Pratt, S. C., and Cawthorne, M. A.,** In vivo and in vitro studies of cromakalim (BRL 34915) and glibenclamide in the rat, *Br. J. Pharmacol.,* 93 (Suppl), 126P, 1988.

117. **Newgreen, D. T., Longmore, J., and Weston, A. H.,** The effect of glibenclamide on the action of cromakalim, diazoxide and minoxidil sulphate on rat aorta, *Br. J. Pharmacol.,* 96, 116P, 1989.

118. **Inoue, T., Ito, Y., and Takeda, K.,** The effects of 2-nicotinamidoethylnitrate on smooth muscle cells of the dog mesenteric artery and trachea, *Br. J. Pharmacol.,* 80, 459, 1983.

118a. **Good, D. M. and Small, R. C.,** unpublished observations.

Chapter 4

CALCIUM AND POTASSIUM CHANNELS IN AIRWAY SMOOTH MUSCLE

R. Towart

TABLE OF CONTENTS

I.   Introduction 96

II. Airway Smooth Muscle — Overview of Excitation/Contraction
     Coupling 97

III. Ion Channels in Airway Smooth Muscle 97
     A.   Sodium Channels 97
     B.   Chloride Channels 98
     C.   Calcium and Potassium Channels 98

IV. Receptor-Operated Calcium Channels 98

V.   Voltage-Sensitive Calcium Channels 100

VI. Potassium Channels 100

VII. The Clinical Status of Channel Modulators in Airway Disease 103
     A.   Calcium Antagonists 103
     B.   Potassium Channel Activators 103

VIII. Conclusions 106

Abbreviations 106

References 106

I. INTRODUCTION

It is already clear from the preceding chapters that calcium ions play a vital role in controlling the tone and contractility of airway smooth muscle. Similarly, it has been shown that the transmitters or mediators which contract the smooth muscle cause at least a temporary increase in the intracellular concentration of free calcium ions in the smooth-muscle cells, leading to activation of the actomyosin complex and contraction. This increase in calcium concentration may be brought about in two fundamentally different ways, either by mobilization of calcium already in the cell, stored in *intracellular* compartments such as the SR as already described, or by entry of *extracellular* calcium.

It is the purpose of this chapter to describe what is known about the mechanisms of this entry, through the calcium channels in airway smooth muscle, and how these calcium channels may be modulated by drugs or disease, leading to changes in response. A series of new drugs, the "calcium antagonists" or "calcium entry blockers",[1-3] has revolutionized cardiovascular medicine in recent years. Have these drugs a role in airway hyperreactivity diseases, or are they merely useful tools for the pulmonary physiologist?

Similarly, alterations in the conductivity of some of the *potassium channels* in airways can markedly affect the smooth-muscle reactivity. Here, too, a promising new range of drugs, termed "potassium channel openers",[4,5] is becoming available. How do they affect airway responses?

The cell membrane contains a large number of macromolecules designed to preserve its "milieu intérieur" and to control communication between the inside and the outside. Receptors, ion channels, and carrier macromolecules receive signals, tranduce signals, and maintain the "milieu". Just as many compounds affect the receptors and markedly modulate their activity, many compounds are now known to affect the ion channels with differing properties have been described, not all will be expressed in any one tissue. Thus a question of immediate importance in this chapter is, do the membranes of the smooth-muscle cells contain the ion channels in question, and if so, does modulation of these produce detectable effects?

Finally, it should be noted that various calcium, potassium, and other ion channels are almost certainly present in the membranes of the many *other* types of cells which make up the lung tissue. Their discussion is beyond the scope of this chapter, but it is worth noting that the classical calcium antagonists have very little effect on neurons or nervous transmission[6] and affect mediator release from mast cells or basophils only at very high concentrations.[7,8] Little has been published about the possible effects of potassium channel openers on these systems, but there is preliminary evidence that cromakalim can in some cases reduce airway tone by presynaptic effects as well as direct action.[9]

Earlier reviews in this area have argued that the ubiquitous role of the calcium ion in airway contraction, secretion, and inflammation would make a calcium entry blocker with selectivity for airway tissue a potentially useful antiasthmatic drug.[10-12] Unfortunately, the effects of calcium antagonists on airways, whether *in vitro, in vivo,* or clinically, have been modest.[13,14] Several more recent reviews have tried to reconcile these disappointing results with the newer ideas on the mechanisms of action of calcium channel blockade.[15-17] Present evidence suggests that no "classical" calcium antagonists such as diltiazem, verapamil, or DHP, which block the L-type voltage-sensitive calcium channels,[18] are likely to be of clinical use in relaxing airway smooth muscle. Nevertheless, some other approaches, such as blocking receptor-operated calcium channels or hyperpolarizing the muscle by activating potassium channels, are becoming viable therapeutic options and will be discussed below.

II. AIRWAY SMOOTH MUSCLE — OVERVIEW OF EXCITATION/CONTRACTION COUPLING

Airway smooth-muscle contraction probably plays an important role in the functioning of the normal lung, with a rhythmic cycle of reflex relaxation and constriction during inspiration and expiration.[19] The intense bronchoconstriction observed when dust or other irritants are inhaled is a normal defense mechanism, but is obviously a liability to the patient with airway disease, especially asthma. The contractile state of any smooth muscle depends on a variety of neuronal, hormonal, and environmental influences, and may be modulated by inflammatory and other mediators. These "first messengers" bind to their specific receptors on the smooth-muscle cell membrane, normally coupled via a guanine nucleotide exchange ("G") protein,[20] to alter the concentration of "second messengers" such as inositol phosphates[21] or cyclic nucleotides, as described in Chapter 2.

Many possible mechanisms have been proposed for linking receptor stimulation to calcium mobilization,[22] but three major pathways are now recognized.

1. IP_3-induced release of calcium stored intracellularly in the sarcoplasmic reticulum (SR)[21,23]
2. Entry of calcium ions via activation of ROC, possibly stimulated by IP_4[24]
3. Entry of calcium via activation of VSC[17,25]

In general, an increase in $[Ca]_i$ will *contract* smooth muscle, and a decrease in $[Ca]_i$ will relax it, although the mutual interactions of several second messengers may cause spatial or temporal inhomogeneities[25] or even oscillations in calcium concentrations.[26,27] The relative amounts originating intra- and extracellulary vary depending on the tissue, the agonist, and the species,[28] although much of the calcium required for contraction of *airway* smooth muscle seems to be released from intracellular stores.[29] Nevertheless, the entry of extracellular calcium can be measured during airway smooth-muscle contraction, and at least part of this entry is sensitive to calcium channel-blocking drugs (see below).

As alluded to above, several other tissues involved in the pathophysiology of airway diseases, e.g., mucous glands, epithelia, mast cells, and granulocytic leukocytes, depend on ion movements, especially calcium, for their activity (see References 8,30 for reviews). In general, classical calcium channel blockers have little effect in these tissues, and the actions of potassium channel openers are not yet known. In principle, however, the techniques described below could also be used to identify and isolate calcium channels in those tissues and to screen for or design drugs which could selectively reduce mucus secretion from submucosal glands or mediator release from mast cells, or curb inflammation by modulating the activity of the other airway proinflammatory cells.

III. ION CHANNELS IN AIRWAY SMOOTH MUSCLE

For many years now the transmembrane movement of certain ions has been regarded as vital to simulus-response coupling in excitable tissue. Significant transmembrane gradients of Na^+, K^+, Ca^{2+}, and Cl^- are maintained, directly or indirectly, via energy-dependent pumps and transporters. The asymmetric distributions of these ions are subsequently exploited by excitable tissue, in that membrane-associated ion channels, controlled by receptors or by membrane potential, allow rapid stimulus-response coupling for the initiation or propagation of electrical signals or for contraction or secretion (see Chapter 2).

A. SODIUM CHANNELS

Sodium-carrying channels are of course vital for neuronal function, but sodium channel blockers such as tetrodotoxin have little effect on smooth muscle in general, and in airway smooth muscle in particular[31] (but see Reference 32).

B. CHLORIDE CHANNELS

Chloride-carrying channels play a major role in epithelial transport, and a genetic defect in chloride transport is now known to be responsible for cystic fibrosis,[33] but this topic is outside the scope of the present chapter. Chloride channels have not been investigated in airway smooth muscle to my knowledge, and the possible effects of modulation are unknown.

C. CALCIUM AND POTASSIUM CHANNELS

The pioneering electrophysiological studies of Kirkpatrick[34] and Coburn and Yamaguchi[35] in the 1970s suggested the existence of *calcium channels* in airway smooth muscle, and studies reviewed below have shown that at least one type of potassium channel is also present. Work in the early 1980s showed that airway smooth muscle was essentially similar to other smooth muscle in that, as perceptively described by Bolton,[36] contraction could be activated by calcium release from intracellular SR sites, or by entry of extracellular calcium ions through ROCs or VSCs. In contrast to their effects on many other smooth muscles, however, the calcium entry blockers (see Figure 1), which are now known to block one type of VSC, had little effect on airway smooth muscle.[13,14,17] Reasons for this lack of effect include the fact that much of the activator calcium originates intracellularly,[29,37] that calcium antagonist-resistant ROCs (see below) are probably responsible for much of the calcium originates intracellularly,[29,37] that calcium antagonists themselves are less potent on airway smooth muscle.[22,39] Initial electrophysiological studies with isolated bronchial cells also suggest a high threshold for VSC activation (see Section V, below). The calcium antagonist were effective at blocking VSCs and mechanical activity only when contractions were induced by depolarization (e.g., by elevated potassium)[40] or by potassium channel blockers such as TEA.[41] This area has been reveiwed and discussed at length.[12,14,15,17,22]

Our understanding of these phenomena has greatly improved in recent years. Major advances have been made in the elucidation of the role of the various VSCs, especially that of the DHP-sensitive "L-channel",[42,43] and although there seems little chance that "classical" calcium antagonists can be used therapeutically in airways,[15] effects on membrane potential and thus indirectly on calcium handling and contraction are being found using the new potassium channel activators.[4,5]

IV. RECEPTOR-OPERATED CALCIUM CHANNELS

There is little *direct* evidence for ROCs in airway smooth muscle, and most ^{45}Ca studies cannot detect a significant influx of calcium ions in connection with agonist stimulation.[17,44] Most studies in which receptor-mediated contractions are refractory to block of VSCs by calcium antagonists can be explained by release of mainly intracellular calcium. Nevertheless, repeated or prolonged stimulation in calcium-free solution leads to diminished contraction,[17,45-47] implying that an influx of calcium ions is important. In some cases the agonist-mediated contraction can be varied by altering the extracellular calcium concentration, despite the presence of VSC blockers,[48] suggesting that a receptor-mediated calcium influx has taken place.

Most information about ROCs has come from other tissues and has attracted much interest.[49-52] An ATP-stimulated calcium channel in smooth muscle has been reported,[53] but the best evidence for the existence of ROCs has come from patch clamp studies on platelet membranes.[54] Though selective for calcium ions and blocked by nickel ions, these channels are unaffected by membrane potential or by DHPs. Possible second messengers for ROCs are IP_4 and/or IP_3,[51,52] or phosphatidic acid.[50] Although the existence of ROCs was postulated more than 10 years ago,[36] little progress in the field had been made until recently, because of the lack of stable activators or blockers. The recent development of novel photoaffinity and thio-analogs of IP_3 and IP_4[55] is encouraging, as is the news of an inhibitor of platelet

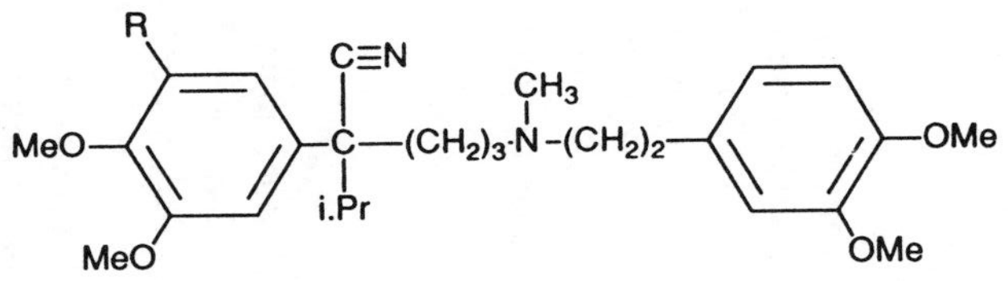

Verapamil (R= H-)

Gallopamil (R= MeO-)

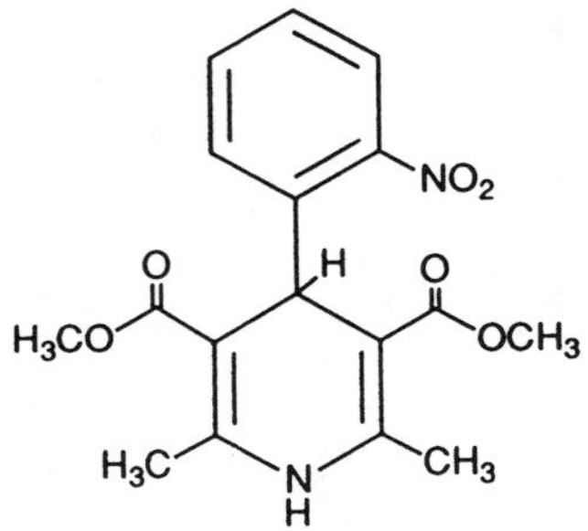

Nifedipine

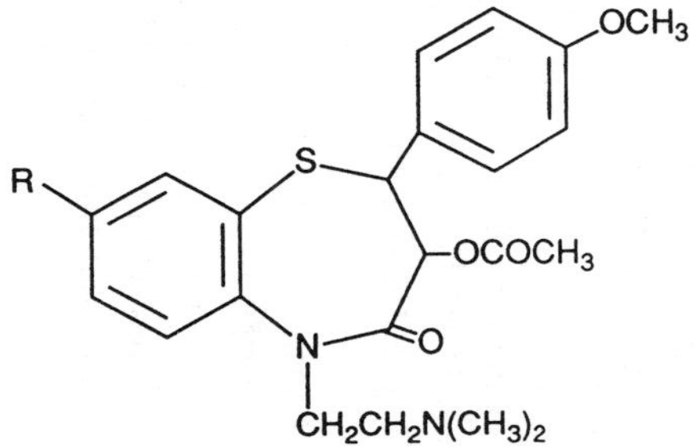

Diltiazem (R= H-)

TA 3090 (R= Cl-)

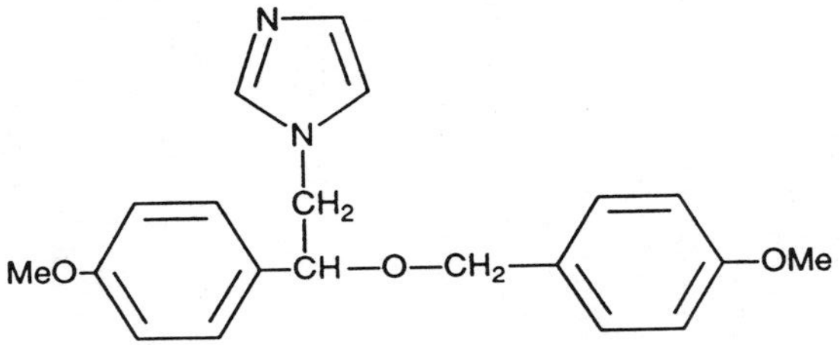

SKF 96365

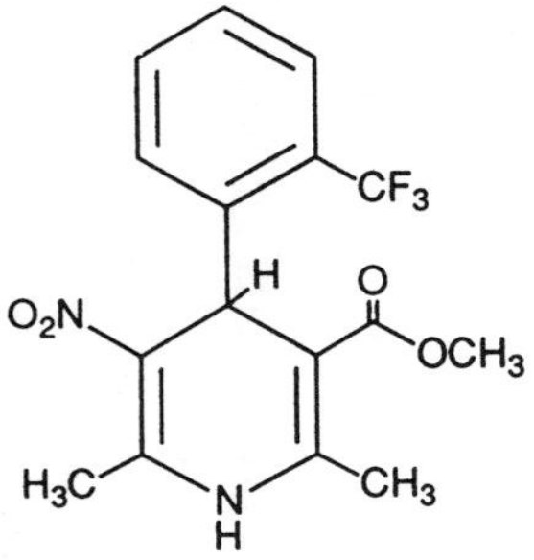

BAY K 8644

FIGURE 1. Some drugs which act on calcium channels. Verapamil, diltiazem, and nifedipine block the L-type voltage-sensitive calcium channel; BAY K 8644 activates it. SKF 96365 blocks receptor-operated calcium channels of platelets; its effects on smooth muscle are not yet known.

ROCs, SKF 96365, 1-(3-[*p*-methoxyphenyl]-propyloxy)-*p*-methoxyphenethyl-1H-imidazole hydrochloride (see Figure 1).[56] If receptor-mediated calcium entry in airway smooth muscle uses an ROC similar to those already described, then drugs blocking ROC-mediated calcium entry into airway tissue may be able to be developed. Specific agents which bind to the ROCs will also permit the isolation, purification, and sequencing of these channel(s), as has been done for the DHP-sensitive VSC.[57]

V. VOLTAGE-SENSITIVE CALCIUM CHANNELS

At least three different types of VSC have been described: the N-channel ("neuronal"), sensitive to conotoxin; the T-channel ("transient"), sensitive to amiloride; and the L-channel ("long"), sensitive to the classical calcium antagonists such as the DHPs.[18,58,59] The L-channel is widely distributed, especially in smooth and cardiac muscles, and plays a fascinating role as a voltage sensor in skeletal muscle.[60] Its biochemical structure has been widely investigated and its amino acid sequence determined.[57,59] It is blocked by calcium antagonists, activated by calcium agonists such as BAY K 8644 (see Figure 1),[61] and may even be modulated by endogenous ligands.[59,62]

It is not known whether or not airway smooth muscle contains N- or T-type VSCs (which have mainly been described in neuron),[58] but it clearly contains DHP-sensitive L-type channels. Until recently the evidence for this was indirect and consisted of the functional effects of calcium antagonists, blocking depolarization-induced contractions,[40,63,64] the potentiating effects of the calcium agonist BAY K 8644,[65,66] or the existence of DHP binding sites on the muscle membranes.[67,68] Marthan et al.[69] have now used the whole-cell patch clamp method to demonstrate calcium currents in smooth-muscle cells enzymatically isolated from human bronchus. These had the characteristics of VSCs and were unaffected by tetrodotoxin, but were blocked by cobalt and the DHP PN 200-110 and enhanced by BAY K 8644. Interestingly, the VSC threshold membrane potential measured in this study was higher than those found in other tissues with spiking smooth muscle, and the authors speculate that this high threshold in a nonspiking tissue such as airway smooth muscle could reduce the role of VSCs in contraction and give an explanation for the small effects observed with the calcium channel blockers.

In animal airway muscle (e.g., guinea pig trachealis) the VSCs are apparently involved in the electrical activity: spontaneous slow waves are associated with mechanical activity and are blocked by calcium withdrawal or by calcium antagonists.[64,70] However, the significance of these findings to normal or hyperreactive human airways is unknown: the human muscle that has been examined is electrically quiescent,[71] contractions induced by acetylcholine or by histamine are mainly independent of membrane potential,[71] and calcium antagonists have minimal effects on normal or asthmatic lung function. VSCs are, however, very important in indirectly mediating the actions of the potassium channel modulators (see below).

VI. POTASSIUM CHANNELS

Although there are plainly several different types of calcium channel, there seem to be *many* types of potassium channel. To date, 15 or so different types have been described,[72] although many may share common structural features.[73] Essentially they can be categorized as voltage-operated, calcium-activated, receptor-operated, and others, such as ATP-sensitive or volume-sensitive.[72,74,75] Many of these are blocked by Ba^{2+} or by TEA, or by the scorpion venom charybdotoxin, and many more selective blockers are becoming available for specific channel types.[72,74]

The roles of potassium channels are extremely diverse.[72] Their purpose is not normally to transduce direct signals, but rather to limit or terminate the effects of other signals or events, i.e., to stabilize the cell membrane. The high intracellular potassium concentrations can be used to stimulate K^+ efflux to counteract the effects of Na^+ or Ca^{2+} entry into the cells. Thus, for example, Boyle et al.[78] find that stimulation of guinea pig trachealis by histamine or acetylcholine evokes hyperpolarizing transients caused by the opening of membrane potassium channels activated by the increased intracellular calcium concentration.

It has been clear for many years that airway smooth muscle contains potassium channels, as blockers such as Ba^{2+} or TEA stimulate both electrical and mechanical activity (see Chapter 3 and References 34,64,70). More direct evidence is now coming from electrophysiological data using patch clamp methods to investigate single cells.[69,76,77] These outward currents are reduced by TEA or Ba^{2+}, or when Cs^+ is substituted for K^+, and can be separated into a voltage-sensitive and a calcium-activated component.[69]

There is normally a "tonic" activation of membrane potassium channels; i.e., they are not all either totally open or totally closed. Therefore, blocking the channels will cause increased excitability, leading to depolarization, whereas increasing the number of open channels will hyperpolarize the cells and cause decreased excitability. Perhaps because of their diversity and the lack until recently of selective modulators, the pharamacology of potassium channels had been little studied, but over the last few years it has gradually been discovered that potassium channel modulation is responsible for the smooth-muscle effects of various drugs. The prototype activator, or "opener", of potassium channels is the new antihypertensive agent cromakalim[79] (BRL 34915), whose activity rests mainly in its $(-)-$isomer, BRL 38277[80] (see Figure 2). Newer drugs with similar structures and actions include RP 49356,[81] EMD 52692,[82] and Ro 31-6930.[83] Pinacidil,[84] nicorandil,[85] diazoxide,[86] and minoxidil[87] are older drugs which owe some or all of their effects to potassium channel activation. The mechanism of action has been largely investigated using vascular smooth muscle (e.g., Reference 79), but most of the findings hold true for airway smooth muscle. Thus, in guinea pig trachealis, cromakalim reduces spontaneous electrical activity, hyperpolarizes the cell with the membrane potential moving towards -80 mV, the equilibrium potential for potassium, and reduces mechanical activity.[88] An efflux of ^{86}Rb, as a marker for potassium ions, is observed.[86,88] In vascular smooth muscle the reduction in mechanical activity can be thought of as being due to a decreased activation of voltage-sensitive calcium channels,[74] but this explanation is not adequate to explain the results in airway smooth muscle, where block of VSCs has little effect. Additional mechanisms that have been postulated include a reduction in the refilling of intracellular calcium stores, and a stimulation of Na^+/Ca^+ exchange, again leading to lower intracellular calcium available for contraction.[89,90] It may also be that because the potassium channel openers, in contrast to the calcium blockers, cause hyperpolarization, the spectrum of VSCs inactivated by the change in membrane potential is different from that blocked by the calcium antagonists. Whatever the exact mechanism, it is now clear that cromakalim and the other potassium channel openers relax airway smooth muscle *in vitro*,[88] *in vivo*,[90] and clinically (see Section VII.B, below).

It is not yet clear which of the many potassium channels are affected by cromakalim and its analogs. Its effects are not affected by apamin,[88] which blocks low-conductance, Ca^{2+}-activated potassium channels.[74] There is at present evidence for effects on other calcium-dependent potassium channels[91] and also for effects on ATP-sensitive channels.[92,93] Ideally, this question could be answered by using cromakalim or a more potent analog as a probe for the potassium channels affected. However, no binding of labeled cromakalim could be detected *in vitro* or *in vivo*.[94]

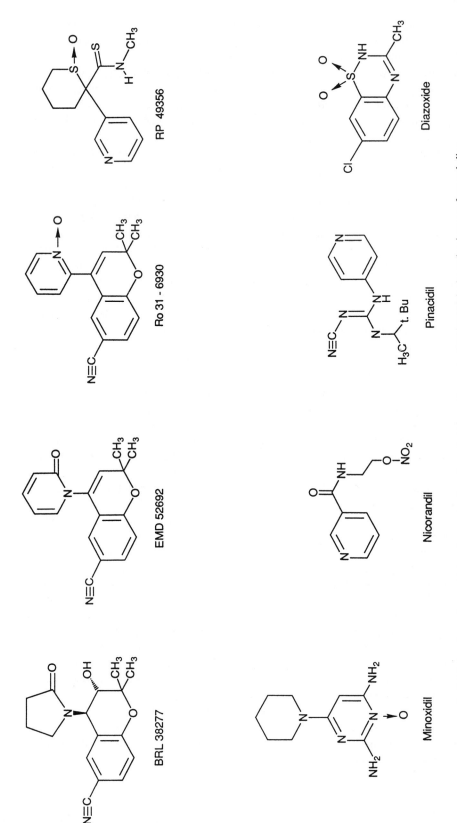

FIGURE 2.   Some drugs which activate potassium channels in smooth muscle. BRL 38277 is the active isomer of cromakalim.

VII. THE CLINICAL STATUS OF CHANNEL MODULATORS IN AIRWAY DISEASE

A. CALCIUM ANTAGONISTS

The importance of calcium channel-blocking drugs in cardiovascular medicine has led to a large number of clinical and animal studies attempting to find a rationale for the use of these compounds in asthma (e.g., References 13,15). Although one of the first studies published claimed useful results with nifedipine,[95] subsequent studies with nifedipine, verapamil, diltiazem, or their analogs, orally or inhaled, acutely or chronically, have been disappointing (for earlier studies see Reference 13; for more recent studies see References 96-101). No evidence has emerged for additive or synergistic effects of calcium antagonists with other bronchodilators.[102] One group has claimed that the "new" verapamil analog, gallopamil, is effective in inhibiting antigen-induced bronchoconstriction in humans[103] and in blocking antigen-induced, late-phase bronchoconstriction in the sheep model,[104] but other studies with gallopamil have shown that the beneficial effects are modest and of short duration,[105-107] so these studies need confirmation. However, an almost universal conclusion has been that, in contrast to beta receptor-blocking drugs, no danger of bronchospasm exists, and that the calcium antagonists are safe antianginal drugs in patients with co-existing asthma.[100,102]

The undoubted success of the original three calcium antagonists in cardiovascular disease has encouraged the development of "second-generation" drugs, with real or supposed pharmakokinetic or therapeutic advantages:

1. *Nifedipine,* which is being followed by other DHPs, e.g., benidipine, darodipine, felodipine, flordipine, franidipine, isradipine, lacidipine, niguldipine, nilvadipine, nitrendipine, nisoldipine, etc. (see Figure 3; the new DHP amlodipine is interesting because of its long duration of action)
2. *Verapamil* by other phenylalkylamines, e.g., anipamil, devapamil, gallopamil, etc.
3. *Diltiazem* by other benzothiazepines, e.g., TA 3090, SA 2572, nictiazem, etc.

Two related developments are the reports of "chimeric molecules", which combine structural elements of known calcium antagonists and of another drug class in one molecule,[108-110] and the discovery of calcium antagonists with novel chemical structures unrelated to the drugs discussed above (e.g., tetrandine,[111] MCI-176,[112] MDL 12330A,[113] and HOE 166;[114] see Figure 4). It is safe to predict that many of these new calcium channel modulators will be tested, experimentally and clinically, to investigate their potential bronchorelaxant properties.

To my knowledge, only one patient has claimed bronchoselectivity for a calcium antagonist,[115] and I know of no calcium channel blocker presently being developed with sufficient airway selectivity for asthma. As discussed above, and on the present clinical and experimental evidence, it would seem unlikely that classical-type calcium antagonists can be useful therapeutically in airway disease.

B. POTASSIUM CHANNEL ACTIVATORS

The novel potassium channel openers described above (see Section VI, above) seem more promising as antiasthmatic drugs. Clinical results in airway disease have not yet been reported for the newer agents, some of which are more potent than cromakalim,[83] but these are awaited with interest.

Initial clinical trials showed that cromakalim was an effective antihypertensive drug with a long duration of action, and as it was known to relax guinea pig trachea[88] it was tested on human airways.[116] An oral dose of 2 mg inhibited histamine-induced bronchoconstriction

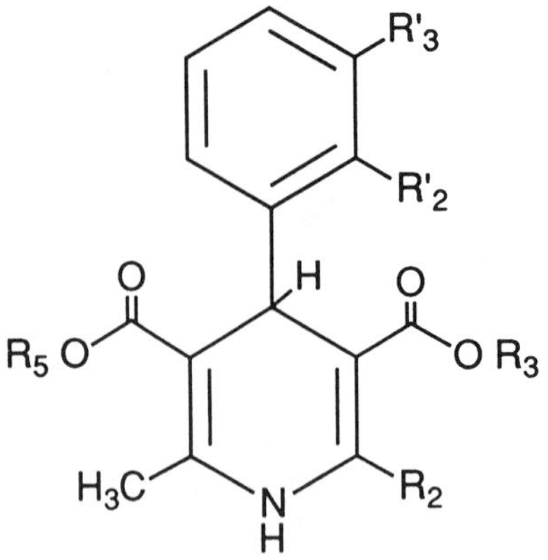

	R_2	R_3	R_5	R'_2	R'_3
Nifedipine	-CH$_3$	-CH$_3$	-CH$_3$	-NO$_2$	-H
Amlodipine	-CH$_2$O(CH$_2$)$_2$NH$_2$	-C$_2$H$_5$	-CH$_3$	-Cl	-H
Benidipine	-CH$_3$	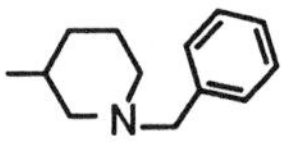 (piperidine-benzyl group)	-CH$_3$	-H	-NO$_2$
Felodipine	-CH$_3$	-C$_2$H$_5$	-CH$_3$	-Cl	-Cl
Franidipine	-CH$_3$	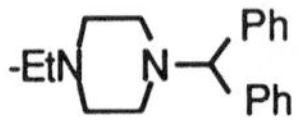 -EtN(piperazine)N-C(Ph)(Ph)	-CH$_3$	-H	-NO$_2$
Niguldipine	-CH$_3$	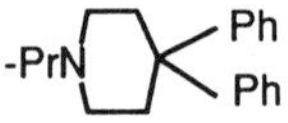 -PrN(piperidine)C(Ph)(Ph)	-CH$_3$	-H	-NO$_2$
Nilvadipine	-CN	-CH(CH$_3$)$_2$	-CH$_3$	-H	-NO$_2$
Nisoldipine	-CH$_3$	-CH$_2$CH(CH$_3$)$_2$	-CH$_3$	-NO$_2$	-H
Nitrendipine	-CH$_3$	-C$_2$H$_5$	-CH$_3$	-H	-NO$_2$
Darodipine	-CH$_3$	-C$_2$H$_5$	-C$_2$H$_5$	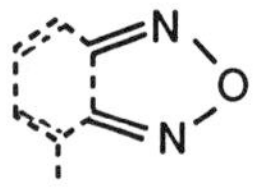 (benzofurazan group)	
Isradipine	-CH$_3$	-CH(CH$_3$)$_2$	-CH$_3$		

FIGURE 3.   Structures of some new dihydropyridines (see Reference 119).

5 h after dosing, but without effects on blood pressure in healthy volunteers.[116] The long-lasting effects suggested a use in nocturnal asthma, and a trial has shown it to be effective in patients with "morning dipping".[117] Subsequent trials are going to be carried out using the active (−)−isomer of cromakalim, BRL 38277.[80] A preliminary report has suggested that as chronic chromakalim did not diminish eosinophil accumulation in broncho-alveolar lavage fluid of guinea pigs with idiopathic eosinophilia,[118] potassium channel openers might be more useful as symptomatic rather than prophylactic antiasthmatic drugs, but these findings will have to be confirmed clinically.

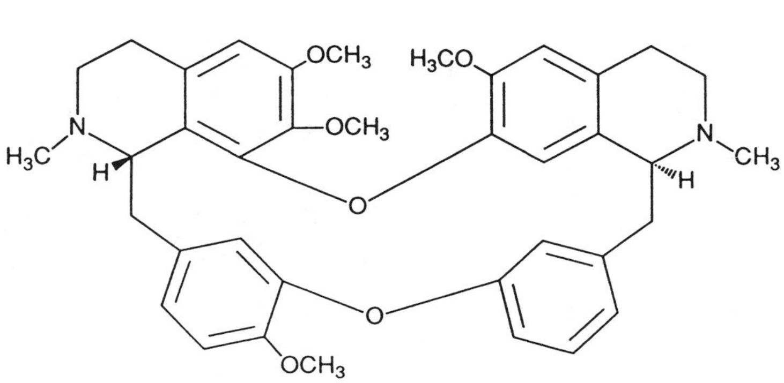

FIGURE 4. Structures of some new putative calcium channel blockers.

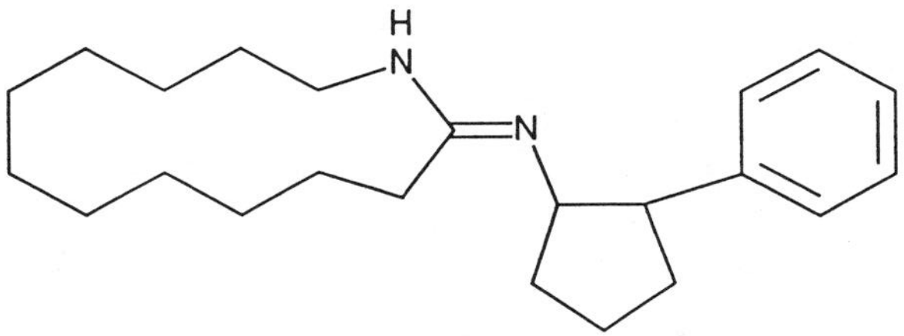

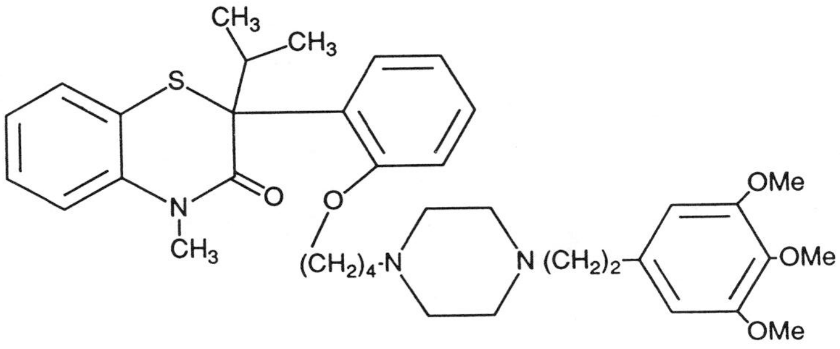

MCI - 176

HOE 166

(+) - Tetrandine

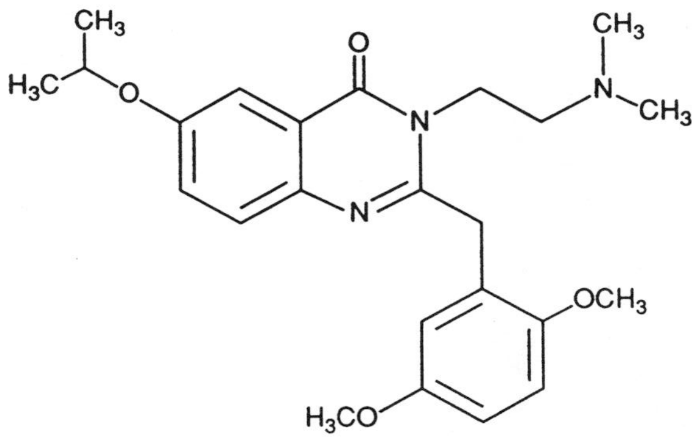

MDL 12,330A

VIII. CONCLUSIONS

After many years of indirect studies, calcium and potassium ion channels of the airway smooth muscle (including human bronchi) are at last being examined directly. New toxins and drugs — both blockers and activators — are being developed which interact with these channels and modulate the electrical and mechanical responses of the smooth muscle. They are proving to be useful tools for pulmonary physiology, but more importantly some, like the potassium channel openers, are showing promise as new and useful therapeutic agents.

ABBREVIATIONS

ATP — adenosine triphosphate
DHP — dihydropyridine
IP$_3$ — inositol (1,4,5)-triphosphate
IP$_4$ — inositol (1,3,4,5)-tetrakisphosphate
ROC — receptor-operated calcium channel
SR — sarcoplasmic reticulum
TEA — tetraethylammonium
VSC — voltage-sensitive calcium channel

REFERENCES

1. **Fleckenstein, A.,** Specific pharmacology of calcium in myocardium, cardiac pacemakers and vascular smooth muscle, *Annu. Rev. Pharmacol. Toxicol.,* 17, 49, 1977.
2. **Schwartz, A. and Triggle, D. J.,** Cellular action of calcium channel blocking drugs, *Annu. Rev. Med.,* 35, 325, 1984.
3. **Vanhoutte, P. M. and Paoletti, R.,** The WHO classification of calcium antagonists, *Trends Pharmacol. Sci.,* 8, 4, 1987.
4. **Small, R. C., Foster, R. W., and Boyle, J. P.,** K$^+$-Channel opening as a mechanism for relaxing airways smooth muscle, *Agents Actions Suppl.,* 23, 89, 1988.
5. **Hamilton, T. C. and Weston, A. H.,** Cromakalim, nicorandil and pinacidil: novel drugs which open potassium channels in smooth muscle, *Gen. Pharmacol.,* 20, 1, 1989.
6. **Blaustein, M. P.,** Calcium and synaptic function, in *Calcium in Drug Actions, Handbook Exp. Pharmacol.,* Baker, P. F., Ed., Springer-Verlag, Berlin, 1988, 275.
7. **Ennis, M., Ind, P. W., Pearce, F. L., and Dollery, C. T.,** Calcium antagonists and histamine secretion from rat peritoneal mast cells, *Agents Actions,* 13, 144, 1983.
8. **Chand, N., Perhach, J. L., Diamantis, W., and Sofia, R. D.,** Heterogeneity of calcium channels in mast cells and basophils and the possible relevance to pathophysiology of lung diseases: a review, *Agents Actions,* 17, 407, 1985.
9. **McCaig, D. J. and de Jonckheere, B.,** Effect of cromakalim on bronchoconstriction induced by stimulation of the vagus nerve in isolated guinea-pig trachea, *Br. J. Pharmacol.,* 96, 252p, 1989.
10. **Middleton, E. J.,** Antiasthmatic drug therapy and calcium ions: a review of pathogenesis and the role of calcium, *J. Pharm. Sci.,* 69, 243, 1980.
11. **Triggle, D. J.,** Calcium, the control of smooth muscle function and bronchial hyperreactivity, *Allergy,* 38, 1, 1983.
12. **Goodman, F. R.,** Calcium channel blockers and respiratory smooth muscle, in *New Perspectives on Calcium Antagonists,* Weiss, G. B., Ed., Williams & Wilkins, Baltimore, 1981, 217.
13. **Barnes, P. J.,** Clinical studies with calcium antagonists in asthma, *Br. J. Clin. Pharmacol.,* 20 (Suppl.), 2, 289s, 1985.
14. **Towart, R. and Rounding, H. P.,** Calcium antagonists and airways smooth muscle, in *Asthma, Clinical Pharmacology and Therapeutic Progress,* Kay, A. B., Ed., Blackwell Scientific, Oxford, 1986, 128.
15. **Hendles, L. and Harman, E.,** Should we abandon the notion that calcium channel blockers are potentially useful for asthma?, *J. Allergy Clin. Immunol.,* 79, 853, 1987.

16. **Ahmed, T., D'Brot, J., and Abraham, W.,** The role of calcium antagonists in bronchial reactivity, *J. Allergy Clin. Immunol.,* 81, 133, 1988.

17. **Fedan, J. S., Hay, D. W. P., and Raeburn, D.,** Ca^{2+} and respiratory smooth muscle function: is there a role for calcium entry blockers in asthma therapy?, *Curr. Top. Pulm. Pharmacol. Toxicol.,* 3, 53, 1987.

18. **Triggle, D. J. and Janis, R. A.,** Calcium channel ligands, *Annu. Rev. Pharmacol. Toxicol.,* 27, 347, 1987.

19. **Nunn, J. F.,** *Applied Respiratory Physiology,* 2nd ed., Butterworths, London, 1977, 52.

20. **Gilman, A. G.,** G proteins: transducers of receptor-generated signals, *Annu. Rev. Biochem.,* 56, 615, 1987.

21. **Berridge, M. J.,** Inositol lipids and calcium signalling, *Proc. R. Soc. London,* 234, 359, 1988.

22. **Triggle, D. J.,** Calcium ions and respiratory smooth muscle function, *Br. J. Clin. Pharmacol.,* 20 (Suppl. 2), 213s, 1985.

23. **Berridge, M. J.,** Inositol triphosphate and diacylglycerol: two interacting second messengers, *Annu. Rev. Biochem.,* 56, 159, 1987.

24. **Downes, C. P.,** Inositol phosphates: a family of signal molecules?, *Trends Neurol. Sci.,* 11, 336, 1988.

25. **Rasmussen, H. and Barrett, P. Q.,** Calcium messenger system: an integrated view, *Physiol. Rev.,* 64, 938, 1984.

26. **Berridge, M. J. and Galione, A.,** Cytosolic calcium oscillators, *FASEB J.,* 2, 3074, 1988.

27. **Weissberg, P. L., Little, P. J., and Bobik, A.,** Spontaneous oscillations in cytoplasmic calcium concentration in vascular smooth muscle, *Am. J. Physiol.,* 256, C951, 1989.

28. **Godfraind, T., Miller, R., and Wibo, M.,** Calcium antagonism and calcium entry blockade, *Pharmacol. Rev.,* 38, 321, 1986.

29. **Nouailhetas, V. L. A., Lodge, N. J., Twort, C. H. C., and van Breeman, C.,** The intracellular calcium stores in the rabbit trachealis, *Eur. J. Pharmacol.,* 157, 165, 1988.

30. **Richardson, P. S., Mian, N., and Balfre, K.,** The role of calcium ions in airway secretion, *Br. J. Clin. Pharmacol.,* 20 (Suppl. 2), 275s, 1985.

31. **Walsh, J. V. and Singer, J. J.,** Identification and characterisation of major ionic currents in isolated smooth muscle cells using the voltage-clamp technique, *Pfluegers Arch.,* 408, 83, 1987.

32. **Souhrada, M. and Souhrada, J. F.,** A transient calcium influx into airways smooth muscle cells induced by immunization, *Respir. Physiol.,* 67, 323, 1987.

33. **Quinton, P. M.,** Defective epithelial ion transport in cystic fibrosis, *Clin. Chem.,* 35, 726, 1989.

34. **Kirkpatrick, C. T.,** Excitation and contraction in bovine tracheal smooth muscle, *J. Physiol. (London),* 244, 263, 1975.

35. **Coburn, R. F. and Yamaguchi, T.,** Membrane potential-dependent and -independent tension in the canine tracheal muscle, *J. Pharmacol. Exp. Ther.,* 201, 276, 1977.

36. **Bolton, T. B.,** Mechanisms of action of transmitters and other substances on smooth muscle, *Physiol. Rev.,* 59, 606, 1979.

37. **Raeburn, D., Roberts, J. A., Rodger, I. W., and Thomson, N. C.,** Agonist-controlled contractile responses of human bronchial muscle in vitro: effects of Ca^{2+} removal, La^{3+} and PY 108068, *Eur. J. Pharmacol.,* 121, 251, 1986.

38. **Fujiwara, T., Itoh, T., and Kuriyama, H.,** Regional differences in the mechanical properties of rabbit airway smooth muscle, *Br. J. Pharmacol.,* 94, 389, 1988.

39. **Yousif, F. B. and Triggle, D. J.,** Inhibitory actions of a series of Ca^{2+} channel antagonists against agonist and K^+ depolarisation induced responses in smooth muscle: an assessment of selectivity of action, *Can. J. Physiol. Pharmacol.,* 64, 273, 1986.

40. **Foster, R. W., Small, R. C., and Weston, A. H.,** The spasmogenic action of potassium chloride in guinea-pig trachealis, *Br. J. Pharmacol.,* 80, 553, 1983.

41. **Foster, R. W., Small, R. C., and Weston, A. H.,** Evidence that the spasmogenic action of TEA in guinea-pig trachealis is both direct and dependent on the influx of calcium ion, *Br. J. Pharmacol.,* 79, 255, 1983.

42. **Janis, R. A., Silver, P. J., and Triggle, D. J.,** Drug action and cellular calcium regulation, *Adv. Drug Res.,* 16, 309, 1987.

43. **Kamp, T. J. and Miller, R. J.,** Voltage-sensitive calcium channels and calcium antagonists, *ISI Atlas Sci. Pharmacol.,* 1, 133, 1987.

44. **Raeburn, D. and Rodger, I. W.,** Lack of effect of leukotriene D_4 on Ca-uptake in airway smooth muscle, *Br. J. Pharmacol.,* 83, 499, 1984.

45. **Creese, B. R. and Denborough, M. A.,** Sources of calcium for contraction of guinea-pig isolated tracheal smooth muscle, *Clin. Exp. Pharamacol. Physiol.,* 8, 175, 1981.

46. **Langlands, J. M., Kardasz, A. M., Rodger, I. W., and Watson, J.,** Lack of turnover of inositol phosphates in guinea-pig and rat parenchyma may be due to its dependence on extracellular calcium during contraction, *Biochem. Soc. Trans.,* 16, 35, 1988.

47. **Mitchell, R. W., Koenig, S. M., Kelly, E., and Leff, A. R.,** Augmented shortening during quasi-isotonic contraction to agonist-mediated Ca^{++} entry in canine tracheal smooth muscle in vitro, *Am. Rev. Respir. Dis.,* 137, A306 (Abstr.), 1988.

48. **Gunst, S. J. and Pisoni, J. M.,** Effects of extracellular calcium on canine tracheal smooth muscle, *J. Appl. Physiol.,* 61, 706, 1986.

49. **Rink, T. J.,** A real receptor-operated calcium channel?, *Nature (London),* 334, 649, 1988.

50. **Exton, J. H.,** Mechanisms of action of calcium-mobilizing agonists: some variations on a young theme, *FASEB J.,* 2, 2670, 1988.

51. **Gallacher, D. V.,** Control of calcium influx in cells without action potentials, *News Physiol. Sci.,* 3, 244, 1988.

52. **Hallam, T. J. and Rink, T. J.,** Receptor-mediated calcium entry: diversity of function and mechanism, *Trends Pharmacol. Sci.,* 10, 8, 1989.

53. **Benham, C. D. and Tsien, R. W.,** A novel receptor-operated Ca^{2+}-permeable channel activated by ATP in smooth muscle, *Nature (London),* 328, 275, 1987.

54. **Zschauer, A., van Breeman, C., Bühler, F. R., and Nelson, M. T.,** Calcium channels in thrombin-activated human platelet membrane, *Nature (London),* 334, 703, 1988.

55. **Nahorski, S. R. and Potter, B. V. L.,** Molecular recognition of inositol polyphosphates by intracellular receptors and metabolic enzymes, *Trends Pharamcol. Sci.,* 10, 139, 1989.

56. **Merrit, J. E., Armstrong, W. P., Hallam, T. J., Jaxa-Chamiec, A., Leigh, B. K., Moores, K. E., and Rink, T. J.,** SK&F 96365, a novel inhibitor of receptor-mediated calcium entry and aggregation in quin2-loaded human platelets, *Br. J. Pharmacol.,* in press.

57. **Tanabe, T., Takeshima, H., Mikami, A., Flockerzi, V., Takahashi, H., Kangawa, K., Kojima, M., Matsuo, H., Hirose, T., and Numa, S.,** Primary structure of the receptor for calcium channel blockers from skeletal muscle, *Nature (London),* 328, 313, 1987.

58. **Miller, R. J.,** Multiple calcium channels and neuronal function, *Science,* 235, 46, 1987.

59. **Greenberg, D. A.,** Recent advances in calcium channel pharmacology, *Drug News Perspect.,* 1, 167, 1988.

60. **Rios, E. and Brum, G.,** Involvement of dihydropyridine receptors in excitation-contraction coupling in skeletal muscle, *Nature (London),* 325, 717, 1987.

61. **Schramm, M., Thomas, G., Towart, R., and Franckowiak, G.,** Novel dihydropyridines with positive inotropic action through activation of Ca^{2+} channels, *Nature (London),* 303, 535, 1983.

62. **Callewaert, G., Hanbauer, I., and Morad, M.,** Modulation of calcium channels in cardiac and neuronal cells by an endogenous peptide, *Science,* 243, 663, 1989.

63. **Farley, J. M., and Miles, P. R.,** The sources of calcium for acetylcholine-induced contractions of dog tracheal smooth muscle, *J. Pharmacol. Exp. Ther.,* 207, 340, 1978.

64. **Ahmed, F., Foster, R. W., and Small, R. C.,** Some effects of nifedipine in guinea-pig isolated trachealis, *Br. J. Pharmacol.,* 84, 861, 1985.

65. **Allen, S. L., Foster, R. W., Small, R. C., and Towart, R.,** The effects of the dihydropyridine BAY K 8644 in guinea-pig isolated trachealis, *Br. J. Pharmacol.,* 86, 171, 1986.

66. **Marthan, R., Armour, C. L., Johnson, P. R. A., and Black, J. L.,** The calcium channel agonist BAY K 8644 enhances the responsiveness of human airway to KCl and histamine but not to carbachol, *Am. Rev. Respir. Dis.,* 135, 185, 1987.

67. **Cheng, J. B., Bewtra, A., and Townley, R. G.,** Identification of calcium antagonist receptor binding sites using (^{3}H)-nitrendipine in bovine tracheal smooth muscle membranes, *Experientia,* 40, 267, 1984.

68. **Triggle, D. J. and Janis, R. A.,** Nitrendipine: binding sites and mechanism of action, in *Nitrendipine,* Scriabine, A. et al., Eds., Urban & Schwarzenberg, Baltimore, 1984, 32.

69. **Marthan, R., Martin, C., Amédée, T., and Mironneau, J.,** Calcium channel currents in isolated muscle cells from human bronchus, *J. Appl. Physiol.,* 66, 1706, 1989.

70. **Small, R. C.,** Electrical slow waves and tone of guinea-pig isolated trachealis muscle: effects of drugs and temperature changes, *Br. J. Pharmacol.,* 77, 45, 1982.

71. **Small, R. C. and Foster, R. W.,** Electrophysiology of the airway smooth muscle cell, in *Asthama: Basic Mechanisms and Clinical Management,* Barnes, P. J., Rodger, I. W., and Thomson, N. C., Eds., Academic Press, London, 1988, 35.

72. **Castle, N. A., Haylett, D. G., and Jenkinson, D. H.,** Toxins in the characterisation of potassium channels, *Trends Neurol. Sci.,* 12, 59, 1989.

73. **MacKinnon, R., Reinhart, P. H., and White, M. M.,** Chaybdotoxin block of shaker K^+ channels suggests that different types of K^+ channels share common structural features, *Neuron,* 1, 997, 1988.

74. **Cook, N. S.,** The pharmacology of potassium channels and their therapeutic potential, *Trends. Pharmacol. Sci.,* 9, 21, 1988.

75. **Bernardi, H., Bidard, J. N., Fosset, M., Hugues, M., Mourre, C., Rehm, H., Romey, G., Schmidt-Antomarchi, H., Schweitz, H., de Weille, J. R., and Lazdunski, M.,** Molecular properties of potassium channels, *Arzneim.-Forsch.,* 39, 159, 1989.

76. **McCann, J. D. and Welsh, M. J.,** Calcium-activated potassium channels in canine airway smooth muscle, *J. Physiol. (London),* 372, 113, 1986.

77. **McCann, J. D. and Welsh, M. J.,** Neuroleptics antagonise a calcium-activated potassium channel in airway smooth muscle, *J. Gen. Physiol.,* 89, 339, 1987.

78. **Boyle, J. P., Davies, J. M., Foster, R. W., Good, D. M., Kennedy, I., and Small, R. C.,** Spasmogen action in guinea-pig isolated trachealis: involvement of membrane K$^+$ channels and the consequences of K$^+$ channel blockade, *Br. J. Pharmacol.,* 93, 319, 1988.

79. **Hamilton, T. C., Weir, S. W., and Weston, A. H.,** Comparison of the effects of BRL 34915 and verapamil on electrical and mechanical activity in rat portal vein, *Br. J. Pharmacol.,* 88, 103, 1986.

80. **Buckingham, R. E., Clapham, J. C., Coldwell, M. C., Hamilton, T. C., and Howlett, D. R.,** Stereospecific mechanisms of action of the novel antihypertensive agent BRL 34915, *Br. J. Pharmacol.,* 87, 78p, 1986.

81. **Mondot, S., Mestre, M., Caillard, C. G., and Cavero, I.,** RP 49356: a vasorelaxant with potassium channel activating properties, *Br. J. Pharmacol.,* 95, 813p, 1988.

82. **Gericke, R., Lues, I., de Peyer, J., and Haeusler, G.,** Electrophysiological and pharmacological characterisation of EMD 52693, a new potassium channel activator, *Arch. Pharmacol.,* 339, (Suppl.), R62 (Abstr.) 247, 1989.

83. **Paciorek, P. M., Cowlrick, I. S., Perkins, R. S., Taylor, J. C., Wilkinson, G. F., and Waterfall, J. F.,** Actions of Ro 31-6930, a novel potassium channel opener, on guinea-pig tracheal smooth muscle preparations, *Br. J. Pharmacol.,* in press.

84. **Nielsen-Kudsk, J. E., Mellemkjaer, S., Siggard, C., and Neilsen, C. B.,** Effects of pinacidil on guinea-pig airway smooth muscle contracted by asthma mediators, *Eur. J. Pharmacol.,* 157, 221, 1988.

85. **Allen, S. L., Foster, R. W., Morgan, G. P., and Small, R. C.,** The relaxant action of nicorandil in guinea-pig isolated trachealis, *Br. J. Pharmacol.,* 87, 117, 1986.

86. **Gater, P. R.,** Effects of K$^+$ channel openers on bovine tracheal muscle, *Br. J. Pharmacol.,* in press.

87. **Meisheri, K., Cipkus, L. A., and Taylor, C. J.,** Mechanism of action of minoxidil sulphate-induced vasodilatation: a role for increased K$^+$ permeability, *J. Pharmacol. Exp. Ther.,* 245, 751, 1988.

88. **Allen, S. L., Boyle, J. P., Cortijo, L., Foster, R. W., Morgan, G. P., and Small, R. C.,** Electrical and mechanical effects of BRL 34915 in guinea-pig trachealis, *Br. J. Pharmacol.,* 89, 395, 1986.

89. **Weston, A. H.,** New developments in potassium-channel pharmacology, *Drug News Perspect.,* 1, 205, 1988.

90. **Arch, J. R. S., Buckle, D. R., Bumstead, J., Clarke, G. D., Taylor, J. F., and Taylor, S. G.,** Evaluation of the potassium channel activator cromakalim (BRL 34915) as a bronchodilator in the guinea-pig: comparison with nifedipine, *Br. J. Pharmacol.,* 95, 763, 1988.

91. **Nakao, K., Okabe, K., Kitamura, K., Kuriyama, H., and Weston, A. H.,** Characteristics of cromakalim-induced relaxations in the smooth muscle cells of guinea-pig mesenteric artery and vein, *Br. J. Pharmacol.,* 95, 795, 1988.

92. **Buckingham, R. E., Hamilton, T. C., Howlett, D. R., Mootoo, S., and Wilson, C.,** Inhibition by glibenclamide of the vasorelaxant action of cromakalim in the rat, *Br. J. Pharmacol,* 97, 57, 1989.

92. **Escande, D., Thuringer, D., Lanville, M., Courteix, J., and Cavero, I.,** RP 49356 is a potent opener of ATP-modulated potassium channels in cardiac myocytes, *Br. J. Pharmacol.,* 95, 814p, 1988.

94. **Coldwell, M. C. and Howlett, D. R.,** Specificity of action of the novel antihypertensive agent, BRL 34915, as a potassium channel activator, *Biochem. Pharmacol.,* 36, 3663, 1987.

95. **Cerrina, J., Denjean, A., Alexandre, G., Lockhart, A., and Duroux, P.,** Inhibition of exercise-induced asthma by a calcium antagonist, nifedipine, *Am. Rev. Respir. Dis.,* 123, 156, 1981.

96. **Foresi, A., Corbo, G. M., Ciappi, G., Valente, S., and Polidori, G.,** Effect of two doses of inhaled diltiazem on exercise-induced asthma, *Respiration,* 51, 241, 1987.

97. **Patakas, D., Maniki, E., Tsara, V., and Dascalopoulou, E.,** Nifedipine treatment of patients with bronchial asthma, *J. Allergy Clin. Immunol.,* 79, 959, 1987.

98. **Rafferty, P., Varley, J. G., Edwards, J. S., and Holgate, S. T.,** Inhibition of exercise-induced asthma by nifedipine: a dose-response study, *Br. J. Clin. Pharmacol.,* 24, 479, 1987.

99. **Gordon, E. H., Wong, S. C., and Klaustermeyer, W. B.,** Comparison of nifedipine with a new calcium channel blocker, flordipine, in exercise-induced asthma, *J. Asthma,* 24, 261, 1987.

100. **Christopher, M. A., Harman, E., Pieper, J., and Hendeles, L.,** Effect of maintenance therapy with calcium blockers for chronic asthma, *Am. Rev. Respir. Dis.,* 137 (Suppl.) 37, 1988.

101. **Patel, K. and Peers, E.,** Felodipine, a new calcium antagonist, modifies exercise-induced asthma, *Am. Rev. Respir. Dis.,* 138, 54, 1988.

102. **Greenspon, L. W. and Levy, S. F.,** The effect of aerosolized verapamil on the response to isoproterenol in asthmatics, *Am. J. Respir. Dis.,* 137, 722, 1988.

103. **Ahmed, T., Kim, C. S., and Danta, I.,** Inhibition of antigen-induced bronchoconstriction by a new calcium antagonist, gallopamil: comparison with cromolyn sodium, *J. Allergy Clin. Immunol.,* 81, 852, 1988.

104. **D'Brot, J., Abraham, W. A., and Ahmed, T.,** Effect of calcium antagonist gallopamil on antigen-induced early and late bronchoconstriction responses in allergic sheep, *Am. Rev. Respir. Dis.,* 139, 915, 1989.

105. **Patel, K. R. and Tullet, W. M.,** Comparison of two calcium channel blockers, verapamil and gallopamil (D 600) in exercise-induced asthma, *Eur. J. Respir. Dis.,* 67, 269, 1985.

106. **Massey, K. L., Hill, M., Harman, E., Rutledge, D. R., Ahrens, R., and Hendeles, L.,** Dose response of inhaled gallopamil (D 600), a calcium channel blocker, in attenuating airway reactivity to methacholine and exercise, *J. Allergy Clin. Immunol.,* 81, 912, 1988.

107. **Massey, K. L., Harman, E., and Hendeles, L.,** Duration of protection of calcium channel blockers against exercise-induced bronchospasm: comparison of oral diltiazem and inhaled gallopamil, *Eur. J. Clin. Pharmacol.,* 34, 555, 1988.

108. **Marsh, J. D., Dionne, M. A. M., Chiu, M., and Smith, T. W.,** A dihydropyridine calcium channel blocker with phosphodiesterase inhibitory activity: effects on cultured vascular smooth muscle and cultured heart cells, *J. Mol. Cell. Cardiol.,* 20, 1141, 1988.

109. **Marciniak, G., Delgado, A., Leclerc, G., Velly, J., Decker, N., and Schwartz, J.,** New 1,4-dihydropyridine derivatives combining calcium antagonism and alpha-adrenolytic properties, *J. Med. Chem.,* 32, 1402, 1989.

110. **Ennis, C., Granger, S. E., Middlefell, V. C., Philpot, M. E., and Shepperson, N. B.,** Pharmacologic effects of Wy 27569: a combined calcium channel blocker and thromboxane synthetase inhibitor, *J. Cardiovasc. Pharmacol.,* 13, 511, 1989.

111. **King, V. F., Garcia, M. L., Himmel, D., Reuben, J. P., Lam, Y. T., Pan, J., Han, G., and Kaczorowski, G. J.,** Interaction of tetrandine with slowly-inactivating calcium channels, *J. Biol. Chem.,* 263, 2238, 1988.

112. **Hara, Y., Ichihara, K., and Abiko, Y.,** MCI-176, a novel calcium channel blocker, attenuates the ischemic myocardial acidosis induced by coronary artery occlusion in dogs, *J. Pharmacol. Exp. Ther.,* 245, 305, 1988.

113. **Rampe, D., Triggle, D. J., and Brown, A. M.,** Electrophysiologic and biochemical studies on the putative Ca^{2+} channel blocker MDL 12330A in an endocrine cell, *J. Pharmacol. Exp. Ther.,* 243, 402, 1987.

114. **Qar, J., Barhanin, J., Romey, G., Henning, R., Lerch, U., Oekonomopulos, R., Urbach, H., and Lazdunski, M.,** A novel high affinity class of Ca^{2+} channel blockers, *Mol. Pharmacol.,* 33, 363, 1988.

115. **Wehinger, E. and Towart, R.,** Sulphonydihydro pyridines, *Ger. Offen.,* DE 3501695, 1986.

116. **Baird, A., Hamilton, T., Richards, D., Tasker, T., and Williams, A. J.,** Cromakalim, a potassium channel activator inhibits histamine induced bronchoconstriction in healthy volunteers, *Br. J. Clin. Pharmacol.,* 25, 144p, 1988.

117. **Williams, A. J., Vyse, T., Richards, D. H., and Lee, T.,** Cromakalim, a potassium channel activator inhibits histamine induced bronchoconstriction and nocturnal bronchoconstriction in patients with asthma, *N.E.J. Allergy Proc.,* 9, 249, 1988.

118. **Sanjar, S., Morley, J., Chapman, I., and Kings, M.,** K^+-Channel activation in tests for prophylactic anti-asthma drug efficacy in the guinea-pig, *Am. Rev. Respir. Dis.,* 139 (Suppl.), A467, 1989.

119. **Prous, J. R.,** Lacidipine, *Drugs of the Future,* 14, 317, 1989.

Chapter 5

EVALUATION OF AIRWAY SMOOTH MUSCLE FUNCTION
IN VITRO

R. G. Goldie, K. M. Lulich, P. J. Henry, and J. W. Paterson

TABLE OF CONTENTS

I.   Introduction 112

II.   Standard Central Airway Preparations 112

III.   The Lung Parenchyma Strip as a Peripheral Airway Model 113

IV.   Comparison of Isometric and Isotonic Measurements 115

V.   Alternative Airway Preparations 117
        A.   Airway Tube Preparations 117
        B.   Isolated Smooth-Muscle Cell Preparations 118

VI.   Functional Antagonism 118
        A.   Important Determinants of Functional Antagonism 119
        B.   Use of Functional Antagonism to Estimate Affinity and
                Efficacy 120

VII.   Epithelium-Modulated Airway Responsiveness to Drugs 120
        A.   Transfer and Bioassay of Epithelium-Derived Inhibitory Factor 121

VIII.   Summary 122

References 123

I. INTRODUCTION

Isolated airway preparations have been used for many years in the assessment of drug- or mediator-induced responses of airway smooth muscle. Generally, tracheal tissue from various laboratory animals including the rat, cat, dog, rabbit, and most commonly the guinea pig has been used to measure the spasmogenic and spasmolytic activity of drugs and mediators from a wide variety of chemical groups. The general aim of these studies has been to improve our understanding of the mechanism(s) underlying the control of airway tone and of the action of drugs which influence airway smooth-muscle tone. In addition, many studies have attempted to assess the role of airway smooth muscle in lung function in health and disease. Results have often provided considerable insight with respect to human airway smooth-muscle responses to drugs. The following is an analysis of the importance of various factors relevant to the use of isolated airway preparations for evaluating drug-induced airway smooth-muscle responsiveness *in vitro*.

II. STANDARD CENTRAL AIRWAY PREPARATIONS

Airway tissue is prepared for study using an essentially standard regime, although important modifications to the general guidelines have been made to improve an evolving methodology. Isolated airway preparations may be suspended under an applied tension in a chamber containing a physiological salt solution which is gassed (usually with 5% CO_2 in 95% oxygen) and maintained at constant temperature (usually 37°C), or the tissue can be superfused with this fluid.[1] Either way, the tissue is mounted such that the smooth-muscle fibers are oriented to allow efficient detection of changes in airway muscle tension via a force/displacement transducer. The transducer may be an electronic device which transforms mechanical displacements into electrical signals that can then be amplified, integrated, and displayed as a permanent pen recording, or it may be a simple lever for direct, mechanically amplified measurements.

Initially, tracheal tissue was prepared as a series of interlinked rings to form an airway chain.[2] This method was superseded by the use of "cross-cut" tracheal chains or spirals[3] and by small closed[4] or open ring preparations.[5] These preparations have been primarily developed to simplify procedures. However, each of these variants provides essentially similar information concerning the potency and efficacy of drugs with respect to alterations in airway smooth-muscle tone.

Interestingly, in the case of some agonists, the method used to prepare the isolated airway tissue is apparently critical to the response pattern observed. For example, adenosine and ATP relaxed open ring preparations of guinea pig trachea cut in transverse section, but contracted spiral tracheal strips obtained from the same animal.[6] These differences in response probably reflect differences in the number of appropriately oriented transverse or longitudinal smooth-muscle bundles in these preparations.

Other modifications to so-called "standard" tracheal preparations have also been shown to cause significant changes in airway smooth-muscle response to drugs. For example, removal of the guinea pig tracheal cartilage has been shown to reduce the contractile potency and maximal contractile effect of KCl and histamine.[7] Conversely, the relaxant potency and maximal effect of verapamil was significantly enhanced in cartilage-free preparations. It was shown that these effects were most likely due to the loss of a source of extracellular calcium. In addition, removal of the fibroelastic layer surrounding pig tracheal smooth muscle enhanced histamine-induced contractions.[8] This was shown to be due to the loss of an indomethacin-sensitive system producing a relaxant prostanoid in response to histamine.

It has also been shown that large human bronchial preparations (approximately 6 mm I.D.) produced significantly lower levels of tension in response to various contractile agonists than did smaller preparations (approximately 2 mm I.D.) from the same airway.[9] This may have been related to differences in the relative proportions of muscle to nonmuscle components in these airways and the mechanical impediment of the greater mass of surrounding bronchial cartilage in the larger airway preparations.[10] Alternatively, it might reflect differences in muscle fiber properties or fiber orientation at different levels in the bronchial tree.

It is well established that airway structure changes markedly down the respiratory tree. Tracheal muscle exists as a narrow strip spanning the gap between otherwise continuous cartilage rings. In contrast, bronchial airway smooth muscle is a continuous band present in the circumference of the airway between cartilaginous plates and the mucosa. Similarly, in noncartilaginous bronchioles, airway smooth muscle forms a continuous submucosal strip.

It is perhaps not surprising then that regional differences have been reported with respect to the responsiveness of guinea pig airways to various relaxants and spasmogens. For example, it has recently been shown that the maximal contractile response to the muscarinic cholinoreceptor agonist carbachol and the maximal relaxant effect of the β-adrenoreceptor agonist isoprenaline were 27 and 39% greater, respectively, in trachea than in bronchus.[11] In addition, histamine-induced contractions were significantly smaller at both sites than those produced by carbachol. Conversely, leukotriene(LT)D_4 and prostaglandin (PG) D_4 were equiactive in trachea and bronchus. However, these data are at variance with other results showing that histamine and carbachol were equiactive in guinea pig tracheal spirals.[12] A major difference between these studies was that Wasserman and Mukherjee[11] equilibrated airway preparations under an initial resting tension of 10 g, while 2 g was used in the earlier investigations. Clearly, then, different equilibration preload conditions, resulting in different preparation lengths in the relaxed state, can result in different response profiles to agonists.

Regional differences in airway smooth-muscle responsiveness to drugs might also reflect different receptor densities at various levels within the respiratory tree. Radioligand binding and autoradiographic studies have now established that the density of beta-adrenoreceptors increases from the trachea to the most peripheral airways in rabbit,[13] pig,[14] and human lung.[15] In contrast, in the ferret airway smooth muscle, muscarinic cholinoreceptors were most numerous in the trachea and bronchi, were sparse in proximal bronchioles, and virtually absent in distal bronchioles.[16]

The great majority of studies concerning the function of airway smooth muscle have been conducted using guinea pig tracheal smooth muscle. It is important to question whether or not tracheal airway smooth muscle in general and guinea pig trachea in particular provide appropriate and representative models of respiratory smooth muscle in human central airways.

Clear species differences are also evident with respect to airway responsiveness to both relaxant and contractile agonists. For example, rat, cat, and rabbit trachea are insensitive to histamine,[17] while guinea pig trachea[17] and pig and human bronchus[18] contract powerfully. Furthermore, 5-hydroxytryptamine (5HT) relaxed human bronchus, but failed to initiate any response in pig bronchus.[18] While guinea pig trachea seems to provide an essentially adequate model for human airways with respect to its responsiveness to most agonists, some major differences are also evident between these tissues. For example, the spasmogenic potencies of neurokinin A and substance P in human bronchus are approximately 10- and 100-fold less, respectively, than those observed in guinea pig trachea.[19] This correlates well with the relative densities of specific binding sites for substance P in these tissues.[20]

III. THE LUNG PARENCHYMA STRIP AS A PERIPHERAL AIRWAY MODEL

The lung parenchyma strip from the cat was developed to measure *in vitro* pharmacological activity of peripheral airways.[21] Since that time, other workers have used lung parenchyma strips from many species, including guinea pig, rat, cat, dog, pig, sheep, cow, horse, and man.[22]

It is often assumed that the drug-induced effects observed were due solely to the response of the smooth muscle of airways proximal to alveoli, i.e., bronchioles, terminal bronchioles, and respiratory bronchioles. However, the status of the lung parenchyma strip as a preparation for assessing peripheral airways pharmacology has been challenged. As mammalian lung parenchyma is morphologically complex, a lung strip preparation contains many different cell types, several of which are potentially contractile.[23] These include vascular smooth-muscle cells and interstitial cells in alveolar walls.[24]

It has been shown that bovine lung parenchyma strip has pharmacological characteristics in common with both pulmonary vascular and airway smooth muscle.[25] Several other authors have also suggested that peripheral blood vessels may also contribute to drug-induced responses.[18,26-28] Considerable numbers of muscular blood vessels have been described in lung strips from different animal species[12,21,23,27] and man.[18]

Interstitial cells in alveolar walls have been implicated as a third population of potentially contractile cells capable of contributing to drug-induced responses of lung parenchyma strips. Adrenaline-induced contraction of parenchyma strip has been attributed to stimulation of alveolar interstitial myofibroblasts.[24] Ultra-thin preparations of guinea pig lung parenchyma which contained no conducting airways or blood vessels contracted to histamine and carbachol.[12] These authors concluded that alveolar contractile interstitial cells and/or alveolar duct smooth muscle[23] were responsible for these responses. The contractile response of the human lung parenchyma strip to noradrenaline has also been attributed to stimulation of nonvascular α-adrenoreceptors, possibly in alveolar contractile cells.[26] It has been established that alveolar contractile cells in amphibian lung contract and relax to a wide range of agonists.[29,30] However, it has not been shown that similar interstitial cells in mammalian lung which also contain actin fibrils respond appropriately to applied agonists. Indeed, many noncontractile cells also contain actin fibrils.[31]

Theoretically, net responses of the lung strip might arise in a variety of ways. Firstly, a given agonist may have a selective effect on a single, potentially reactive component. If that component consists of bronchiolar smooth muscle or alveolar contractile cells, then the lung strip could be said to be responding as a true peripheral airways preparation. The same might be said if several peripheral airways elements were responding to the agonists simultaneously and in like fashion, that is, if each component was contracting or if each was relaxing. The net response of the lung strip would then be related to the sum of resultant responses of the reacting components.

For an agonist which had opposing effect in two separate pulmonary cell populations, the possibility arises that the net response of the lung strip could be zero, given that an increase in tension produced in one element could be counteracted by a decrease in tension in cells elsewhere. Faced with this result, one might incorrectly conclude that the agonist was inactive in peripheral airways. Alternatively, the net response of the lung strip might be relaxation or contraction, if the proportions of different reactive components differ between lung strips. This situation becomes even more complex if the agonist causes changes in tension within both airways and vascular reactive elements. Once again, responses may be of the same type or in opposing directions. In the extreme case, an agonist may only contract vascular smooth muscle, and then the lung strip might be better described as a preparation of peripheral blood vessels. It is not surprising, therefore, that the status of the lung strip, as the model for assessing only peripheral airways pharmacology, has been challenged.

It has also been pointed out that the effects of drugs in lung strips from different species might be expected to differ, given the likelihood that lung strips of similar size, taken from animals of different sizes, will contain quite different amounts and proportions of the various contractile components. In fact, lung strips from some animals of quite different sizes, e.g., guinea pig, rabbit, cat, and dog, respond to a wide range of agonists in qualitatively similar ways, although rat lung strips demonstrate a unique pattern of pharmacological responses.[22]

Correlations have been sought between pharmacological responses of human lung parenchyma strips and quantitative estimates of the proportions of the three major contractile components.[32] Both 5HT and noradrenaline caused contraction, relaxation, or had little effect in human lung strips, confirming previous findings.[18] These results are consistent with the notion that different lung strips from the same or from different specimens of lung contain different proportions of at least two contractile components, one of which contracted while the other relaxed to 5HT and to noradrenaline. The size and direction of responses of human lung strips to 5HT and noradrenaline may therefore be related to the relative volume densities of these contractile elements.

It was shown that on average, human lung strips that contracted to 5HT contained a significantly greater proportion of blood vessels and a significantly lesser proportion of larger airways than the preparations that relaxed. However, all of these lung strips contained similar amounts of parenchymal tissue. Importantly, a highly significant correlation existed between the size and direction of 5HT-induced responses of lung strips and the ratio of the volume densities of blood vessel wall to airways wall in tissue. Presumably, preparations that contracted to 5HT were responding to predominantly vascular preparations. Responses of contractile cells within alveolar parenchyma probably did not contribute significantly to 5HT-induced responses. Indeed, no direct evidence was obtained to suggest that 5HT caused either relaxation or contraction of elements within alveolar tissue, although the possibility cannot be excluded. A similar relationship held for responsiveness of human lung strips to noradrenaline. Results with both 5HT and noradrenaline suggest that human lung strips can be screened to separate those preparations which are most likely to behave as airway preparations from those which may manifest primarily vascular responses to drugs. It seems likely that this is also true for lung strip preparations from other species.

A structure-function analysis has also been performed in human lung parenchyma strips with respect to responsiveness to carbachol.[33] It was concluded that the contractile effect of this agonist reflected a true peripheral airway response. In contrast, the contractile effect of LTC_4 in rat lung strips seemed to primarily involve nonairway components.[28] Clearly, if there is a need to measure drug-induced responsiveness of peripheral bronchi or bronchioles, such airways should be examined directly,[34] rather than relying on potentially inappropriate data from lung parenchyma strips.

IV. COMPARISON OF ISOMETRIC AND ISOTONIC MEASUREMENTS

Responses in airway smooth muscle are usually measured isometrically, although an isotonic method can also be used.[35-38] Isometric recording involves measurement of the tension developed in tissue of fixed length, in contrast to isotonic recording, where a constant load is applied and the change in preparation length is measured. In most cases, the method of recording is chosen according to convenience and the purpose of the experiment, although isotonic recording may measure responses more closely resembling physiological responses in bronchial airway smooth muscle, since this tissue shortens considerably when contracted.[39] Furthermore, changes in airway resistance may be determined more by changes in airway smooth-muscle length than by changes in airway smooth-muscle tension.[40]

Changes in tension have also been measured in a tracheal segment *in situ*[41] in order to determine whether or not the responses observed reflected changes in standard nonisometric measurements of lung function *in vivo* such as changes in pulmonary resistance (R_L) and dynamic lung compliance (Cdyn). On the basis of potency measurements, it was found that tracheal tension *in situ* was a more sensitive and selective measure of airway contraction than R_L and Cdyn. It was suggested that a significant contributing factor to this difference was that the airway smooth muscle was not at an optimal resting length for contraction when the pulmonary responses were measured *in vivo*. In contrast, in the tracheal segment the smooth muscle was initially preset to an optimal resting length so that optimal contractile responses could be obtained. It was also concluded that significant changes in airway smooth-muscle tone may precede nonisometric changes to a constrictor stimulus *in vivo*.[41]

The active isotonic tension generated in a given length of canine tracheal smooth muscle has been reported to be generally lower than that recorded isometrically.[35] The possibility that such differences were of importance with regard to the results obtained in pharmacological experiments has recently been investigated by comparing the isometric and isotonic responses of human bronchiolar strips to a number of drugs.[36] When isotonic measurements were made, methacholine was 1.4 times less potent than when contractions were measured isometrically. Thus, for methacholine in human bronchiolar strips, smooth-muscle tension developed slightly before shortening could be detected, perhaps because intrinsic mechanical resistances had to be overcome. These results are in agreement with other findings.[41] A similar trend was observed for histamine, LTC$_4$, PGF$_{2\alpha}$, isoprenaline, and theophyline, although the differences between the two methods were not statistically significant. On this basis, it was concluded that in conventional pharmacological studies of airway smooth muscle, the choice between an isometric or isotonic recording is of little practical importance.[36]

Isometric and isotonic contractions produced by acetylcholine and potassium in canine isolated tracheal smooth muscle have also been compared.[37] Concentration-effect curves to potassium using isometric and isotonic measurements were superimposable. However, the mean concentration-effect curve for acetylcholine was to the left of the mean isometric curve, and the maximal isometric contraction to acetylcholine was considerably greater than that to potassium. These authors suggested that the limit for isotonic shortening was reached at doses of acetylcholine which could still produce additional isometrically recorded responses. When this was corrected for by normalizing the acetylcholine-induced responses in terms of the dose of acetylcholine which produced contractions equal to the maximal contractions produced by potassium, mean acetylcholine concentration-effect curves obtained isotonically and isometrically were superimposable.

Drug-induced isometric and isotonic responsiveness in both spirally cut and intact ring preparations of rabbit bronchi have also been compared.[38] It was found that carbachol was more potent in both types of preparation when measurements were made isotonically rather than isometrically. In contrast, the potency of histamine was similar using either recording system in spiral and ring preparations. In both types of preparation, the maximal response produced by carbachol was greater than that produced by histamine. The greater potency of carbachol determined isotonically may be due to mechanical limitations to isotonic shortening occurring at higher doses of agonist, while isometric changes may be measured across a wider concentration range.[37]

A significant correlation between the maximal contractile response to carbachol and airway smooth-muscle volume or percentage airway smooth muscle in both the spiral and ring preparations has also been reported when isometric responses were measured.[38] However, there was no significant correlation between the maximum contraction and airway smooth-muscle volume or percentage airway smooth muscle present in either preparation when isotonic measurements were made. A similar trend was observed with histamine. These authors suggested that isometric measurements could be more representative of the airway smooth-muscle changes produced by spasmogens *in vitro* and concluded that the isometric method appeared to be a more satisfactory way of studying the properties of isolated airway smooth muscle.

In summary, advantages have been reported for measuring contractions isometrically rather than isotonically in isolated airway smooth muscle.[34-38,41] We also measure responses isometrically in airway smooth muscle, since we have found this approach convenient and reliable. However, in many cases, essentially similar data are obtained with both recording systems.

V. ALTERNATIVE AIRWAY PREPARATIONS

A. AIRWAY TUBE PREPARATIONS

Several mechanical factors contribute to the extent to which airway narrowing occurs in response to spasmogens *in vivo*. These include the level of active force developed and shortening of airway smooth muscle,[35] airway wall thickness, and transmural forces acting on the airway wall.[42] It is perhaps not surprising then that sensitivities of isolated airway preparations such as spiral strips and open or closed airway rings to spasmogens such as histamine do not correlate significantly with *in vivo* measures of bronchial sensitivity to histamine, such as the PC_{20} (i.e., concentration provoking 20% change in baseline lung function).[43-45]

Several studies have been conducted using isolated airway tube preparations in an attempt to obtain data describing responses to drugs which more closely reflect physiological responsiveness. In the earliest studies, fluid-filled tracheal tubes were used.[46,47] Under a constant resting pressure, these preparations were immersed in aerated Kreb's buffer and relaxant or contractile agents applied to the external environment. Changes in luminal pressure reflected the activity of smooth-muscle relaxants such as isoprenaline, theophyline, and PGE_2, smooth-muscle spasmogens including histamine and 5HT, and of electrically stimulated cholinergic, noradrenergic, or nonadrenergic/noncholinergic nerves.[48] These preparations were reportedly very robust, providing consistent, reproducible responses for several hours. Changes in airway tone were caused by stimulation of airway smooth muscle in the absence of drug effects on the airway epithelium, since drugs were administered to the outside of the airway and had to diffuse through the wall to the underlying muscle. In essence, however, this tube preparation showed sensitivities to drugs similar to those expected from studies using airway strips.

A significant advance was made with the use of the guinea pig tracheal tube with intact parasympathetic and sympathetic nerve supplies *in situ*.[49] This model was improved upon with the development of the fluid-filled, dual innervated, isolated guinea pig tracheal tube preparation.[50] The trachea with an intact right sympathetic nerve chain including the superior cervical and stellate ganglia, as well as the right vagus nerve from below the recurrent laryngeal branch, was mounted horizontally in the Kreb's bathing medium to which drugs could be added. The major advantage of this system over more standard transmural stimulation models is that separate stimulation of cholinergic and noradrenergic nerves can be achieved without the need to use selective blocking drugs to separate responses. Interactions between the two systems can also be studied during simultaneous but separate electrical stimulation.[51] The system has also been combined with single-cell microelectrode recording techniques to examine the relationship between altered membrane potential and airway smooth-muscle response.[52]

More recently, a luminally perfused pig bronchial tube preparation has been developed to investigate airway narrowing in response to spasmogens.[53] Responsiveness of the bronchus was compared with that of strip preparations to assess the influence of preparation geometry. It was shown that under conditions where perfusion pressure was maintained in the range 5 to 6 mm H_2O, resistance rose exponentially in response to luminal histamine or carbachol without reaching a plateau. Responses were maximal for both spasmogens at 43 to 47% muscle shortening, at which point complete airway closure occurred. Furthermore, there were no significant differences in sensitivities (EC_{50} values) to carbachol or histamine in strip preparations (where responses were measured isometrically or isotonically) compared with perfused tube segments. In contrast, under conditions of constant flow, concentration-pressure response curves to histamine and carbachol were sigmoidal and sensitivities to these spasmogens were at least ten times lower than in bronchial strips. It was concluded that airway closure occurred before maximal pharmacological effects could be obtained in bronchial tubes perfused at constant pressure, i.e., that only the first part of the concentration-effect curve as seen in airway strips could be obtained.

In the constant flow preparation, the increase in transmural pressure during airway narrowing is a feature seen *in vivo* with bronchoconstriction,[54] although only the threshold region of the concentration-effect curve corresponded to moderate bronchoconstriction seen *in vivo*. In man, bronchial provocation with spasmogens such as histamine would also lead to airway closure long before full pharmacological effect (i.e., maximal muscle shortening) could occur, if this could be done without endangering the life of the subject.

The perfused bronchial segment may be a more appropriate *in vitro* preparation for modeling *in vivo* bronchial provocation with spasmogens. However, it is most important to use an airway preparation which can provide data to accurately answer particular questions. Thus, standard airway strip or ring preparations can be used with confidence if, for example, the problem essentially involves a straightforward assessment of relative potencies or efficacies of spasmogens or relaxants.

B. ISOLATED SMOOTH-MUSCLE CELL PREPARATIONS

Responsiveness of plasma membrane-damaged isolated vascular smooth-muscle cells to extracellular Ca ions was first described in 1965.[55] Glycerol was used to disrupt the cell membrane, thereby increasing permeability to Ca ions. These "skinned" muscle cells were shown to develop tension in response to Ca ions in a concentration-dependent manner. More recently, detergents have been used to skin smooth-muscle fibers.[56,57] In such preparations, the contractile machinery remains structurally intact, and tension development is comparable with that obtained before detergent treatment.[58,59] However, cell viability as assessed by contraction and relaxation characteristics is short lived.[60] Improved response characteristics and duration of viability have been reported in studies conducted at 37°C[61] rather than at the more commonly used 20 to 25°C.[58,59,62] While these preparations cannot be used to examine cell surface receptor-mediated responses to drugs, they have been extremely useful for studying the mechanisms of smooth-muscle cell relaxation and contraction.[61-65] This technique has also been used to examine aspects of airway smooth-muscle function including the effects of Ca^{++} and calmodulin on tension development,[61] the effect of relaxants on Ca^{++}-induced contractions,[65,66] and regional differences in the mechanical properties of airway smooth muscle.[67]

VI. FUNCTIONAL ANTAGONISM

The level of airway smooth-muscle tone is dependent on the relative contributions made by constrictor and relaxant agonists. The interaction between spasmogenic and spasmolytic agonists is called functional antagonism and is defined as two (or more) agonists acting through independent receptor systems to produce opposite effects along a common effector system. An example of functional antagonism that has been extensively studied in airway smooth muscle is the interaction between constrictor muscarinic agonists (such as acetylcholine, carbachol, and methacholine) and the relaxant β-adrenoreceptor agonists. Several mathematical models have been developed to explain the marked and complex changes in the shape and position of agonist concentration-effect curves observed to occur in the presence of functional antagonists.[68-70] In general, there is an inverse relationship between the initial level of smooth-muscle tone induced by the spasmogen (e.g., cholinoreceptor agonist) and the ability of the functional antagonist (e.g., β-adrenoreceptor agonist) to induce relaxation. This reduction in the ability of the β-adrenoreceptor agonist to induce relaxation is observed as an increase in the EC_{50} value and, under certain circumstances, a decrease in the maximum relaxation response. A basic understanding of the phenomenon of functional antagonism is particularly relevant to pharmacological studies on airway smooth muscle.

Relaxation of airway smooth muscle is an important antiasthmatic effect of β-adrenoreceptor agonists and methylxanthines, such as theophyline.[71] The smooth-muscle relaxant properties of these agents are often determined in isolated central airways preparations and expressed in terms of the ability to either prevent or reverse spasmogen-induced contraction. In order to establish the bronchodilator potency of these agents, it is almost invariably necessary to first constrict the preparation, because central airways preparations from most species of laboratory animals possess little or no natural tone. Even those central airways preparations known to exhibit variable degrees of natural tone (guinea pig trachea and human bronchus) are generally constricted with spasmogen, to induce a more stable level of elevated tone, prior to exposure to relaxant drugs. Tone can be induced in isolated airway smooth-muscle preparations with (1) exogenously added agonists, such as muscarinic agonists, histamine, 5HT, LT, bradykinin, or $PGF_{2\alpha}$, which are added directly to the bathing fluid; there exists marked interspecies differences with respect to the sensitivity to these spasmogens; (2) transmural electrical stimulation, which initiates cholinergically mediated contraction and avoids the need for exogenously added spasmogens; and (3) ionic solutions, such as $BaCl_2$ and KCl.

The use of muscarinic agonists has proven to be the most popular method for inducing tone. In addition to the likelihood that acetylcholine plays a significant role in elevating smooth-muscle tone *in vivo,* the widespread use of muscarinic agonists to induce tone is probably due at least in part to their general ability to induce sustained levels of induced tone in central airways preparations from all mammalian species thus far examined.

A. IMPORTANT DETERMINANTS OF FUNCTIONAL ANTAGONISM

A number of recent studies have made significant contributions to our understanding of those factors which are important in determining the outcome of a functional interaction. It was recognized that the respective capacities of the relaxant and contractile systems were important determinants of the functional antagonism.[69] For example, large interspecies and intersite (central vs. peripheral airways) differences exist in the ability of β-adrenoreceptor agonists to reverse acetylcholine-induced contractions.[72] Tracheal preparations from the rat and guinea pig precontracted with acetylcholine to 75% of the maximum level of tone show markedly different quantitative responses to maximal concentrations of the β-adrenoreceptor agonist, isoprenaline. The maximum reversal of acetylcholine-induced contraction produced with isoprenaline was 140% in guinea pig trachea, but less than 25% in rat trachea, perhaps because of different numbers of β-adrenoreceptors and/or differences in coupling efficiency. Differences in maximum responses induced by isoprenaline were also observed between cervical and thoracic preparations obtained from dog trachea.[73] Thus, in studies investigating the relaxant action of agonists, it is often necessary to determine the relative capacities of the receptor-effector systems for the respective functional antagonists. This can be readily accomplished by completing cumulative concentration-effect curves to the relaxant agonist in preparations constricted with increasing concentrations of spasmogen. From these preliminary studies, we would generally select a concentration of spasmogen such that the level of tone induced is marginally greater than that which can be reversed by the relaxant agonists. Using this approach, experimentally induced changes in relaxant agonist E_{max} as well as potency can be determined without significant loss of relaxant response (which may occur at higher levels of spasmogen-induced tone).

Recent studies have indicated that the capacity of relaxant agonists to functionally antagonize contracted airway smooth-muscle preparations also depends on the choice of spasmogen.[74,75] For example, the tracheal relaxant activity of β-adrenoreceptor agonists and forskolin is significantly greater in tissues preconstricted with metabolites of arachidonic acid ($PGF_{2\alpha}$, LTD_4) than in tissues preconstricted with muscarinic agonists (carbachol, methacholine). Differences in relaxant potency have also been reported in airway smooth-muscle preparations constricted with acetylcholine compared to histamine[76] or 5HT.[23,77] Such differences may reflect differential influences of spasmogens on β-adrenoreceptor-mediated effects[74] or that the spasmogens induce contraction by different mechanisms which are differentially sensitive to antagonism by β-adrenoreceptor agonists.

In addition, studies using isolated tracheal smooth-muscle preparations have shown that the particular pattern of curve shifting for β-adrenoreceptor agonists observed in the presence of increasing concentrations of muscarinic agonist is dependent on the choice of β-adrenoreceptor agonist.[69,78,79] For example, at low levels of methacholine-induced tone the β-adrenoreceptor agonists, isoprenaline and norfenefrine were full relaxants of calf isolated tracheal smooth muscle.[69] The effect of increasing the concentration of methacholine 10-fold was to reduce the potency of isoprenaline and norfenefrine by 40- and 3-fold, respectively. At the higher level of induced tone, isoprenaline was still a full relaxant, whereas norfenefrine, at maximally effective concentrations, induced less than 20% relaxation. It is thought that the differential extent to which the β-adrenoreceptor agonist curves are shifted reflects differences in the efficacies of the agonists. Indeed, the ratio of the maximum shift of the spasmogen-induced curve produced by two β-adrenoreceptor agonists has been proposed to be an unequivocal measure of the relative efficacies of the agonists.[69] This approach was also used to establish differences in the efficacies of fenoterol and salbutamol.[80]

B. USE OF FUNCTIONAL ANTAGONISM TO ESTIMATE AFFINITY AND EFFICACY

Functional antagonism has also been used to estimate affinity and relative efficacy values for β-adrenoreceptor agonists[78,81] and peptidoleukotrienes.[82] In these studies, concentration-effect curves were analyzed using the null equations derived by Furchgott[83] to describe irreversible antagonism, even though there can be no theoretical basis for equating receptor occlusion produced by irreversible antagonists with the complex post-receptor interactions produced by functional antagonists. Furthermore, even the application of null equations which were specifically developed to describe functional interactions[70] are likely to provide variable overestimates of true agonist affinity. At this stage, therefore, there is insufficient evidence that the analysis of functional antagonism data is a valid method for estimating agonist affinity constants or relative efficacy values.

Despite the limitations in obtaining accurate estimates of agonist affinity and efficacy values, the current mathematical models describing functional antagonism may be useful in predicting the displacement of relaxant agonist curves under various conditions. For example, *in vivo*, the airways of asthmatics are hyperreactive to contractile stimuli[84] and hyporesponsive to β-adrenoreceptor agonists *in vitro*.[85] Clearly, the use of these models of functional antagonism to describe the pattern of curve shifting for a series of β-adrenoreceptor agonists with different efficacies under conditions of elevated smooth-muscle tone and reduced β-adrenoreceptor-effector function may be of some predictive value.

VII. EPITHELIUM-MODULATED AIRWAY RESPONSIVENESS TO DRUGS

Until recently, the role of the healthy epithelium in modulating the sensitivity of the airways *in vivo* to inhaled spasmogens was seen largely as passive, i.e., that the airway epithelium provided an effective barrier to the penetration of stimulatory solutes, including allergens, to the underlying smooth muscle, submucosal mast cells, irritant receptors, and C fiber afferent nerves involved in mucosal axon reflexes.[86] In addition, epithelial secretions and the activity of cilia are important to the effective clearance of irritant particles from the bronchi.[87] The suggestion of a more active role for the airway epithelium in modulating smooth-muscle responsiveness to drugs has been prompted by studies examining the effect of the experimental removal of the airway epithelium from isolated airway preparations. Such studies have established that epithelium removal causes enhancement of airway smooth-muscle responsiveness to spasmogens, including histamine and methacholine. This was first demonstrated in canine bronchus[88] and was confirmed in airways from cattle,[89] guinea pigs,[4,90] rabbits,[91] rats,[92] and man.[93] However, the reasons for these effects remain the subject of controversy.

For some agonists in some species, the airway epithelium may act as a site of loss from the biophase, reducing tissue sensitivity. This has been reported for isoprenaline,[94] adenosine,[95] and for various neurokinins, including substance P.[96] It is also possible that the removal of the epithelium facilitates access of bronchoconstrictor substances to submucosal structures, including airway smooth muscle, causing increased reactivity to spasmogens.[1] However, this does not explain the selective enhancement of only some airway spasmogens,[4,92,97] or reduced responsiveness to some relaxant agonists such as isoprenaline.[88]

The airway epithelium may respond to some chemical stimuli by releasing an inhibitory substance(s) capable of attenuating airway responsiveness to these agents. Such a system may function in a manner analogous to that described for vascular smooth muscle and endothelium-derived relaxant factor.[98] Recent work has demonstrated that hyperosmolar stimuli caused concentration-dependent, nonprostanoid-induced relaxation of luminally perfused guinea pig trachea.[99] This response was markedly reduced or abolished when the epithelium was removed, suggesting the involvement of an epithelium-derived inhibitory factor (EpDIF).

While notable species differences have been reported and various methodological differences have perhaps contributed to apparently conflicting results within some species, it remains clear that a large body of independent research has provided confirmation of the phenomenon of epithelium-induced modulation of airway responsiveness to some agents *in vitro*. It is also true that the majority of this data, while consistent with the existence of EpDIF, provides only indirect support for this concept.

A. TRANSFER AND BIOASSAY OF EPITHELIUM-DERIVED INHIBITORY FACTOR

A coaxial sandwich assembly in which the recipient or assay preparation was mounted within the lumen of an EpDIF donor airway tube segment has recently been described.[100] This provided the first direct evidence for the release and transfer of an epithelium-derived inhibitory substance capable of causing relaxation of a recipient endothelium-denuded rabbit aorta.

The bioassay of EpDIF activity from guinea pig trachea in response to acetylcholine has recently been demonstrated using phenylephrine-contracted rat anococcygeus muscle in a coaxial assembly.[101] It has also been shown that histamine and methacholine caused concentration-dependent relaxation of phenylephrine-induced tone in endothelium-denuded rat thoracic aorta strips when these preparations were mounted coaxially within tube segments of epithelium-intact guinea pig trachea or human bronchus[102] (Figure 1). Removal of the epithelium from the donor airway tube segment abolished the relaxant effect of both histamine and methacholine on rat aorta preparations. These studies convincingly establish the ability of airway epithelium to release a smooth-muscle relaxant factor in response to some spasmogens.

Thus, there is a growing body of compelling evidence in support of the idea that some agents can induce the release of a nonprostanoid inhibitory substance from the airway epithelium, which is capable of attenuating spasmogenic potency on airway smooth muscle.

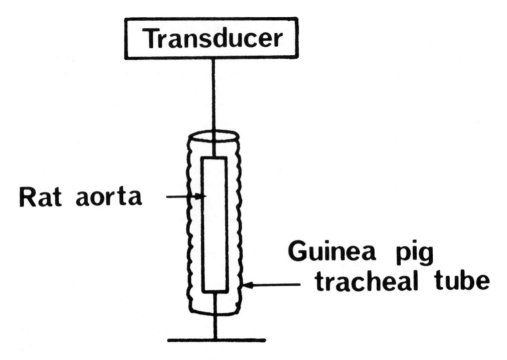

FIGURE 1.   Diagrammatic representation of a coaxial bioassay system in which a guinea pig tracheal tube segment acts as a donor of epithelium-derived inhibitory factor (EpDIF) to be assayed on endothelium-denuded rat aorta strip mounted within the airway lumen.

It has now been shown that guinea pig tracheal and human bronchial EpDIF can directly relax vascular,[102] gastrointestinal,[101] and airway smooth muscle.[99] It is also possible that this autacoid can reduce spasmogen potency in the airway by means additional to functional antagonism at airway smooth muscle. Clearly, the integrity of the airway epithelium must be carefully considered when assessing drug-induced responses of isolated airway preparations.

VIII. SUMMARY

While some studies have demonstrated that human isolated airway preparations can be used successfully in assessments of responses to pharmacological stimuli, the difficulties involved in obtaining viable tissue samples highlight the necessity for drug testing in animal airway models. Guinea pig tracheal tissue is most widely used and its responsiveness to a wide range of agonists generally reflects the responsiveness of human bronchial tissue, although clear and important exceptions have been described.

The choice of airway model should depend upon the question being addressed, giving consideration to species differences, particularly with respect to tissue sensitivity to drugs and agonist receptor characteristics. This decision is particularly important, for example, to the outcome of investigations of functional antagonism. In most circumstances, isometric and isotonic measurements provide essentially similar drug concentration-effect data. In choosing an appropriate model, it may be important to consider possible regional differences in airway responsiveness to drugs. It is now clear that data derived from the lung parenchyma strip does not necessarily describe drug-induced reactivity of peripheral airways. Investigations of peripheral bronchial airway pharmacology should utilize appropriate isolated bronchial strip, ring, or tube preparations. The use of airway tube preparations may provide data which more closely reflect physiological responsiveness to pharmacological stimuli *in vivo*.

Regardless of the model used, it is now realized that the integrity of the eptihelium must also be considered when evaluating airway responsiveness to drugs. This is important since the epithelium can (1) behave as a barrier to drug access to airway smooth muscle, (2) act as a site of loss for some agonists, or (3) generate inhibitory factors which may modify airway smooth-muscle responsiveness to drugs.

REFERENCES

1. **Holroyde, M. C.**, The influence of the epithelium on the responsiveness of guinea-pig isolated trachea, *Br. J. Pharmacol.*, 87, 501, 1986.
2. **Castillo, J. C. and de Beer, E. J.**, The tracheal chain: a preparation for the study of antispasmodics with particular reference to bronchodilator drugs, *J. Pharamacol. Exp. Ther.*, 90, 104, 1947.
3. **Patterson, R.**, The tracheal strip: observations on the response of tracheal muscle, *J. Allergy*, 29, 165, 1958.
4. **Goldie, R. G., Papadimitriou, J. M., Paterson, J. W., Rigby, P. J., Self, H. M., and Spina, D.**, Influence of the epithelium on responsiveness of guinea-pig isolated trachea to contractile and relaxant agonists, *Br. J. Pharmacol.*, 87, 5, 1986.
5. **Akcasu, A.**, The physiologic and pharmacologic characteristics of the tracheal muscle, *Arch. Int. Pharmacodyn.*, 71, 210, 1959.
6. **Satchell, D. and Smith, R.**, Adenosine causes contractions in spiral strips and relaxations in transverse strips of guinea-pig trachea: studies on mechanism of action, *Eur. J. Pharmacol.*, 101, 243, 1984.
7. **Raeburn, D., Hay, D. W. P., Farmer, S. G., and Fedan, J. S.**, Influence of cartilage on reactivity and on the effectiveness of verapamil in guinea-pig isolated airway smooth muscle, *J. Pharmacol. Exp. Ther.*, 242, 450, 1987.
8. **Mitchell, H. W. and Yu, L. L.**, Attenuation of tracheal smooth muscle contraction by connective tissue, *Eur. J. Pharmacol.*, 118, 171, 1985.
9. **Raffestin, B., Cerrina, J., Boullet, C., Labat, C., Benveniste, J., and Brink, C.**, Response and sensitivity of isolated human pulmonary muscle preparations to pharmacological agents, *J. Pharmacol. Exp. Ther.*, 233, 186, 1985.
10. **Horsfield, K.**, The relation between structure and function in the airways of the lung, *Br. J. Dis. Chest*, 68, 145, 1974.
11. **Wasserman, M. A. and Mukherjee, A.**, Regional differences in the reactivity of guinea-pig airways, *Pulm. Pharmacol.*, 1, 125, 1988.
12. **Drazen, J. M. and Schneider, M. W.**, Comparative responses of tracheal spirals and parenchymal strips to histamine and carbachol in vitro, *J. Clin. Invest.*, 61, 1441, 1978.
13. **Barnes, P. J., Jacobs, M., and Roberts, J. M.**, Glucocorticoids preferentially increase fetal alveolar beta-adrenoceptors: autoradiographic evidence, *Pediatr. Res.*, 18, 1191, 1984.
14. **Goldie, R. G., Papadimitriou, J. M., Paterson, J. W., Rigby, P. J., and Spina, D.**, Autoradiographic localization of beta-adrenoceptors in pig lung using [^{125}I]-iodocyanopindolol, *Br. J. Pharmacol.*, 88, 621, 1986.
15. **Carstairs, J. R., Nimmo, A. J., and Barnes, P. J.**, Autoradiographic visualization of beta-adrenoceptor subtypes in the lung, *Am. Rev. Respir. Dis.*, 132, 541, 1985.
16. **Barnes, P. J., Nadel, J. A., Roberts, J. M., and Basbaum, C. B.**, Muscarinic receptors in lung and trachea: autoradiographic localization using [^{3}H]-quinuclidinyl benzilate, *Eur. J. Pharmacol.*, 86, 103, 1983.
17. **Akcasu, A.**, The actions of drugs on the isolated trachea, *J. Pharm. Pharmacol.*, 4, 671, 1952.
18. **Goldie, R. G., Paterson, J. W., and Wale, J. L.**, Pharmacological responses of human and porcine lung parenchyma, bronchus and pulmonary artery, *Br. J. Pharmacol.*, 76, 515, 1982.
19. **Advenier, C., Naline, E., Drapeau, G., and Regoli, D.**, Relative potencies of neurokinins in guinea-pig trachea and human bronchus, *Eur. J. Pharmacol.*, 139, 133, 1987.
20. **Goldie, R. G.**, Receptors in asthmatic airways, *Am. Rev. Respir. Dis.*, 141, S151, 1990.
21. **Lulich, K. M., Mitchell, H. W., and Sparrow, M. P.**, The cat lung strip as a preparation of peripheral airways. A comparison of beta-adrenoceptor agonists, autacoids and anaphylactic challenge on the lung strip and trachea, *Br. J. Pharmacol.*, 58, 71, 1976.

22. **Goldie, R. G., Bertram, J. F., Papadimitriou, J. M., and Paterson, J. W.,** The lung parenchyma strip, *Trends Pharmacol. Sci.,* 5, 7, 1984.

23. **Mitchell, H. W. and Denborough, M. A.,** Anaphylaxis in guinea-pig peripheral airways in vitro, *Eur. J. Pharmacol.,* 54, 69, 1979.

24. **Kapanci, Y., Assimacopoulos, A., Irle, C., Zwahlen, A., and Gabbiani, G.,** Contractile interstitial cells in pulmonary alveolar septa: a possible regulator of ventilation/perfusion ratio?, *J. Cell Biol.,* 60, 375, 1974.

25. **Mirbahar, K. B. and Eyre, P.,** Bovine lung parenchyma strip has both airway and vascular characteristics. (Pharmacological comparisons with bronchus, pulmonary artery and vein), *Res. Commun. Chem. Pathol. Pharmacol.,* 29, 15, 1980.

26. **Black, J. L., Turner, A., and Shaw, J.,** Alpha-adrenoceptors in human peripheral lung, *Eur. J. Pharmacol.,* 72, 83, 1981.

27. **Evans, J. N. and Adler, K. B.,** The lung strip: evaluation of a method to study contractility of pulmonary parenchyma, *Exp. Lung Res.,* 2, 187, 1981.

28. **Szarek, J. L. and Evans, J. N.,** Pharmacologic responsiveness of rat parenchymal strips, bronchi and bronchioles, *Exp. Lung Res.,* 14, 575, 1988.

29. **Bertram, J. B., Goldie, R. G., Robertson, T. A., Papadimitriou, J. M., and Paterson, J. W.,** Ultrastructural and pharmacological observations on contractile tissue of toad (Bufo marinus) lung, *Micron.,* 13, 345, 1982.

30. **Goldie, R. G., Bertram, J. B., Warton, A., Papadimitriou, J. M., and Paterson, J. W.,** A pharmacological and ultrastructural study of alveolar contractile tissue in toad (Bufo marinus) lung, *Comp. Biochem. Physiol.,* 75C, 343, 1983.

31. **Pollard, T. D. and Weihing, R. R.,** Actin and myosin and cell movement, *CRC. Crit. Rev. Biochem.,* 2, 1, 1974.

32. **Bertram, J. F., Goldie, R. G., Papadimitriou, J. M., and Paterson, J. W.,** Correlations between pharmacological responses and structure of human lung parenchyma strips, *Br. J. Pharmacol.,* 80, 107, 1983.

33. **Finney, M. J. B., Berend, N., and Black, J. L.,** Cholinergic responses in the human lung parenchyma strip: a structure-function study, *Eur. J. Respir. Dis.,* 65, 447, 1984.

34. **Finney, M. J. B., Karlsson, J.-A., and Persson, C. G. A.,** Effects of bronchoconstrictors and bronchodilators on a novel human small airway preparation, *Br. J. Pharmacol.,* 85, 29, 1985.

35. **Stephens, N. L. and Van Niekerk, W.,** Isometric and isotonic contractions in airway smooth muscle, *Can. J. Physiol. Pharmacol.,* 55, 883, 1977.

36. **De Jongste, J. C., Mons, H., Van Strik, R., Bonta, I. L., and Kerrebijh, K. F.,** Comparison of isometric and isotonic responses of human small airway smooth muscle in vitro, *J. Pharmacol. Meth.,* 17, 165, 1977.

37. **Mitchell, R. W. and Stephens, N. L.,** Isometric and isotonic dose-response curves to K^+ and acetylcholine in canine airway smooth muscle, *Am. Rev. Respir. Dis.,* 135, A178, 1987.

38. **Armour, C. L., Diment, L. M., and Black, J. L.,** Relationship between smooth muscle volume and contractile responses in airway tissue. Isometric versus isotonic measurement, *J. Pharmacol. Exp. Ther.,* 245, 687, 1988.

39. **Paton, W. D. M.,** The recording of mechanical responses of smooth muscle, in *Methods in Pharmacology,* Vol. 3, Smooth Muscle, Daniel, E. E. and Paton, D. M., Eds., Plenum Press, New York, 1975, chap. 12.

40. **Macklem, P. T.,** Bronchial hyporesponsiveness, *Chest,* 87, 158S, 1985.

41. **Leff, A. R., Munoz, N. M., and Alderman, B.,** Measurement of airway response by isometric and nonisometric techniques in situ, *J. Appl. Physiol.,* 52, 1363, 1982.

42. **Moreno, R. H., Hogg, J. C., and Pare, P. D.,** Mechanics of airway narrowing, *Am. Rev. Respir. Dis.,* 133, 1171, 1986.

43. **Armour, C. L., Lazar, N. M., Schellenberg, R. R., Taylor, S. M., Chan, N., Hogg, J. C., and Pare, P. D.,** A comparison of in vivo and in vitro human airway reactivity to histamine, *Am. Rev. Respir. Dis.,* 129, 907, 1984.

44. **Douglas, J. S., Ridgway, P., and Brink, C.,** Airway responses of the guinea-pig in vivo and in vitro, *J. Pharmacol. Exp. Ther.,* 202, 116, 1977.

45. **Roberts, J. A., Raeburn, D., Rodger, I. W., and Thomson, N. C.,** Comparison of in vivo airway responsiveness and in vitro smooth muscle sensitivity to methacholine in man, *Thorax,* 39, 837, 1984.

46. **Wellens, D.,** Pharmacological reactivity of an isolated tracheal preparation of the guinea-pig, *Med. Pharmacol. Exp.,* 14, 427, 1966.

47. **Farmer, J. B. and Coleman, R. A.,** A new preparation of the isolated intact trachea of the guinea-pig, *J. Pharm. Pharmacol.,* 22, 45, 1970.

48. **Coleman, R. A. and Levy, G. P.,** A non-adrenergic inhibitory nervous pathway in guinea-pig trachea, *Br. J. Pharmacol.,* 52, 167, 1974.

49. **Yip, P., Palombini, B., and Coburn, R. F.,** Inhibitory innervation of the guinea-pig trachealis muscle, *J. Appl. Physiol.,* 50, 374, 1981.

50. **Blackman, J. G. and McCraig, D. J.,** Studies on an isolated innervated preparation of guinea-pig trachea, *Br. J. Pharmacol.,* 80, 703, 1983.

51. **McCraig, D. J.,** Effects of sympathetic stimulation and applied catecholamines on mechanical and electrical responses to stimulation of the vagus nerve in guinea-pig isolated trachea, *Br. J. Pharmacol.,* 91, 385, 1987.

52. **McCraig, D. J.,** Electrophysiology of neuro effector transmission in the isolated, innervated trachea of the guinea-pig, *Br. J. Pharmacol.,* 89, 793, 1986.

53. **Mitchell, H. W., Willet, K. E., and Sparrow, M. P.,** The perfused bronchial segment and the bronchial strip: narrowing versus isometric force by mediators, *J. Appl. Physiol.,* 66, 2704, 1989.

54. **Martin, J. G., Shore, S. A., and Engel, L. A.,** Mechanical load and respiratory muscle action during induced asthma, *Am. Rev. Respir. Dis.,* 128, 455, 1983.

55. **Filo, R. S., Bohr, D. F., and Ruegg, J. C.,** Glycerinated skeletal and smooth muscle: calcium and magnesium dependence, *Science,* 147, 1581, 1965.

56. **Cassidy, P. S., Kerrick, W. G. L., Hoar, P. E., and Malencik, D. A.,** Exogenous calmodulin increases Ca^{++} sensitivity of isometric tension activation and myosin phosphorylation in skinned smooth muscle, *Pfluegers Arch.,* 392, 115, 1981.

57. **Walsh, M. P., Bridenbough, R., Hartshorne, J., and Kerrick, W. G. L.,** Phosphorylation-dependent activated tension in skinned gizzard muscle fibers in the absence of Ca^{++}, *J. Biol. Chem.,* 257, 5987, 1982.

58. **Gordon, A. R.,** Contraction of detergent-treated smooth muscle, *Proc. Natl. Acad. Sci. U.S.A.,* 75, 3572, 1978.

59. **Iino, M.,** Tension responses of chemically skinned fibre bundles of the guinea-pig taenia caeci under varied tonic environments, *J. Physiol. (London),* 320, 449, 1981.

60. **Cornelius, F.,** The regulation of tension in a chemically skinned molluscan smooth muscle, *J. Gen. Physiol.,* 75, 709, 1980.

61. **Sparrow, M. P., Pfitzer, G., Gagelmann, M., and Ruegg, J. C.,** Effect of calmodulin, Ca^{++} and cAMP protein kinase on skinned tracheal smooth muscle, *Am. J. Physiol.,* 246, C308, 1984.

62. **Kerrick, W. G. L. and Hoar, P. E.,** Inhibition of smooth muscle tension by cyclic AMP-dependent protein kinase, *Nature,* 292, 253, 1981.

63. **Ruegg, J. C., Sparrow, M. P., and Mrwa, U.,** Cyclic-AMP mediated relaxation of chemically skinned fibres of smooth muscle, *Pfluegers Arch.,* 390, 198, 1981.

64. **Cassidy, P. S., Hoar, P. E., and Kerrick, W. G. L.,** Inhibition of Ca^{++}-activated tension and myosin light chain phosphorylation in skinned smooth muscle strips by the phenothiazines, *Pfluegers Arch.,* 387, 115, 1980.

65. **Nayler, R. A. and Sparrow, M. P.,** Inhibition of cycling and non-cycling cross bridges in skinned smooth muscle by vanadate, *Am. J. Physiol.,* 250, C325, 1986.

66. **Allen, S. L., Boyle, J. P., Cortijo, J., Foster, R. W., Morgan, G. P., and Small, R. C.,** Electrical and mechanical effects of BRL34915 in guinea-pig isolated trachealis, *Br. J. Pharmacol.,* 89, 395, 1986a.

67. **Fujiwara, T., Itoh, T., and Kuriyama, H.,** Regional differences in the mechanical properties of rabbit airway smooth muscle, *Br. J. Pharmacol.,* 94, 389, 1988.

68. **Ariens, E. G., Simonis, A. M., and van Rossum, J. M.,** Drug receptor interaction: interaction of one or more drugs with different receptor systems, in *Molecular Pharmacology,* Vol. 1, Ariens, E. J., Ed., Academic Press, New York, 1964, 287.

69. **Van den Brink, F. G.,** The model of functional interaction. II. Experimental verification of a new model: the antagonism of β-adrenoceptor stimulants and other agonists, *Eur. J. Pharmacol.,* 22, 279, 1973.

70. **Mackay, D.,** An analysis of functional antagonism and synergism, *Br. J. Pharmacol.,* 73, 127, 1981.

71. **Paterson, J. W., Woolcock, A. J., and Shenfield, G. M.,** Bronchodilator drugs, *Am. Rev. Respir. Dis.,* 120, 1149, 1979.

72. **Niewoehner, D. E., Campe, H., Duane, S., McGowan, T., and Montgomery, M. R.,** Mechanisms of airway smooth muscle response to isoproterenol and theophylline, *J. Appl. Physiol.,* 47, 330, 1979.

73. **Minneman, K. P., Puckett, A. M., Jensen, A. D., and Rinard, G. A.,** Regional variation in beta adrenergic receptors in dog trachea: correlation of receptor density and in vitro relaxation, *J. Pharmacol. Exp. Ther.,* 226, 140, 1983.

74. **Torphy, T. J., Burman, M., Schwartz, L. W., and Wasserman, M.A.,** Differential effects of methacholine and leukotriene D_4 on cyclic nucleotide content and isoproterenol-induced relaxation in the opossum trachea, *J. Pharmacol. Exp. Ther.,* 237, 332, 1986.

75. **Heaslip, R. J., Giesa, F. R., Rimele, T. J., and Grimes, D.,** Sensitivity of the $PGF_{2\alpha}$-versus carbachol-contracted trachea to relaxation by salbutamol, forskolin and prenalterol, *Eur. J. Pharmacol.,* 128, 73, 1986.

76. **Farmer, J. B. and Lehrer, D. N.,** The effect of isoprenaline on the contraction of smooth muscle produced by histamine, acetylcholine or other agonists, *J. Pharm. Pharmacol.,* 18, 649, 1966.

77. **Anderson, R. G., Kovesi, G., and Ericsson, E.,** β-Adrenoceptor stimulation and c-AMP levels in bovine tracheal muscle of old and young animals, *Acta Pharmacol. Toxicol.,* 43, 323, 1978.

78. **Buckner, C. K. and Saini, R. K.,** On the use of functional antagonism to estimate dissociation constants for β-adrenoceptor agonists in isolated guinea pig trachea, *J. Pharmacol. Exp. Ther.,* 194, 565, 1975.

79. **O'Donnell, S. R. and Wanstall, J. C.,** The use of functional antagonism to determine whether β-adrenoceptor agonists must have a lower efficacy than isoprenaline to be trachea selective in vitro in guinea pig, *Br. J. Pharmacol.,* 60, 255, 1977.

80. **O'Donnell, S. R. and Wanstall, J. C.,** Evidence that the efficacy (intrinsic activity) of fenoterol is higher than that of salbutamol on β-adrenoceptors in guinea pig, *Eur. J. Pharmacol.,* 47, 333, 1978.

81. **Broadley, K. J. and Nicholson, C. D.,** Functional antagonism as a means of determining dissociation constants and relative efficacies of sympathomimetic amines in guinea-pig isolated atria, *Br. J. Pharmacol.,* 65, 397, 1979.

82. **Hay, D. W. P., Muccitelli, R. M., Wilson, K. A., Wasserman, M. A., and Torphy, T. J.,** Functional antagonism by salbutamol suggests differences in the relative efficacies and dissociation constants of the peptidoleukotrienes in guinea pig trachea, *J. Pharmacol. Exp. Ther.,* 244, 71, 1988.

83. **Furchgott, R. F.,** The use of β-haloalkyamines in the differentiation of receptors and in the determination of dissociation of receptor agonist complexes, in *Advances in Drug Research,* Vol. 3, Harper, N. J. and Simmonds, A. B., Eds., Academic Press, London, 1966, 21.

84. **Boushey, H. A., Holtzman, M. J., Sheller, J. R., and Nadel, J. A.,** Bronchial hyperreactivity, *Am. Rev. Respir. Dis.,* 121, 389, 1980.

85. **Goldie, R. G., Spina, D., Henry, P. J., Lulich, K. M., and Paterson, J. W.,** In vitro responsiveness of asthmatic and non-diseased bronchus to carbachol, histamine, β-adrenoceptor agonists and theophylline, *Br. J. Clin. Pharmacol.,* 22, 669, 1986.

86. **Barnes, P. J.,** Asthma as an axon reflex, *Lancet,* 1, 242, 1986.

87. **Sleigh, M. A., Blake, J. R., and Liron, N.,** The propulsion of mucus by cilia, *Am. Rev. Respir. Dis.,* 137, 726, 1988.

88. **Flavahan, N. A., Aarhus, L. L., Rimele, T. J., and Vanhoutte, P. M.,** The respiratory epithelium inhibits bronchial smooth muscle tone, *J. Appl. Physiol.,* 58, 834, 1985.

89. **Barnes, P. J., Cuss, F. M., and Palmer, J. B.,** The effect of airway epithelium on smooth muscle contractility in bovine trachea, *Br. J. Pharmacol.,* 86, 685, 1985.

90. **Hay, D. W. P., Farmer, S. G., Raeburn, D., Robinson, V. A., Fleming, W. W., and Fedan, J. S.,** Airway epithelium modulates the reactivity of guinea-pig respiratory smooth muscle, *Eur. J. Pharmacol.,* 129, 11, 1986.

91. **Butler, G. B., Adler, K. B., Evans, J. N., Morgan, D. W., and Szarek, J. L.,** Modulation of rabbit airway smooth muscle responsiveness by respiratory epithelium: involvement of an inhibitory metabolite of arachidonic acid, *Am. Rev. Respir. Dis.,* 135, 1099, 1987.

92. **Frossard, N. and Muller, F.,** Epithelial modulation of tracheal smooth muscle responses to antigenic stimulation, *J. Appl. Physiol.,* 61, 1449, 1986.

93. **Raeburn, D., Hay, D. W. P., Farmer, S. G., and Fedan, J. S.,** Epithelium removal increases the reactivity of human isolated tracheal smooth muscle to methacholine and reduces the effect of verapamil, *Eur. J. Pharmacol.,* 123, 451, 1986.

94. **Farmer, S. G., Fedan, J. S., Hay, D. W. P., and Raeburn, D.,** The effect of epithelium removal on the sensitivity of guinea-pig isolated trachealis to bronchodilator drugs, *Br. J. Pharmacol.,* 89, 407, 1986.

95. **Advenier, C., Devillier, P., Matran, R., and Naline, E.,** Influence of epithelium on the responsiveness of guinea-pig isolated trachea to adenosine, *Br. J. Pharmacol.,* 93, 295, 1988.

96. **Devillier, P., Advenier, C., Drapeau, G., Marsac, J., and Regoli, D.,** Comparison of the effects of epithelium removal and of an enkephalinase inhibitor on the neurokinin-induced contractions of guinea-pig isolated trachea, *Br. J. Pharmacol.,* 94, 675, 1988.

97. **Hay, D. W. P., Farmer, S. G., Raeburn, D., Muccitelli, R. M., Wilson, K. A., and Fedan, J. S.,** Differential effects of epithelium removal on the responsiveness of guinea-pig tracheal smooth muscle to bronchoconstrictors, *Br. J. Pharmacol.,* 92, 381, 1987.

98. **Furchgott, R. F. and Zawadzki, J. V.,** The obligatory role of endothelial cells in the relaxation of arterial smooth muscle cells by acetylcholine, *Nature (London),* 288, 373, 1980.

99. **Munakata, M., Mitzner, W., and Menkes, H.,** Osmotic stimuli induce epithelial-dependent relaxation in the guinea-pig trachea, *J. Appl. Physiol.,* 64, 466, 1988.

100. **Ilhan, M. and Sahin, I.,** Tracheal epithelium releases a vascular smooth muscle relaxant factor: demonstration by bioassay, *Eur. J. Pharmacol.,* 131, 293, 1986.
101. **Guc, M. O., Ilhan, M., and Kayaalp, S. O.,** The rat anococcygeus muscle is a convenient bioassay organ for airway epithelium-derived relaxant factor, *Eur. J. Pharmacol.,* 148, 405, 1988.
102. **Fernandes, L. B., Paterson, J. W., and Goldie, R. G.,** Co-axial bioassay of a smooth muscle relaxant factor released from guinea-pig tracheal epithelium, *Br. J. Pharmacol.,* 96, 117, 1989.

Chapter 6

EPITHELIUM-DERIVED RELAXING FACTOR

Karen Stuart-Smith and Paul M. Vanhoutte

TABLE OF CONTENTS

I.   Introduction 130

II.   The Response to Contractile Agents 130

III.   Electrophysiological Studies 133

IV.   The Response to Isoproterenol 134

V.   The Role of Metabolites of Arachidonic Acid 138

VI.   The Response to Osmotic Stimuli 139

VII.   Bioassay of a Diffusable Epithelium-Derived Relaxing Factor 141

VIII.   The Nature of the Epithelium-Derived Relaxing Factor 141

References 143

I. INTRODUCTION

It is now established beyond doubt that the endothelium of the blood vessel wall can modulate the responsiveness of the underlying vascular smooth muscle, in part by releasing a very powerful vasodilator substance, endothelium-derived relaxing factor. This chapter summarizes the evidence suggesting that a similar situation may exist in the airways, whereby the epithelial cell layer is capable of altering the responsiveness of airway smooth muscle, and discusses why it is likely that this epithelial modulation can be attributed to the secretion by the epithelial cells of a bronchodilator substance (epithelium-derived relaxing factor [EpiDRF]).[1,2]

II. THE RESPONSE TO CONTRACTILE AGENTS

In order to investigate the relationship between epithelial damage and bronchial hyper-reactivity more closely, *in vitro* studies have been performed. In the first such study, the intrapulmonary bronchi of the dog were examined.[3-5] Epithelial damage was mimicked by gentle mechanical rubbing of the luminal surface of the bronchi. This procedure removes the epithelial layer without damaging the underlying structures or compromising the ability of the smooth muscle to contract (Figure 1).[5-7] Paired rings of tissue, with and without epithelium, were placed into organ chambers and their responses to pharmacological stimuli were compared (Figure 2). Removal of the airway epithelium did not alter the sensitivity of the bronchi to potassium chloride, nor did it alter the maximal response to this agonist, providing further evidence that the technique of epithelium removal did not damage the smooth muscle.[5,7] However, tissues without epithelium showed a significant leftward shift of the concentration-effect curve to the contractile agents acetylcholine, histamine, and 5-hydroxytryptamine (Figures 3 and 4). Thus, removal of the airway epithelium enhanced the responsiveness of the bronchial smooth muscle to several bronchoconstrictor agents.[5] Epithelium removal also enhances the effect of various contractile agents on the tracheal smooth muscle of the cow,[8] the guinea pig,[9-12] and the large intrapulmonary bronchi of the rabbit.[13,14]

From this evidence, it has been postulated that the airway epithelium releases a relaxing factor which modulates the responsiveness of the bronchial smooth muscle.[1,2,4,15] To investigate whether or not the effect of the proposed EpiDRF is uniform along the respiratory tree, three orders of intralobar bronchi of the dog were examined.[6] These were the second-order (lobar) bronchus (O.D. 8 to 10 mm), third-order (segmental) bronchus (O.D. 4 to 5 mm), and fourth-order (subsegmental) bronchus (O.D. 1 to 3 mm). For the three orders, removal of the epithelium did not affect the response to potassium chloride. For second- and third-order bronchi, there was a significant leftward shift of the concentration-effect curves for acetycholine, histamine, and 5-hydroxytryptamine (Figure 4). However, the maximal responses to the contractile agents were unaffected. In fourth-order tissues, epithelium removal produced no shift in the response to any of these agonists.

For second- and third-order bronchi, the degree of shift of the concentration-effect curves caused by epithelium removal was similar for the three agonists. The degree of shift was also comparable between orders. This implies that removal of the airway epithelium removes a common signal which would normally exert a tonic restraint on the responsiveness of the underlying bronchial smooth muscle to contractile agents. It may be postulated that this common signal is the basal release of an EpiDRF (Figure 5). The fourth-order bronchi do not show this basal release, as epithelium removal has no effect on the response to contractile agents. These data demonstrate that there is heterogeneity in the basal release of this EpiDRF along the canine respiratory tree.[6]

To determine whether or not this heterogeneity could be observed in another species, third-order (segmental) bronchi and fourth- and fifth-order (subsegmental) bronchi of the

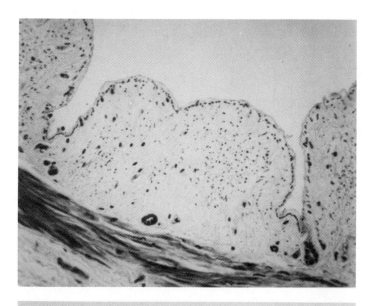

With epithelium **Without epithelium**

FIGURE 1. Demonstration that gentle mechanical rubbing selectively removes the epithelium in canine bronchi. (From Gao, Y. and Vanhoutte, P. M., *J. Appl. Physiol.*, in press. With permission.)

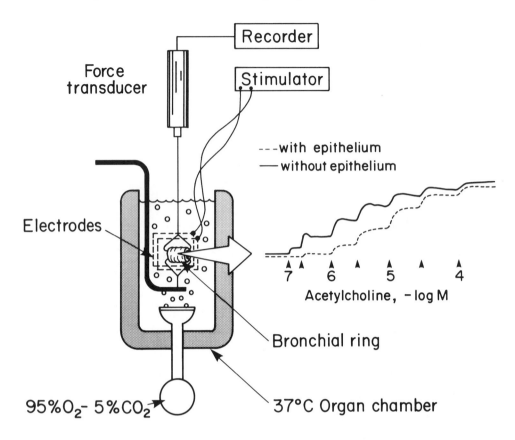

FIGURE 2.   Organ chamber for the study of isolated airways. Arrow points to isometric tension recordings in a ring with epithelium (upper) and a ring without epithelium (lower) of the trachea of the same dog. The preparations were contracted with increasing concentrations of acetylcholine. Note that the ring with epithelium contracts to a lesser degree than the ring without epithelium. (Courtesy of Dr. Michael F. Busk.)

pig were examined.[16] In the pig, removal of the epithelium causes a significant leftward shift in the concentration-response curve for acetylcholine. The shift is most prominent in third- and fourth-order bronchi, and is least in fifth-order tissues. The degree of shift of the concentration-effect curve to histamine is similar in third and fifth-order bronchi and is reduced in fourth-order bronchi. Overall, the shifts in the curves for acetylcholine and histamine are comparable for the three orders. It is likely that in the pig, unlike the dog, the epithelium of bronchi of different diameters exhibits a comparable basal release of relaxing factors. Thus, there is heterogeneity in the basal release of relaxing factors between species. As in the dog, the factor is nonspecific, as similar shifts occur for the concentration-response curves to acetylcholine and histamine with epithelium removal.

The influence of the epithelium also shows considerable heterogeneity along the respiratory tree of the rabbit.[13] In this species, first- and second-order bronchi show a leftward shift of the concentration-effect curve to methacholine when the epithelium is removed; the trachea shows no such shift.[13] This is in contrast to the other species studied so far, where tracheal preparations without epithelium do demonstrate enhanced responsiveness to contractile agents (i.e., the cow[8], the guinea pig,[9,10,12,17] and the dog).[7] For the trachea of the guinea pig, the influence of the epithelium is selective for certain contractile agonists.[12]

This evidence demonstrates that the modulatory effect of basally released EpiDRF shows considerable heterogeneity between pharmacological agents, between orders of bronchi, and between species. The existence of this heterogeneity demonstrates that the effect of epithelium

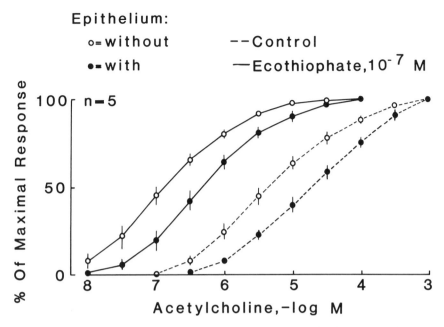

FIGURE 3.   Effects of epithelium removal on responsiveness of canine bronchial rings to acetylcholine in control preparations (broken lines) and following inhibition of acetylcholinesterase with echothiophate ($10^{-7} M$) (solid lines). Data are expressed as percent of maximal response to acetylcholine and are shown as means $\pm$ SEM (n $-$ 5). ●, Rings with epithelium; ○, rings without epithelium. (From Flavahan, N. A., Aarhus, L. L., Rimele, T. J., and Vanhoutte, P. M., *J. Appl. Physiol.*, 58, 834, 1985. With permission.)

removal is not an artifact due to damage of the smooth muscle or the loss of a diffusion barrier, as has been suggested previously.[10] The data are explained best if it is assumed that the epithelium secretes a factor which tends to promote relaxation of the smooth muscle. It is likely that variations in the basal release of this EpiDRF accounts for the heterogeneity in the effect of epithelium removal, and probably reflects the variations in epithelial cell type and secretory properties that are known to occur within the respiratory tree of an individual species, and also between species.[18]

III. ELECTROPHYSIOLOGICAL STUDIES

In canine bronchi (in the presence of antagonists of muscarinic and adrenergic receptors), the resting membrane potential and the depolarization of the smooth muscle in response to potassium are unaltered by epithelium removal.[7] These data confirm the view that mechanical removal of the epithelium does not compromise the contractile properties of the smooth muscle.[5,6,16] The addition of the anticholinesterase, echothiophate, does not alter the resting membrane potential of intact tissues, but induces depolarization in bronchi without epithelium. Furthermore, acetylcholine evoked a greater degree of depolarization in bronchi without epithelium, even when matched contractions are compared[7] (Figure 6). These results imply that the EpiDRF inhibits the depolarization induced by acetylcholine.[7] The mechanism for such an effect is not known. The epithelial factor may influence the sodium/potassium pump in the smooth muscle.[19] It can be postulated that the epithelium exerts its inhibitory effect on membrane potential via this route. Acetylcholine itself might stimulate release of the EpiDRF, as atropine causes a depolarization in bronchi with epithelium, but has no effect in tissues without epithelium.[7] This implies that tonic release of the cholinergic agonist stimulates or enhances the release of relaxing factor, but the origin of the acetylcholine (i.e., smooth muscle, nerve, or epithelium) is not known.

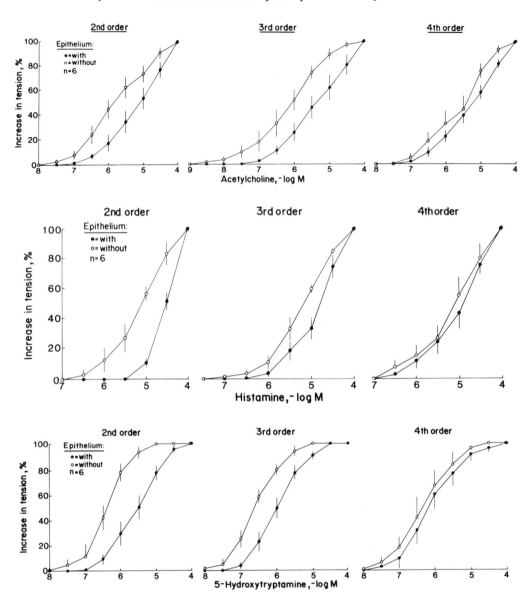

FIGURE 4.   Effect of epithelim removal on concentration-effect curve to acetylcholine (top), histamine (middle), and 5-hydroxytryptamine (bottom) in second-, third-, and fourth-order canine bronchi. Data (means ± SEM) are expressed as percent of response to acetylcholine (10^{-4} M), histamine (10^{-4} M), and 5-hydroxytryptamine (10^{-4} M), respectively. ●, Rings with epithelium; ○, rings without epithelium. (From Stuart-Smith, K. and Vanhoutte, P. M., *J. Appl. Physiol.*, 63, 2510, 1987. With permission.)

IV. THE RESPONSE TO ISOPROTERENOL

In the dog, removal of the airway epithelium reduces the responsiveness of the smooth muscle to the β-adrenergic agonist isoproterenol[5,6] (Figure 7). Similar results have been obtained in the cow,[8] and the pig.[16] In canine airways, second- and third-order bronchi show this effect of epithelium removal only at high concentrations of isoproterenol. However, for fourth-order bronchi, tissues without epithelium exhibit a substantial reduction in the response to the β-adrenergic agonist such that in these smaller canine airways relaxation to isoproterenol is virtually dependent on the presence of the epithelium[6] (Figure 7). These results

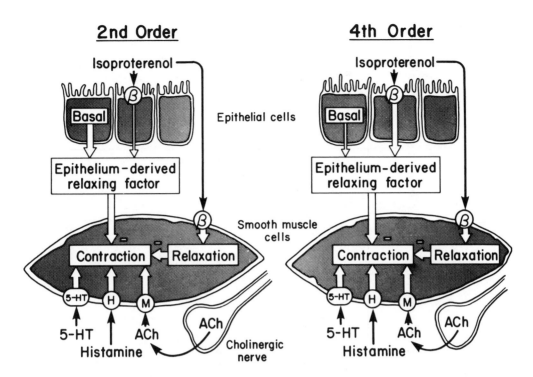

2nd Order

Isoproterenol

Epithelial cells

Basal

Epithelium-derived
relaxing factor

Smooth muscle
cells

Contraction ← Relaxation

5-HT   H   M

5-HT ↑ ACh
Histamine

ACh

Cholinergic
nerve

4th Order

Isoproterenol

Basal

Epithelium-derived
relaxing factor

Contraction ← Relaxation

5-HT   H   M

5-HT ↑ ACh
Histamine

ACh

FIGURE 5. Schematic showing the basal vs. stimulated release of epithelium-derived relaxing factor. β, beta-adrenoreceptor; 5-HT, 5-hydroxytryptamine, serotonergic receptor; ACh, acetylcholine; H, histaminergic receptor; M, muscarinic receptor. (From Vanhoutte, P. M., *Thorax*, 43(a), 665, 1988. With permission.)

are in direct contrast to the response to contractile agents, where there is no effect of epithelium removal in fourth-order bronchi and thus no basal release of EpiDRF(s). These observations suggest that in the presence of isoproterenol, the airway epithelium is stimulated to release a relaxing factor, which enhances the relaxation of the smooth muscle to the β-adrenergic agonist. This effect of isoproterenol must be more prominent in the smaller canine airways (Figure 7). Epithelium removal also reduces the relaxation to isoproterenol in the intrapulmonary bronchi of the pig.[16] However, in contrast to the dog, the influence of the epithelium is much more uniformly distributed along the porcine respiratory tree, again demonstrating heterogeneity in the influence of the epithelium between species.

The stimulated release of the factor is probably mediated via β-adrenoreceptors on the epithelial cells. Epithelial β-adrenoreceptors have been demonstrated histologically in the airways of several species.[20-24] There is considerable evidence that these β-adrenoreceptors can modulate the secretory functions of the epithelium.[25-27] Heterogeneity in the isoproterenol-induced release of EpiDRFs may reflect variations in the distribution and/or sensitivity of the receptors between regions of the respiratory tree and between species.[6,16] These variations in the stimulated release of the EpiDRF may parallel regional differences in the response of the underlying smooth muscle to isoproterenol. In the dog, bronchi without epithelium show decreasing sensitivity to the β-adrenergic agonist with decreasing diameter; in the pig, the relaxations are more uniform.[6,16] It may be postulated that the influence of the epithelium is greatest where the responsiveness of the underlying smooth muscle is reduced. In canine airways, this occurs in the fourth-order bronchi.

Further evidence for this hypothesis comes from the observation that, during a contraction to 5-hydroxytryptamine or to low concentrations of acetylcholine (less than the ED_{40} for the contractile agonist), canine bronchi are very sensitive to isoproterenol, and there is no difference between tissues with and without epithelium.[56a] However, at high degrees of

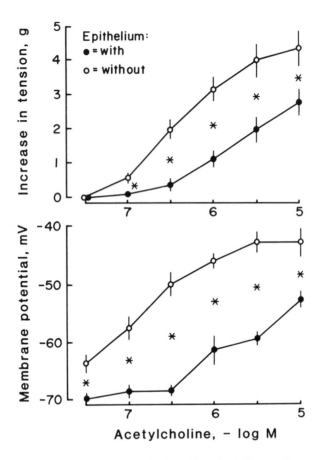

FIGURE 6.   Responses of canine bronchial strips (with and without epithelium) to increasing concentrations of acetylcholine. Top: changes in tension; each group contains seven preparations from different animals. Bottom: changes in membrane potential; each group contains 7 to 14 successful impalements of cells from the same 7 preparations. The asterisks denote a statistically significant difference between the two groups. (From Gao, Y. and Vanhoutte, P. M., *J. Appl. Physiol.*, 65, 2170, 1988. With permission.)

cholinergic tone, bronchi without epithelium show a markedly reduced relaxation to the β-adrenergic agonist. This phenomenon has been reported previously.[28,29] By contrast, in tissues with epithelium, the response to isoproterenol is not attenuated by raising the level of contraction to acetylcholine.[56a] Thus, the influence of the epithelium on relaxations to isoproterenol is affected by the contractile agent used to induce active force, and the degree of contraction achieved. It appears that the contribution of the EpiDRF is most prominent when the responsiveness of the underlying smooth muscle to isoproterenol is reduced; in this case, at high levels of cholinergic tone.

In the trachea of the guinea pig, removal of the airway epithelium has been reported either to enhance[10,30] or reduce[9] relaxations to isoproterenol. In those studies in which the sensitivity of the tissue to isoproterenol was augmented by epithelium removal, the addition of corticosterone abolished the difference between intact and denuded tissues.[30] It was proposed that the epithelium represents a site of extraneuronal uptake for isoproterenol, thus reducing its action on the smooth muscle.[30] However, since experiments in the dog and the pig were performed in the presence of inhibitors of both neuronal and extraneuronal uptake, differences in the epithelial metabolism of isoproterenol cannot explain these data.[6,16] The

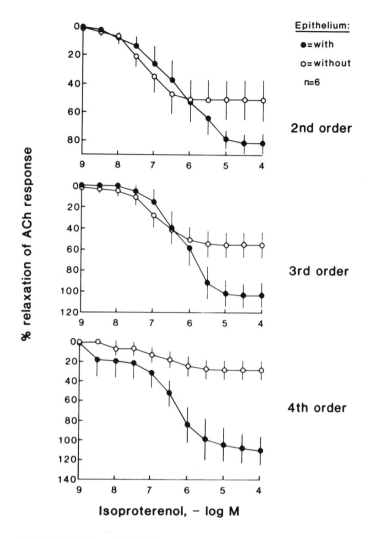

FIGURE 7. Effect of epithelium removal on concentration-effect curve to isoproterenol in second-order (top), third-order (middle), and fourth-order (bottom) canine bronchi. Rings were contracted to equal tensions using concentration producing 50% of maximal response (ED_{50}). Data (means ± SEM) are expressed as percent relaxation of response to acetylcholine; n = 6. ●, Rings with epithelium; ○, rings without epithelium. (From Stuart-Smith, K. and Vanhoutte, P. M., *J. Appl. Physiol.*, 63, 2510, 1987. With permission.)

contradictory results obtained by different workers might be explained in part by the fact that responses to isoproterenol were obtained at different levels of contraction to cholinergic agonists. In those studies in which the relaxation was enhanced by epithelium removal, responses were obtained either on basal tone or at comparatively low levels of muscarinic contraction.[10,30] In the experiments where epithelium removal reduced relaxations to isoproterenol, the tissues were contracted with a supramaximal concentration of the muscarnic agonist.[9] Thus, it may be that in the guinea pig, like the dog, the effect of the EpiDRF on responses to isoproterenol is greatest at high degrees of cholinergic tone. Clearly, when interpreting the effect of removal of the airway epithelium on the responsiveness of bronchial smooth muscle, the experimental conditions under which the tissues are studied must be taken into account.

V. THE ROLE OF METABOLITES OF ARACHIDONIC ACID

Both prostaglandins and leukotrienes play an important role in bronchial smooth-muscle reponsiveness.[31,32] Prostaglandins E_1 and E_2 and prostacyclin are potent bronchodilators.[33-35] Leukotrienes C_4 and D_4, the components of slow-reacting substance of anaphylaxis,[36] are bronchoconstricting agents.[37,38] The airway epithelium metabolizes arachidonic acid to yield products of both cyclooxygenase and lipoxygenase.[26,39-41] Therefore, it is logical to speculate that epithelium-derived metabolites of arachidonic acid might influence the responsiveness of the underlying smooth muscle. In canine airways in the presence of contraction induced by 5-hydroxytryptamine, exogenous arachidonic acid evokes relaxations which are dependent on the presence of the epithelium[42,43] (Figure 8). Epithelium-dependent relaxations to arachidonic acid have also been described in the trachea of the guinea pig[44-46] and in the large intrapulmonary bronchi of the rabbit.[14]

In all species studied so far, epithelium-dependent relaxations to arachidonic acid are abolished by indomethacin, thus implicating a product of cyclooxygenase in the response.[14,42,43,45,46] The most likely candidate is prostaglandin E_2. This substance is a potent bronchodilator[34] and is produced in the airway epithelial cells of several species (i.e., the dog,[26,40,47] the cow,[48] and the rabbit).[14] In the dog, addition of arachidonic acid stimulates the release of prostaglandin E_2 from second- and fourth-order bronchi with epithelium; bronchi without epithelium do not show stimulated release of this product of cyclooxygenase[43] (Figure 9). This is strong evidence that prostaglandin E_2 is the mediator of epithelium-dependent relaxations to arachidonic acid in canine airways. However, there is heterogeneity in the response to arachidonic acid along the canine respiratory tree. Second- and third-order bronchi with epithelium show a marked relaxation to this substance, whereas the response is significantly reduced in fourth-order tissues[43] (Figure 8). This is not due to a loss of sensitivity to prostaglandin E_2 in the smaller airways, as the relaxation induced by exogenous prostaglandin E_2 is similar in the three orders.[43] Furthermore, fourth-order bronchi with epithelium produce significantly more prostaglandin E_2 in reponse to arachidonic acid than do second-order tissues.[43] These data suggest that differences in response to arachidonic acid cannot be explained simply by differences in the release of, and sensitivity to, prostaglandin E_2. Airway epithelial cells are known to release several other products of cyclooxygenase and lipoxygenase.[39,41,48] The presence of these metabolites may modify the epithelium-dependent relaxation to arachidonic acid. In particular, leukotrienes may be produced by both the epithelium and the smooth muscle in reponse to exogenous arachidonic acid. These substances have a direct contractile effect which is greater in the smaller airways.[31] The reduced relaxation to arachidonic acid in the fourth-order bronchi of the dog could then be explained if the relaxing effect of prostaglandin E_2 were counterbalanced by the bronchoconstrictor effect of the leukotrienes.[43] A similar phenomenon may occur for the trachea of the guinea pig.[45] In the presence of indomethacin (which inhibited the epithelium-dependent relaxation) the trachea with epithelium contracts in response to arachidonic acid. This effect is blocked by nordihydroguaiaretic acid, suggesting the involvement of products of lipoxygenase, most likely leukotrienes.[45] Therefore, although the probable mediator of epithelium-dependent relaxations to arachidonic acid is prostaglandin E_2, other products of cyclooxygenase and lipoxygenase may considerably modify the response.

It has been suggested that epithelium-derived prostaglandin E_2 may explain other epithelium-dependent phenomenon in the airways, such as the leftward shift in the concentration-effect curve to contractile agents seen on removal of the epithelium.[14] In the intrapulmonary bronchi of the rabbit, the enhanced responsiveness to the cholinergic agonist bethanecol caused by epithelium removal was mimicked in the intact tissues by addition of the inhibitor of cyclooxygenase, indomethacin.[14] This implies that the EpiDRF in the rabbit is a product of cyclooxygenase, probably prostaglandin E_2.[14] However, the effect of the epithelium on

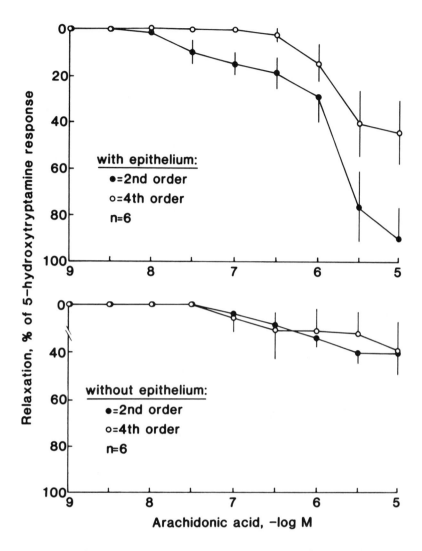

FIGURE 8.   Effect of epithelium removal on concentration-effect curve to arachidonic acid in second- and fourth-order canine bronchi. Rings were contracted using 30% effective dose for 5-hydroxytryptamine. Values (means ± SEM) are expressed as percent of response to 5-hydroxytryptamine. ●, Rings with epithelium; ○, rings without epithelium. (From Stuart-Smith, K. and Vanhoutte, P. M., *J. Appl. Physiol.*, 65, 2170, 1988. With permission.)

responses to contractile agents is not affected by indomethacin in the dog,[5,7] the guinea pig,[10,46] or the cow.[8] Similarly, the influence of the epithelium on responses to isoproterenol in canine airways is not blocked by indomethacin.[56a] It appears that, although prostaglandin E_2 is a substance derived from the airway epithelium, which causes relaxation of bronchial smooth muscle, it does not account for other epithelium-dependent phenomena and cannot be considered to be the EpiDRF.

VI. THE RESPONSE TO OSMOTIC STIMULI

A novel *in vitro* preparation of the guinea pig trachea has been developed, in which either the serosal or the epithelial surface of the airway may be stimulated independently; changes in tracheal tension are measured as the drop in pressure between the inlet and outlet of the trachea under constant flow.[49] In this preparation, application of a hypertonic solution

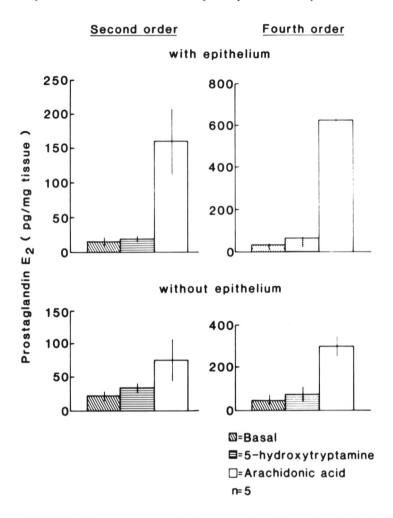

FIGURE 9.   Release of prostaglandin E_2 under basal conditions and evoked by 5-hydroxytryptamine and arachidonic acid in perfused second- and fourth-order canine bronchi with and without epithelium. (From Stuart-Smith, K. and Vanhoutte, P. M., *J. Appl. Physiol.*, 55, 2170, 1988. With permission.)

of potassium chloride to the serosal surface of the trachea evokes a concentration-dependent contraction. If the hypertonic solution is then administered to the inner (epithelial) surface, a concentration-dependent relaxation of the trachea results. Removal of the epithelium abolished the relaxation.[49] In trachea which have been contracted with carbachol, the addition of a hypertonic solution of potassium chloride, urea, or mannitol to the epithelial side of the preparation causes profound relaxation. This demonstrates that the epithelium-dependent relaxation is related to the osmolality of the solution and not the potassium chloride per se. Thus, the guinea pig trachea exhibits epithelium-dependent relaxations to osmotic stimuli.[49] The epithelium-dependent relaxations are not affected by either tetrodotoxin, propanolol, or indomethacin, implying the presence of an EpiDRF whose action is independent of nerve stimulation or prostaglandin release.

The asthmatic state may represent an abnormal response to hyperosmotic stimuli, such as dry air or hyperventilation, which tend to disrupt the epithelial cell.[50] In the normal individual, a hyperosmotic stimulus might cause the epithelial cells to produce an EpiDRF which would protect the airways from the effects of exercise, dry air, or hyperventilation. The epithelium of an asthmatic individual might be altered such that no relaxing factor is present. Bronchoconstriction might then result.

VII. BIOASSAY OF A DIFFUSABLE EPITHELIUM-DERIVED RELAXING FACTOR

The results obtained with arachidonic acid indicate that the airway epithelium can release substances (in this case, prostaglandins) which diffuse to the bronchial smooth muscle and initiate a response. However, it has proved considerably more difficult to demonstrate the diffusion of a nonprostanoid EpiDRF from the epithelium to the smooth muscle. Early superfusion studies showed that perfusate from the bronchial epithelium of the dog could cause direct relaxation of bronchial smooth muscle[1,4] (Figure 10). Unfortunately, these results could not be repeated by other workers.[10] The superfusion system, in which fluid from a preparation with intact epithelium drops onto a bioassay tissue without epithelium, has several inherent problems, including a relatively long transit time between the two preparations, fluctuations in temperature, and dilution of the epithelium-derived factor itself. Greater success has been achieved using protocols in which the intact and denuded tissues are in contact with each other in the organ chamber: the so-called "sandwich" preparation and the coaxial bioassay system. In the first such study, the bioassay material was a segment of the aorta of the rabbit, which had been denuded of endothelium.[51] The aortic segment was passed through a ring of guinea pig trachea with or without epithelium. In the presence of trachea without epithelium, the blood vessel showed no relaxation to acetylcholine. By contrast, when the epithelium was present, the aortic segment demonstrated a concentration-dependent relaxation to the cholinergic agonist.[51] Thus, this coaxial system indicated that the airway epithelium could release a diffusable factor which could influence the responses of vascular smooth muscle.[51] It was nonprostanoid, as the effect was not blocked by indomethacin. Similar results were obtained using the thoracic aorta of the rat as a bioassay material. In the presence of guinea pig trachea with epithelium, the aorta relaxed in response to histamine and methacholine. The effect was not altered by indomethacin.[52] In another coaxial system, a strip of guinea pig trachea without epithelium was placed inside a ring of tracheal tissue with or without epithelium, and the response of the denuded strip to ovalbumin was recorded.[12] There was an eightfold increase in the sensitivity of the denuded strip to ovalbumin when it was placed inside a ring without epithelium, as compared to results obtained in the presence of an intact ring. These results demonstrate the diffusion of a factor from an epithelium-intact to an epithelium-denuded airway.[12] Using a "sandwich protocol", it can be shown that the hyperresponsiveness to substance P seen in guinea pig trachea without epithelium is abolished by applying the luminal surface of an intact airway to the luminal surface of the denuded tissue.[11] In a novel preparation, the hyperresponsiveness of de-epithelialized canine trachealis to acetylcholine and histamine is abolished when a strip of canine mucosa is placed close to, but not in contact with, the airway smooth muscle.[53] These results demonstrate that the airway epithelium releases a diffusable, nonprostanoid factor which influences the responses of both vascular and bronchial smooth muscle.

VIII. THE NATURE OF THE EPITHELIUM-DERIVED RELAXING FACTOR

At present, the identity and mechanism of action of the airway EpiDRF are not known. Indeed, it is not clear whether or not basal and stimulated effects of the epithelium are mediated via the same factor. Only a few definite statements can be made. The factor is nonprostanoid in nature, although this does not exclude a role for other metabolites of arachidonic acid.[43] The influence of the epithelium is temperature sensitive and seems to require extracellular calcium.[54] Part of its action may be to inhibit bronchial smooth muscle depolarization.[7] The sodium/potassium pump has been implicated in epithelium-dependent phenomena, but whether it is the epithelial or the smooth-muscle pump which is important remains uncertain.[19]

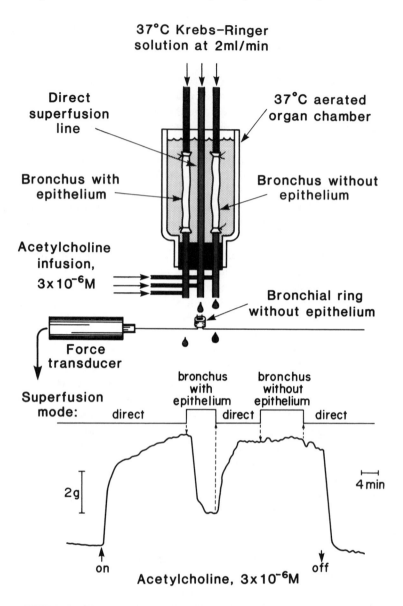

FIGURE 10.   Bioassay experiment in which a ring of canine bronchus without epithelium (contracted with acetylcholine) is superfused with Krebs-Ringer bicarbonate solution flowing either through a bronchus with epithelium (first arrow; note the marked relaxation), a stainless steel tube (direct; note the reversal of the relaxation), or a bronchus without epithelium (note the absence of relaxation). This demonstrates that the bronchial epithelium can release a potent inhibitory factor. (From Vanhoutte, P. M., *Can. J. Physiol. Pharmacol.*, 65, 448, 1987. With permission.)

In blood vessels, nitric oxide has been identified as one of the endothelium-derived relaxing factors.[55] This substance is released from endothelial cells and initiates relaxation of vascular smooth muscle via a cyclic GMP-dependent phenomenon.[56] However, nitric oxide does not cause relaxation of the fourth-order bronchus of the dog.[56a] Furthermore, although the relaxation to sodium nitroprusside is greater in fourth-order bronchi with epithelium, this effect does not appear to be mediated via cyclic GMP[56a] (Figure 11). It can be concluded that the EpiDRF is not nitric oxide. In addition, the relaxation to forskolin in canine bronchi is not affected by epithelium removal, indicating that the EpiDRF does not function via cyclic AMP-dependent mechanisms.[56a]

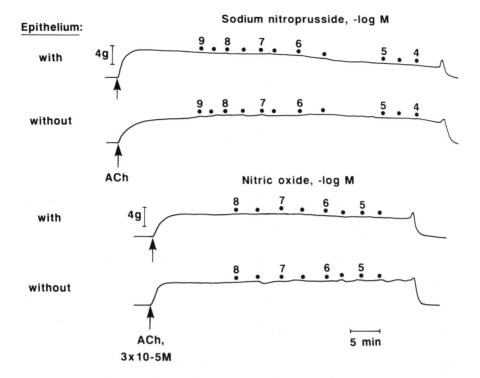

FIGURE 11. Representative tracing of the effect of epithelium removal on the response to sodium nitroprusside and nitric oxide in canine bronchi. Top: response to sodium nitroprusside. Bottom: response to nitric oxide. Each tissue was contracted to the ED_{80} value for acetylcholine. (Stuart-Smith, K. and Vanhoutte, P. M., *J. Appl. Physiol.*, in press. With permission.)

Lastly, it must be emphasized that the effect of the epithelium on bronchial smooth-muscle responsiveness is heavily influenced by the species studied, the branch of the respiratory tree, and the experimental conditions. This very heterogeneity in the EpiDRF(s) may provide clues to its nature and mechanism of action.

REFERENCES

1. **Vanhoutte, P. M.,** Airway epithelium and bronchial reactivity, *Can. J. Physiol. Pharmacol.*, 65, 448, 1987.
2. **Vanhoutte, P. M.,** Epithelium derived relaxing factor: myth or reality?, *Thorax*, 43(9), 665, 1988.
3. **Aarhus, L. L., Rimele, T. J., and Vanhoutte, P. M.,** Removal of the epithelium causes bronchial supersensitivity to acetylcholine and 5-hydroxytryptamine, *Fed. Proc., Fed. Am. Soc. Exp. Biol.*, 43, 955, 1984.
4. **Flavahan, N. A. and Vanhoutte, P. M.,** The respiratory epithelium releases a smooth muscle relaxing factor, *Chest*, 87, 189S, 1985.
5. **Flavahan, N. A., Aarhus, L. L., Rimele, T. J., and Vanhoutte, P. M.,** Respiratory epithelium inhibits bronchial smooth muscle tone, *J. Appl. Physiol.*, 58, 834, 1985.
6. **Stuart-Smith, K. and Vanhoutte, P. M.,** Heterogeneity in the effects of epithelium removal in the canine bronchial tree, *J. Appl. Physiol.*, 63, 2510, 1987.
7. **Gao, Y. and Vanhoutte, P. M.,** Removal of the epithelium potentiates acetylcholine in depolarizing canine bronchial smooth muscle, *J. Appl. Physiol.*, in press.
8. **Barnes, P. J., Cuss, F. M., and Palmer, J. B.,** The effect of airway epithelium on smooth muscle contractility in bovine trachea, *Br. J. Pharmacol.*, 86, 685, 1985.

9. **Goldie, R. G., Papadimitriou, J. M., Paterson, J. W., Rigby, P. J., Self, H. M., and Spina, D.,** Influence of the epithelium on the responsiveness of guinea-pig trachea to contractile and relaxant agonists, *Br. J. Pharmacol.,* 87, 5, 1986.

10. **Holroyde, M. C.,** The influence of epithelium on the responsiveness of guinea-pig isolated trachea, *Br. J. Pharmacol.,* 87, 501, 1986.

11. **Tschirhart, E. and Landry, Y.,** Airway epithelium releases a relaxant factor: demonstration with substance P, *Eur. J. Pharmacol.,* 132, 103, 1986.

12. **Hay, D. W. P., Farmer, S. G., Raeburn, D., Muccitui, R. M., Wilson, K. A., and Fedan, J. S.,** Differential effects of epithelium removal on the responsiveness of guinea-pig tracheal smooth muscle to broncho-constrictors, *Br. J. Pharmacol.,* 92, 381, 1987.

13. **Raeburn, D., Hay, D. W. P., Robinson, V. A., Farmer, S. G., Fleming, W. W., and Fedan, J. S.,** The effect of verapamil is reduced in isolated airway smooth muscle preparations lacking the epithelium, *Life Sci.,* 38, 809, 1986.

14. **Butler, G. B., Adler, K. B., Evans, J. N., Morgan, D. W., and Szarek, J. L.,** Modulation of rabbit airway smooth muscle reponsiveness by respiratory epithelium, involvement of an inhibitory metabolite of arachidonic acid, *Am. Rev. Respir. Dis.,* 135, 1099, 1987.

15. **Cuss, F. M. and Barnes, P. J.,** Epithelial mediators. Airway smooth muscle and disease workshop, *Am. Rev. Respir. Dis.,* 136, 532, 1987.

16. **Stuart-Smith, K. and Vanhoutte, P. M.,** The airway epithelium modulates the responsiveness of porcine bronchial smooth muscle, *J. Appl. Physiol.,* 65, 721, 1988.

17. **Flavahan, N. A., Slifman, N. R., Gleich, G. J., and Vanhoutte, P. M.,** Human eosinophil major basic protein causes hyperreactivity of respiratory smooth muscle: role of the epithelium, *Am. Rev. Respir. Dis.,* in press.

18. **Weibel, E. R.,** Lung cell biology, in *Handbook of Physiology, The Respiratory System, Circulatory and Nonrespiratory Functions,* Sect. 3, Vol. I, American Physiological Society, Bethesda, MD, 1985, 47.

19. **Lamport, S. J. and Fedan, J. S.,** Temperature-dependent modulatory effect of epithelium on the reactivity of guinea-pig isolated trachealis, Abstract, *FASEB,* Las Vegas, NV, May 1988, A1057.

20. **Jones, R. and Reid, L. M.,** Beta-agonists and secretory cell number and intracellular glycoprotein in airway epithelium: the effect of isoproterenol and salbutamol, *Am. J. Pathol.,* 95, 407, 1979.

21. **Rugg, E. L., Barnett, D. B., and Nahorski, S. R.,** Co-existence of beta 1 and beta 2 adrenoceptors in mammalian lung: evidence from direct binding studies, *Mol. Pharmacol.,* 14, 996, 1978.

22. **Barnes, P. J., Basbaum, C. B., Nadel, J. A., and Roberts, J. M.,** Localization of beta-adrenoceptors in mammalian lung by light microscopic autoradiography, *Nature (London),* 299, 444, 1982.

23. **Xue, Q. F., Maurer, R., and Engel, G.,** Selective distribution of beta-and alpha$_1$-adrenoceptors in rat lung visualized by autoradiography, *Arch. Int. Pharmacodyn. Ther.,* 266, 308, 1983.

24. **Goldie, R. G., Papadimitriou, J. M., Paterson, J. W., Rigby, P. J., and Spina, D.,** Autoradiographic localization of beta-adrenoceptors in pig lung using {^{125}I} iodocyanopinolol, *Br. J. Pharmacol.,* 88, 621, 1986.

25. **Davis, B., Marin, M. G., Yee, J. W., and Nadel, J. A.,** Effect of terbutaline on movement of Cl$^-$ and Na$^+$ across the trachea of the dog in vitro, *Am. Rev. Respir. Dis.,* 120, 547, 1979.

26. **Smith, P. L., Welsh, M. J., Stoff, J. S., and Frizzell, R. A.,** Chloride secretion by canine tracheal epithelium: role of intracellular cAMP levels, *J. Memb. Biol.,* 70, 217, 1982.

27. **Welsh, M. J.,** Single apical membrane anion channels in primary cultures of canine tracheal epithelium, *Pfluegers Arch.,* 407, S116, 1986.

28. **Torphy, T. J., Rinard, G. A., Rietow, M. G., and Mayer, S. E.,** Functional antagonism of canine tracheal smooth muscle: inhibition by methacholine of the mechanical and biochemical responses to iso-proterenol, *J. Pharmacol. Exp. Ther.,* 227, 694, 1983.

29. **Torphy, T. J., Zheng, C., Peterson, S. M., Fiscus, R. R., Rinard, G. A., and Mayer, S. E.,** Inhibitory effect of methacholine and drug-induced relaxation, cyclic AMP accumulation, and cyclic AMP-dependent protein kinase, activation in canine tracheal smooth muscle, *J. Pharmacol. Exp. Ther.,* 233, 409, 1985.

30. **Farmer, S. G., Fedan, J. S., Hay, D. W. P., and Raeburn, D.,** The effects of epithelium removal on the sensitivity of guinea-pig isolated trachealis to bronchodilator drugs, *Br. J. Pharmacol,* 89, 407, 1986.

31. **Bakhle, Y. S. and Ferreira, S. H.,** Lung metabolism of eicosanoids, prostaglandins, prostacyclin, thromboxane and leukotrienes, in *Handbook of Physiology,* Sect. 3, The Respiratory System, Vol. I, Circulatory and Nonrespiratory Functions, Fishman, A. P. and Fisher, A. B., Eds., American Physiological Society, Bethesda, MD, 1985, 365.

32. **Morris, H. G.,** Physiology and pharmacology of prostaglandins and leukotrienes in bronchial asthma, in *Brochial Asthma: Mechanisms and Therapeutics,* Weiss, E. B., Segal, M. S., and Stein, M., Eds., Little, Brown, Boston, 1985, 160.

33. **Shore, S. A., Powell, W. S., and Martin, J. G.,** Endogenous prostaglandins modulate histamine-induced contraction in canine tracheal smooth muscle, *J. Appl. Physiol.,* 58, 859, 1985.

34. **Gardiner, P. J.,** Characterization of prostanoid relaxant inhibitory receptors (4) using a highly selective agonist, TR4979, *Br. J. Pharmacol.,* 87, 45, 1986.

35. **Stuart-Smith, K. and Vanhoutte, P. M.,** Epithelium, contractile tone and responses to relaxing agonists in canine bronchi, *J. Appl. Physiol.,* in press.

36. **Murphy, R. C., Hammarström, S. and Samuelsson, B.,** Leukotriene C: a slow-reacting substance from murine mastocytoma cells, *Proc. Natl. Acad. Sci. U.S.A.,* 76, 4275, 1979.

37. **Burka, J. F. and Saad, M. H.,** Mediators of arachidonic acid-induced contractions of indomethacin-treated guinea-pig airways: leukotrienes C_4 and D_4, *Br. J. Pharmacol.,* 81, 465, 1984.

38. **Samhoun, M. N. and Piper, P. J.,** Actions of leukotrienes in nonhuman respiratory tissues, in *The Leukotrienes: Their Biological Significance,* Piper, P. J., Ed., Raven Press, New York, 1986, 151.

39. **Holtzman, M. J., Aizawa, H., Nader, J. A., and Goetzl, E. J.,** Selective generation of leukotriene B_4 by tracheal epithelial cells from dogs, *Biochem. Biophys. Res. Commun.,* 114, 1071, 1983.

40. **Leikauf, G. D., Ueki, I. F., Widdicombe, J. H., and Nadel, J. A.,** Alteration of chloride secretion across canine tracheal epithelium by lipoxygenase products of arachidonic acid, *Am. J. Physiol.,* 250, F47, 1986.

41. **Eling, T. E., Danilowicz, R. M., Henke, D. C., Sivarajah, K., Yankaskas, J. R., and Boucher, R. C.,** Arachidonic acid metabolism by canine tracheal epithelial cells: product formation and relationship to chloride secretion, *J. Biol. Chem.,* 261, 12841, 1986.

42. **Flavahan, N. A., Danser, A. J., and Vanhoutte, P. M.,** Arachidonic acid and calcium ionophore cause epithelium-dependent relaxation of canine bronchial smooth muscle, *Proc. Int. Union Physiol. Sci.,* (Abstr.), Vancouver, BC, Canada, July 13 to 18, 1986, 18.

43. **Stuart-Smith, K. and Vanhoutte, P. M.** Arachidonic acid evokes epithelium-dependent relaxations in canine airways, *J. Appl. Physiol.,* 65, 2170, 1988.

44. **Nijkamp, F. P. and Folkerts, G.,** Reversal of arachidonic acid-induced guinea-pig tracheal relaxation into contraction after epithelium-removal, *Eur. J. Pharmacol.,* 131, 315, 1987.

45. **Farmer, S. G., Hay, D. W. P., Raeburn, D., and Fedan, J. S.,** Relaxation of guinea-pig tracheal smooth muscle is converted to contraction following epithelium removal, *Br. J. Pharmacol.,* 92, 231, 1987.

46. **Tschirhart, E., Frossard, N., Bertrand, C., and Landry, Y.,** Arachidonic acid metabolites and airway epithelium-dependent relaxant factor, *J. Pharmacol. Exp. Ther.,* 243, 310, 1987.

47. **Welsh, M. J.,** Effect of phorbol ester and calcium ionophore on chloride secretion in canine tracheal epithelium, *Am. J. Physiol.,* 253 (Cell Physiol. 22), C828, 1987.

48. **Leikauf, G. D., Driscoll, K. E., and Wey, H. E.,** Ozone-induced augmentation of eicosanoid metabolism in epithelial cells from bovine trachea, *Am. Rev. Respir. Dis.,* 137, 435, 1988.

49. **Munakata, M., Mitzner, W., and Menkes, H.,** Osmotic stimuli induce epithelial-dependent relaxation in the guinea-pig trachea, *J. Appl. Physiol.,* 64, 466, 1988.

50. **Hogg, J. C., and Eggleston, P. A.,** Is asthma an epithelial disease?, *Am. Rev. Respir. Dis.,* 129, 207, 1984.

51. **Ilnan, M. and Sahin, I.,** Tracheal epithelium releases a vascular smooth muscle relaxant factor: demonstration by bioassay, *Eur. J. Pharmacol.,* 131, 293, 1986.

52. **Goldie, R. G., Fernandes, L. B., and Paterson, J. W.,** Release and transfer of airway epithelium-derived relaxant factor (EpDRF) in a co-axial bioassay system, Abstract, American Thoracic Society, Las Vegas, NV, May 8 to 11, 1988, 101.

53. **Manning, P. J., Jones, G. L., Lane, C. G., Daniel, E. E., and O'Byrne, P. M.,** Decreased contractility occurs when epithelium is near, but not attached, to airway smooth muscle, Abstract, American Thoracic Society, Las Vegas, NV, May 8 to 11, 1988, 308.

54. **Lev, A., Christensen, G. C., Ryan, J. P., Wang, M., and Kelsen, S. G.,** Respiratory epithelial modulation of airway smooth muscle contraction is calcium and temperature dependent, Abstract, American Thoracic Society, Las Vegas, NV, May 8 to 11, 1988, 309.

55. **Palmer, R. M. J., Ferrige, A. G., and Moncada, S.,** Nitric oxide release accounts for the biological activity of endothelium-derived relaxing factor, *Nature (London),* 327, 524, 1987.

56. **Ignarro, L. J., Byrns, R. E., Buga, G. M., Wood, K. S., and Chandhuri, G.,** Pharmacological evidence that endothelium-derived relaxing factor is nitric oxide: use of pyrogallel and superoxide dismutase to study endothelium-dependent and nitric oxide-elicited vascular smooth muscle relaxation, *J. Pharmacol. Exp. Ther.,* 244, 181, 1988.

56a. **Stuart-Smith, K. and Vanhoutte, P. M.,** *J. Appl. Physiol.,* in press.

Chapter 7

IN VIVO MEASUREMENT OF AIRWAY RESPONSES IN EXPERIMENTAL ANIMALS

Krishna P. Agrawal

TABLE OF CONTENTS

I.   Introduction 148

II.   Methods of Measuring Respiratory Flow Resistance and Dynamic
       Lung Compliance 149
       A.   Measurement of Lung Resistance and Dynamic Compliance 149
              1.   Principles 149
                     a.   Measurement of Dynamic Compliance 149
                     b.   Measurement of Lung Resistance by Subtracting
                            Elastic Recoil Pressure 149
                     c.   Measurement of Lung Resistance by Canceling
                            Elastic Recoil Pressure 149
              2.   Procedures 149
                     a.   Measurement of Transpulmonary Pressure, Tidal
                            Volume, and Airflow 149
                     b.   Recording and Analysis of Data 151
       B.   Measurement of Functional Residual Capacity and
              Determination of Specific Lung Conductance 153
              1.   Principles 153
              2.   Procedures 154
       C.   Direct Measurement of Specific Airway Conductance 154
              1.   Principles 154
              2.   Procedures 155
                     a.   Measurement of Body Box Signal and Airflow 155
                     b.   Analysis of Data 155

III.   Measurement of Airway Response 157
       A.   Airway Challenge 157
       B.   Bronchoconstrictor Dosage 158
       C.   Measurement of Changes in Flow Resistance and Dynamic
              Compliance 158
       D.   Dose-Response Curve and Determination of Airway
              Responsiveness 159

IV.   Selection of a Suitable Method for Measuring Airway Responses in
       Different Experimental Animals 159
       A.   Guinea Pigs 160
       B.   Rats 162
       C.   Dogs 163
       D.   Monkeys 163
       E.   Sheep 163

Acknowledgment 164

References 165

I. INTRODUCTION

Airways respond to various stimuli by change in their caliber, either generalized or predominantly confined to central or peripheral (small) airways. Central airways usually account for most of the flow resistance of the airways and changes in their caliber are best monitored by measuring airway resistance.[1] Fall in dynamic lung compliance, on the other hand, has been found to be a sensitive measure of small-airway obstruction.[2]

The first method for *in vivo* measurement of flow resistance and dynamic compliance in experimental animals was described by Amdur and Mead[3] for guinea pigs in 1958. It is based on the principles of Neergaard and Wirz,[4,5] and is similar to the method described by Cook et al.[6] for the newborn infant. It has been extensively used for measuring airway responses in almost all the experimental animals. However, some workers have preferred the original method of Neergaard and Wirz[4] or the electrical subtraction method of Mead and Whittenberger[7] for measuring lung resistance because separate measurements of inspiratory and expiratory flow resistance are possible using them.

These methods, however, measure lung resistance, i.e., airway resistance as well as viscous resistance of the lung tissue, which is about 13% of total lung resistance when measured under similar conditions.[8] This will add a fixed resistance of similar magnitude in series with airway resistance, which is undesirable while measuring airway responses. The oscillation method of measuring flow resistance is even worse in this regard because it measures total respiratory resistance, 30 to 40% of which is contributed by chest wall and lung tissue.[8-13] This method would therefore underestimate changes in airway resistance and will not be described here.

DuBois et al.[14] developed the panting method of measuring airway resistance in man and suitably modified it for use in cats during quiet breathing to compare the values of airway resistance with total respiratory resistance.[9] However, this method was never put to use. The next attempt in this direction was made by Johanson and Pierce,[15] who developed a noninvasive method for measuring airway conductance in anesthetized rats. They also showed that direct measurement of specific airway conductance was possible without measuring thoracic gas volume in anesthetized rats. Their method needed submersion of the body plethysmograph in water at body temperature and was cumbersome to use. Another noninvasive technique for measuring specific airway resistance (or conductance) in anesthetized guinea pigs was developed by Pennock et al.[16] It also required measurements at body temperature, achieved by circulating heated water around the plethysmograph. Although developed for bronchial challenge studies, the method was not suitable for this purpose. A simple and more convenient method for directly measuring specific airway conductance in intact conscious guinea pigs was developed a little later in this laboratory and used successfully to measure airway response to histamine.[17]

Antigen challenge in sensitized guinea pigs, sheep, and basenji greyhound dogs results in increased functional residual capacity (FRC) due to peripheral bronchoconstriction and air trapping.[18-21] Measurement of FRC is therefore sometimes carried out to observe the severity of peripheral bronchoconstriction. The value of FRC is also needed for calculating specific airway (sGaw) and lung conductance (sG_L) from airway and lung conductance (Gaw and G_L).

The basic principles of these methods, the experimental procedures involved in them, and their application in measuring airway responses in experimental animals are described in this chapter.

II. METHODS OF MEASURING RESPIRATORY FLOW RESISTANCE AND DYNAMIC LUNG COMPLIANCE

A. MEASUREMENT OF LUNG RESISTANCE AND DYNAMIC COMPLIANCE
1. Principles

Transpleural pressure (P_{TP}) changes during respiration have two components (Figure 1A). One, $P_{TP(E)}$, is related to elastic recoil of the lung and is proportional to the lung volume. The other, $P_{TP(R)}$, is related to resistance to flow of air in the airways and "viscous" resistance of the lung tissue and is proportional to airflow.

The magnitude of P_{TP} is equal to the sum of these two pressures. These pressures can be separated and related to tidal volume (V_T) and airflow ($\dot{V}$) to determine dynamic lung compliance (Cdyn) and lung resistance (R_L), respectively.

a. Measurement of Dynamic Compliance

Using the records of P_{TP} and V_T, Cdyn is calculated by dividing V_T by the transpulmonary pressure difference between end tidal points, $\Delta P_{TP(E)}$, because at these instants airflow is zero, as is $P_{TP(R)}$.

b. Measurement of Lung Resistance by Subtracting Elastic Recoil Pressure

Flow resistance-related pressure $P_{TP(R)}$ may be determined by graphically subtracting the elastic recoil pressure $P_{TP(E)}$ from P_{TP}. When divided by airflow at that instant it provides the value of lung resistance.[5] Measurement is usually carried out at midinspiration. Subtraction of $P_{TP(E)}$ from P_{TP} may also be carried out continuously by electrically subtracting a signal proportional to lung volume and equal to the elastic recoil pressure from P_{TP} (Figure 1B).[7]

c. Measurement of Lung Resistance by Canceling Elastic Recoil Pressure

At equal volume points on inspiratory and expiratory limbs, elastic recoil pressures are equal and the difference between inspiratory and expiratory P_{TP}, $\Delta P_{TP(R)}$, will be solely related to the difference between inspiratory and expiratory flows, $\Delta \dot{V}$. The ratio of these two will provide the value of average lung resistance. These measurements are carried out near mid-tidal volume.[3,25,26]

2. Procedures
a. Measurement of Transpulmonary Pressure, Tidal Volume, and Airflow

Transpulmonary pressure is measured as the pressure difference between airway opening and pleural cavity. Pleural pressure changes are measured either directly by putting a catheter in the pleural cavity or indirectly using an esophageal balloon. V_T is measured either as chest volume change or as air volume respired. Chest volume change is determined plethysmographically, while respired air volume is measured either by integrating the flow signal or by breathing into a spirometer. Airflow is measured either by connecting a pneumotachograph to the airway opening or by differentiating the respired air volume. Quite often, the chest volume flow is used as a measure of airflow.

Figure 2 shows a commonly used setup for measuring R_L and Cdyn in unanesthetized

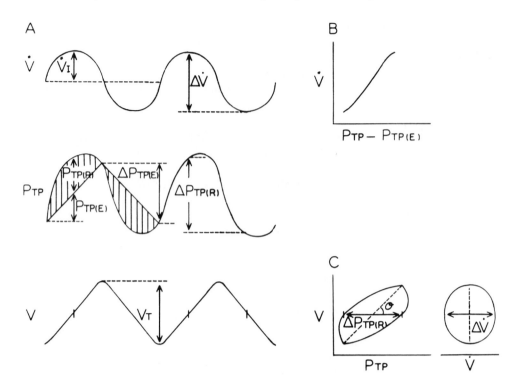

FIGURE 1.   (A) Diagrammatic records of airflow ($\dot{V}$), transpulmonary pressure (P_{TP}), and volume (V) signals, graphic analysis of P_{TP} into flow-resistive (shown by vertical bars) and elastic recoil-related components, $P_{TP(R)}$ and $P_{TP(E)}$, and their relationship with flow and volume changes. $\Delta P_{TP(E)}$ = transpulmonary pressure difference between end tidal points; $\Delta P_{TP(R)}$ = transpulmonary pressure difference between midtidal points; $\dot{V}_I$ = flow at midinspiration; $\Delta\dot{V}$ = flow difference between midtidal points; V_T = tidal volume. (B) $P_{TP}/\dot{V}$ plot after subtracting a signal proportional to lung volume and equal to $P_{TP(E)}$ from P_{TP}. (C) V/P_{TP} and $V/\dot{V}$ plots to determine $V/P_{TP(E)}$ slope (tan θ), $\Delta P_{TP(R)}$, and $\Delta\dot{V}$.

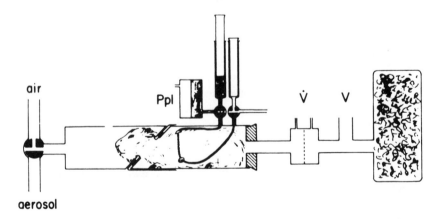

FIGURE 2.   The body plethysmograph for measuring flow ($\dot{V}$), volume (V), and intrapleural pressure (P_{pl}) in an unanesthetized, spontaneously breathing guinea pig. Exposure to air or histamine aerosol is regulated by the stopcock at the entrance to the exposure hood. (From Douglas, J. S., Dennis, M. W., Ridgway, P., and Bouhuys, A., *J. Pharmacol. Exp. Ther.*, 180, 98, 1972. With permission.)

guinea pig.[27] It is based on the technique of Amdur and Mead[3] and differs only in interposing a pneumotachograph between the body plethysmograph and the 5-l reservoir. Briefly, a PE 60 polyethylene catheter with two to three holes in the middle 1 cm is placed in the pleural cavity under light ether or sodium pentobarbital anesthesia, nonsurgically with the help of a stiff wire. The animal is then placed in a body plethysmograph and the ends of the catheter are connected to three-way stopcocks through two cannulae in the wall of the plethysmograph. An airtight seal is made at the neck and the plethysmograph is connected to a 5-l reservoir through a Fleisch no. 0000 pneumotachograph. Transpulmonary pressure changes in the pleural catheter, in the reservoir, and across the pneumotachograph.

Using this setup we determine chest volume flow rather than airflow. This would give erroneous results during airway obstruction due to increased compression-decompression of alveolar air, which would cause larger chest volume change than respired volume, and greater volume flow than airflow.[28,29] The measured value of R_L would therefore be lower than the actual value.

Some investigators have measured V_T and airflow by attaching a spirometer to an endotracheal tube.[20] The spirometer provides the volume signal, which, on differentiation, gives airflow. This arrangement would also introduce some error because the volume records needed for determining Cdyn are those of the lung or thoracic cage. Respired volume can substitute for them only in the absence of airway obstruction. In the presence of airway obstruction, respired volume will be less than chest or lung volume changes, and the measured fall in Cdyn will be greater than actual.

For correct measurements of R_L and Cdyn, airflow measurement should be carried out at the airway opening, and volume changes should be recorded using a body plethysmograph as shown in Figure 3.[30] In this setup the animal is seated in a body plethysmograph, breathing outside it. Chest volume changes are directly measured by a spirometer attached to the plethysmograph, airflow is measured by a pneumotachograph attached to the proximal end of the endotracheal tube, and intrapleural pressure changes are measured by an esophageal balloon. The method is noninvasive and suitable for long-term, repetitive studies. The resistance of the endotracheal tube should be subtracted from the measured values of R_L.

b. Recording and Analysis of Data

Recording and analysis of the data should meet the requirements of the experiment. If monitoring of Cdyn or R_L is needed during the course of the experiment and an on-line analysis system is not available, an X-Y storage oscilloscope may be used for display of the signals. X-Y plots of P_{TP} and V_T are needed for monitoring Cdyn (Figure 1C).[25,26] The slope of V/P_{TP} loop (shown by the broken line) provides the value of Cdyn. For R_L measurements, P_{TP} and airflow signals are fed to X-Y axes, respectively, and a signal proportional to lung volume is electrically subtracted from P_{TP} till the X-Y loop is closed. The alternative is to subtract a signal equal to V/Cdyn from P_{TP} (Figure 4). The slope of this closed loop gives the value of $1/R_L$, i.e., G_L. It may be noticed that the rising and falling limbs of the open loop have a slope similar to that of the closed loop. This is because at end tidal points there is hardly any change in lung volume and P_{TP} is related almost totally to the flow changes. These limbs may therefore be used for measuring R_L.

On-line analysis systems are needed for simultaneous and breath-by-breath measurements of Cdyn and R_L. An analog computer for this purpose was designed by Dennis et al.[32] and successfully used by Douglas et al.[27,33] for measuring airway responses in guinea pigs. A somewhat similar analog computer was later developed by Giles et al.[34] It is commercially available from Buxco Electronics, Sharon, CT, and has been successfully used for breath-by-breath analysis of R_L and Cdyn in dogs, monkeys, rats, and guinea pigs.[34-37]

An on-line analog computer (8816A) is also available from Hewlett Packard®, Palo Alto, Ca, for measuring R_L using the electrical subtraction method of Mead and Whittenberger.[7] It carries out breath-by-breath analysis of Cdyn and R_L.

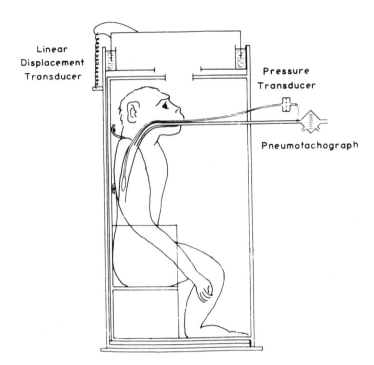

FIGURE 3. The volume displacement body plethysmograph for measuring air-flow, volume, and pleural pressure changes in an anesthetized, spontaneously breathing monkey, showing esophageal balloon and endotracheal tube in place. (From Pare, P. D., Michoud, M. C., and Hogg, J. C., *J. Appl. Physiol.*, 41, 668, 1976. With permission.)

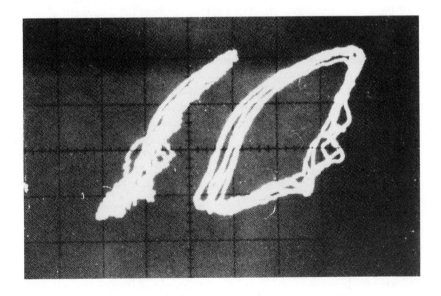

FIGURE 4. X-Y plot of transpulmonary pressure and airflow in an unanesthetized, sponta-neously breathing dog before (right) and after (left), subtracting a signal equal to volume/compliance from transpulmonary pressure. (From Drazen, J. M., Loring, S. H., and Regan, R., *J. Appl. Physiol.*, 40, 110, 1976. With permission.)

For analyzing data after the experiment, time-based records are obtained on a polygraph (Figure 1A) and X-Y plots on a film or paper (Figures 1C and 4). From the time-based records, Cdyn is calculated by dividing the V_T by the transpulmonary pressure difference at end tidal points.

$$Cdyn = V_T/\Delta P_{TP(E)} \tag{1}$$

To calculate Cdyn from the V/P_{TP} plot, the slope of the line joining the end tidal points is determined by measuring the angle θ and taking its tangent. The value of Cdyn is then obtained as follows:

$$Cdyn = \tan\theta \cdot \frac{ml/div.\ of\ V}{cm\ H_2O/div.\ of\ P_{TP}} \tag{2}$$

To calculate inspiratory R_L from the time-based records, flow resistance-related pressure $P_{TP(R)}$ is determined by subtracting elastic recoil-related pressure $P_{TP(E)}$ from P_{TP} and dividing by airflow V_I at midinspiration.

$$R_L\ (insp) = P_{TP(R)}/\dot{V}_I \tag{3}$$

The analysis may be carried out graphically as shown in Figure 1A, or first $P_{TP(E)}$ is determined by dividing the volume change by Cdyn, which is then subtracted from P_{TP} to provide the value of $P_{TP(R)}$. Expiratory R_L could be determined by carrying out similar measurements during the expiratory phase.

The average value of R_L is calculated by dividing the transpulmonary pressure difference, $P_{TP(R)}$ by the difference between inspiratory and expiratory flows at equal volume (midtidal) points, using time-based records of X-Y plots.

$$R_L\ (avg) = \Delta P_{TP(R)}/\Delta\dot{V} \tag{4}$$

V/P_{TP} and $V/\dot{V}$ plots may also be used for separate measurements of inspiratory and expiratory R_L. In that case, pressure and flows are measured either on inspiratory or on expiratory sides of the lines joining the end tidal points. To calculate inspiratory and expiratory R_L from the pressure flow loops shown in Figure 4, the slopes are measured over inspiratory or expiratory phase. The average value of R_L may be determined measuring the average slope of the loop. Measurements are usually made over the linear portion. With the axes as shown in Figure 4, the slope of the loop (with respect to the X axis) provides the value of $1/R_L$. If the slope is measured with respect to the Y axis, it will give the value of R_L.

B. MEASUREMENT OF FUNCTIONAL RESIDUAL CAPACITY AND DETERMINATION OF SPECIFIC LUNG CONDUCTANCE

1. Principles

The method is based on Boyle's law and was described by DuBois et al.[38]

If, for an alveolar pressure drop of ΔP, lung volume V increases by ΔV without any inflow of air, then according to Boyle's law,

$$(P - \Delta P)(V + \Delta V) = P \cdot V \tag{5}$$

Where P is barometric pressure (P_B) minus water vapor pressure (P_{H_2O}) at body temperature.

Solving Equation 5 and dropping the term $\Delta P \cdot \Delta V$, we get

$$\Delta P \cdot V = (P_B - P_{H_2O}) \cdot \Delta V \tag{6}$$

or

$$V = (P_B - P_{H_2O})\Delta V/\Delta P \tag{7}$$

When the airflow of an animal breathing spontaneously in a body plethysmograph is interrupted, the mouth pressure becomes equal to alveolar pressure and ΔP can be recorded at the mouth. This, when related to box volume change (which is equal to lung volume change ΔV), as shown in Equation 7, we get the value of V.

To measure FRC, airflow is interrupted at end expiration.

2. Procedures

A typical setup is shown in Figure 3. The airway opening is occluded at end expiration either by a cork or by using a solenoid value interposed between the endotracheal tube and the pneumotachograph. The pressure change during first inspiratory effort is plotted against the box signal on an X-Y storage oscilloscope. The slope of $\Delta V/\Delta P$ is used to calculate FRC according to Equation 7.

R_L is measured as described in Section II.A. Its reciprocal when divided by FRC gives the value of sG_L.

C. DIRECT MEASUREMENT OF SPECIFIC AIRWAY CONDUCTANCE
1. Principles

If, for a small change in alveolar pressure, ΔP, airflow changes by $\Delta \dot V$, then

$$Raw = \Delta P/\Delta \dot V$$

and

$$Gaw = \Delta \dot V/\Delta P$$

If the measurement is carried out at FRC, then

$$sGaw = \Delta \dot V/\Delta P \cdot FRC \tag{8}$$

Substituting $(P_B - P_{H_2O}) \cdot \Delta V$, for $\Delta P \cdot FRC$ from Equation 6,

$$sGaw = \Delta \dot V/(P_B - P_{H_2O}) \cdot \Delta V \tag{9}$$

ΔV can be determined by making the animal breathe inside a whole-body plethysmograph as the difference between chest volume change (V_1) and air volume respired (V_2).

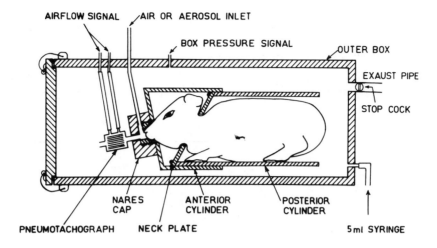

FIGURE 5.   The body plethysmograph for measuring airflow and differential box pressure in an unanesthetized, spontaneously breathing guinea pig. The box pressure calibration port is used for bias current leak after detaching the 5-ml syringe. (From Agrawal, K. P., *Respir. Physiol.*, 43, 23, 1981. With permission.)

2. Procedures
a. Measurement of Body Box Signal and Airflow

The body plethysmographic setup for measuring body box signal and airflow in a guinea pig is shown schematically in Figure 5.[17] The inner two-chambered box is used for housing the animal, isolating its head from the body and attaching the pneumotachograph to the nares. The pneumotachograph is large sized (Fleisch no. 0) and has a very low resistance (0.0025 cm $H_2O \cdot ml^{-1} \cdot s$). A bias current of air is passed through an inlet between the nares and the pneumotachograph to prevent rebreathing. Airflow is measured after zero suppression of the bias current signal.

To measure the difference between the chest volume change and respired volume, $\Delta(V_1 - V_2)$ or ΔV, this two-chambered box is placed inside an outer box. A leak is provided in the outer box for the bias current of air (1 l/min) with a time constant of 0.5 s, which is about ten times the transition period from expiration to inspiration or inspiration to expiration (about 0.05 s).[39]

Box pressure changes are calibrated as volume changes using a syringe. Sharp injections of air are given in the box with the animal inside it, at reduced gain and simulating rapid adiabatic pressure changes occurring during quick transition from one phase of respiration to the other.

b. Analysis of Data

Figure 6 shows the records of airflow, box signal, and volume obtained by integrating airflow. The box signal has two components — one related to the airflow and the other related to the temperature-humidity artifact. At end tidal points, quick transition occurs from one phase of respiration to the other, resulting in a large change in airflow. These are shown in phases I and III in Figure 6. Over these periods there is minimal change in lung volume and therefore the temperature-humidity artifact is negligible. During the remaining part of the respiratory cycle, phases II and IV, lung volume changes are maximal, as are the temperature-humidity artifacts. Airflow is almost constant during these periods.

The relationship between airflow and flow-related box signal is determined by obtaining an X-Y plot of box signal and airflow on a storage oscilloscope as shown in Figure 7. Limbs I and III show the relationship between airflow and airflow-related box signal during transition

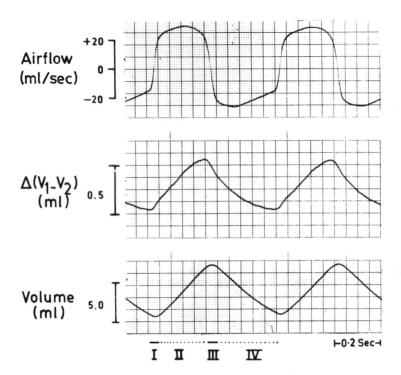

FIGURE 6.   Airflow, $\Delta(V_1 - V_2)$, and tidal volume traces of a guinea pig, breathing inside the body plethysmograph. The solid and broken lines below the records show various phases of a respiratory cycle. During phase I, transition from expiration to inspiration occurs in the airflow waveform. It is accompanied by a slight increase in $\Delta(V_1 - V_2)$. Change in volume is bidirectional and is very small. Phase II shows almost constant inspiratory flow and gradually increasing $\Delta(V_1 - V_2)$ along with inspiration. Phase III shows transition of airflow from inspiration to expiration with a fall in $\Delta(V_1 - V_2)$ and a negligible change in volume. Phase IV shows almost constant expiratory flow and gradually decreasing $\Delta(V_1 - V_2)$ with continued expiration. ($V_1 - V_2$) during phases I and III is practically free from ''temperature-humidity artifact'' because of minimal volume changes. (From Agrawal, K. P., *Respir. Physiol.*, 42, 23, 1981. With permission.)

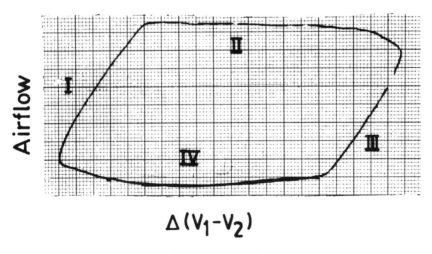

FIGURE 7.   X-Y loop of $\Delta(V_1 - V_2)$ and airflow signals. Limbs I to IV represent phases I to IV shown in Figure 6. (From Agrawal, K. P., *Respir. Physiol.*, 43, 23, 1981. With permission.)

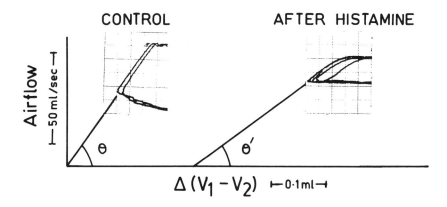

FIGURE 8.   The rising limbs of X-Y loops before and after histamine inhalation. The slopes of these limbs are determined by measuring the angles θ and θ′ using a protractor and taking their tangent values. (From Agrawal, K. P., *Respir. Physiol.*, 43, 23, 1981. With permission.)

from expiration to inspiration (phase I) and from inspiration to expiration (phase III), respectively.

sGaw at FRC is determined by substituting the slope of limb I for $\Delta\dot{V}/\Delta V$ in Equation 9.

$$sGaw = \tan\theta \cdot \frac{ml/s/div\ of\ \dot{V}}{ml/div\ of\ \Delta(V_1 - V_2)} \cdot \frac{1}{P_B - P_{H_2O}} \tag{10}$$

The slope of limb I is measured on the screen using a protractor as shown in Figure 8. Slopes should be measured between 24 and 66° so that a 1° error in their measurement does not cause more than a 5% error in the value of tan θ and therefore of sGaw.

It may be mentioned here that the rising limb of the box signal airflow loop (Figure 7, limb I) is similar to what Brody and DuBois[9] had used for calculating airway resistance in cats.

Lorino et al.[40] have recently developed a computer program for on-line measurement of sGaw using this technique.[43]

III. MEASUREMENT OF AIRWAY RESPONSE

A. AIRWAY CHALLENGE
For eliciting an airway response, the excitatory substance may be delivered parenterally or by inhalation. The jugular vein is commonly used for intravenous infusion. An indwelling catheter is ideal for this purpose. During injection by this route the drug reaches respiratory bronchioles, alveolar ducts, and lung parenchyma via the pulmonary circulation. However, to see the effect of the drug on the tracheobronchial tree, the injection must be made directly in the left atrium so that it reaches the airways via bronchial arteries.

Inhalation challenge is the most commonly used method for studying airway responses. If the head of the animal is outside the body plethysmograph, aerosol can be delivered through a hood as shown in Figure 2. A method for delivering aerosol to a spontaneously breathing guinea pig inside a body plethysmograph is shown in Figure 5. The exhaust is opened during aerosol delivery. Airflow and V_T can be monitored during challenge by suppressing the aerosol current signal. Care should be taken so that the aerosol current plus the airflow of the animal do not exceed the linear range of the pneumotachograph. Monitoring of V_T during the period of airway challenge is essential for estimating the amount of inhaled

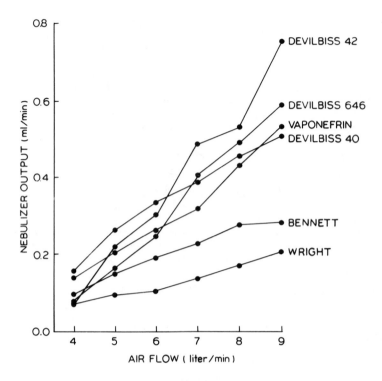

FIGURE 9.   The output of some commonly used nebulizers at different flow rates.
(From Ryan, G., Dolovich, M. B., Obminski, G., Cockcroft, D. W., Juniper, E.,
Hargreave, F. E., and Newhouse, M. T., *J. Allergy Clin. Immunol.*, 67, 156, 1981.
With permission.)

aerosol, if required. The other information needed for this calculation is the output of the
nebulizer, which should be measured for individual nebulizers. This can be done by weighing
the nebulizer before and after the challenge. Output of some of the commonly used nebulizers
at different flow rates is shown in Figure 9.[41] Usual operating flow rates, aerosol particle
size, and outputs of these nebulizers are shown in Table 1.[41]

If the experiment does not specifically require measurement of airway response to
parenterally administered drugs, airway challenge should be carried out by inhalation route.
The method is noninvasive, and repeated measurements are possible for checking long-term
reproducibility. Not only that, long-term effects of various treatments which influence airway
responsiveness can be evaluated using a noninvasive method of measuring airway responsiveness.

B. BRONCHOCONSTRICTOR DOSAGE

The starting dose of a bronchoconstrictor should be sufficiently low so that a minimal
response is obtained in the most sensitive animal. In guinea pigs, 30 s inhalation during
spontaneous breathing of an aerosol of a 0.16 mg/ml histamine solution generated by a
DeVilbiss 646 nebulizer at 20 psi is a fairly low starting dose. Challenges are made by
doubling concentrations of the drug till the desired response is obtained or a maximum of
either the drug or the response is reached.

C. MEASUREMENT OF CHANGES IN FLOW RESISTANCE AND DYNAMIC
COMPLIANCE

An on-line analysis system should be used for breath-by-breath analysis of changes in
R_L and Cdyn if these parameters are to be measured simultaneously. Measurement of changes

TABLE 1
Nebulizer Output and Particle Size

| | Operating flow rate (l/min) | Nebulizer output (ml/min) (mean ± 1 SD) | Aerosol particle size | |
			AMMD (μm)	g
Wright				
A	7	0.130 ± 0.006	1.32	2.11
B	7	0.121 ± 0.006	0.75	1.20
C	7	0.134 ± 0.005	1.48	2.34
DeVilbiss 40				
A	6	0.378 ± 0.015	1.85	2.50
B	6	0.378 ± 0.012	3.50	3.00
C	6	0.384 ± 0.012	1.50	2.70
DeVilbiss 42				
A	6	0.299 ± 0.011	4.40	3.28
B	6	0.290 ± 0.016	2.90	2.24
DeVilbiss 646				
A	6	0.313 ± 0.009	2.70	2.87
B	6	0.247 ± 0.021	2.75	2.39
C	6	0.282 ± 0.017	2.37	2.95
Bennett® Twin	7	0.222 ± 0.005	3.60	3.47
Vaponefrin®	6	0.246 ± 0.006	5.20	3.59
Monaghan 670	8	1.59 ± 0.189	4.30	2.10

Note: AMMD = Aerodynamic mass median diameter; g = geometric standard deviation; A, B, C = different nebulizers.

in R_L using the electrical subtraction method, in Cdyn using the V/P_{TP} plot, and in sGaw using the open-loop method may be carried out by simply measuring and comparing the slopes of X-Y plots before and after airway challenge with a protractor attached to the oscilloscope (Figure 8).

D. DOSE-RESPONSE CURVE AND DETERMINATION OF AIRWAY RESPONSIVENESS

To generate a dose-response curve, log doses are plotted on the X axis and resistance or dynamic compliance values expressed as a percentage of the control are plotted on the Y axis. Airway responsiveness is determined by calculating the dose of the drug that produces a threshold change in flow resistance or dynamic compliance, such as a 50 or 100% increase in R_L or sRaw, a 35 or 50% fall in sG_L or sGaw, and a 35 or 50% fall in Cdyn.

When a finite response is obtained as with inhaled ouabain challenge, airway responsiveness may also be determined by calculating the dose to produce a half-maximal response. Agrawal and Hyatt[39] observed good correlations between doses of inhaled ouabain to produce a 15% fall in sGaw (ouabain ED_{15}) and doses to produce a half-maximal response on two occasions 3 d apart in spite of an up to threefold change in sensitivity (Figure 10). This suggests that a threshold dose could be as good a measure of airway responsiveness as a half-maximal dose.

IV. SELECTION OF A SUITABLE METHOD FOR MEASURING AIRWAY RESPONSES IN DIFFERENT EXPERIMENTAL ANIMALS

The selection of the method depends on the purpose of the experiment. If the aim is to

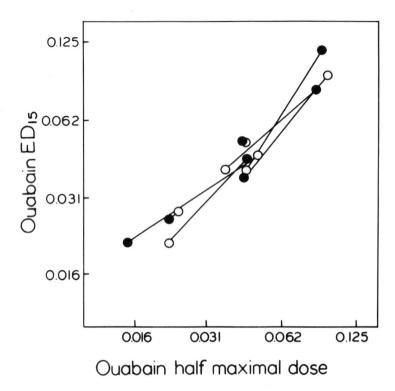

FIGURE 10.   Relationship between the doses of inhaled ouabain producing 50% of the maximum percent fall in sGaw (half maximal dose) and the doses producing a 15% decrease in the baseline value of sGaw (ED$_{15}$), determined twice in seven guinea pigs, 3 d apart (●, day 1, r = 0.96; ○, day 4, r = 0.97). Individual guinea pigs show an up to threefold change in airway sensitivity (●—○), but the relationship between half maximal dose and ED$_{15}$ does not change. (Based on data from Agrawal, K. P. and Hyatt, R. E., *J. Appl. Physiol.*, 60, 2089, 1986. With permission.)

study the responses of airways to an antigen or a given drug, both flow resistance, and dynamic compliance should be measured to determine the site and the extent of airway constriction. On the other hand, if the aim is to determine the airway responsiveness in a given animal or to see the distribution of airway responsiveness in a given species, the sensitivity and reproducibility of the parameter and the suitability of the method for its measurement for long-term studies should be considered. Available information on some animals commonly used as models of experimental asthma — guinea pig, dog, rat, monkey and sheep — is presented here.

A. GUINEA PIGS

In guinea pigs using the method of Amdur and Mead,[3] Stein et al.[42] found a disproportionately larger fall in Cdyn than an increase in R_L in response to inhaled histamine. Douglas et al.[27,33] reported similar results. On the other hand, using the same technique, Amdur[43] observed changes of equal magnitude in both parameters. The discrepancy in their results is difficult to understand.

Using the dose of inhaled histamine to produce a 50% fall in Cdyn (ED$_{50}$ Cdyn) as a measure of airway responsiveness, Douglas et al.[33] observed about a 100 times variation in ED$_{50}$ Cdyn in 131 guinea pigs studied by them (0.1 to 10 mg/ml histamine base). The variation was about 30 times (0.2 to 5.8 mg/ml) in a smaller group (n = 10). Similar results were obtained by Nath et al.[44] and Agrawal and Hyatt,[39] who observed 60 and 30 times variations in the dose of histamine to produce a 50% fall in sGaw. However, the most

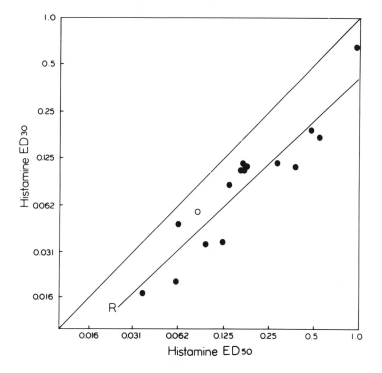

FIGURE 11. Relationship between histamine ED_{50} and ED_{30} in 16 guinea pigs (r = 0.92). The regression line R is shifted to the right and is almost parallel to the line of identity. In animal #12, shown here by the open circle, the value of histamine ED_{30} has been corrected from 0.105 to 0.056. (Based on data from Agrawal, K. P. and Hyatt, R. E., *J. Appl. Physiol.*, 60, 2089, 1986. With permission.)

sensitive guinea pigs in these series needed somewhat higher doses of histamine (0.40 and 0.36 mg/ml) to produce a 50% fall in sGaw. Doses in the range of 0.1 to 0.2 mg/ml produced only a 30% fall in sGaw in the most sensitive animals.[39] A highly significant correlation (r = 0.92) was, however, observed between log doses of histamine to produce 30 and 50% falls in sGaw, and the doses of histamine producing a 50% fall in sGaw were about two times the doses producing a 30% fall as shown in Figure 11.

Douglas et al.[27] studied the reproducibility of doses of inhaled and intravenous histamine for producing a fall of up to about 70% in Cdyn over a few hours. Reproducible results were obtained with inhaled histamine only (the number of animals was not given). Agrawal and Hyatt[39] studied short- as well as long-term reproducibility of the dose of histamine to produce a 50% fall in sGaw and obtained highly reproducible values. Their results are shown in Figure 12. While hardly any change occurred within 2 h, not more than twofold variability was observed over a period of 2 to 4 weeks.

Long-term repeated measurements are, however, not possible using the invasive technique of measuring Cdyn, and therefore Popa et al.[45] and Douglas et al.[46] used a 10% fall in V_T in place of a 50% fall in Cdyn as a threshold response. Moreover, placing a catheter in the pleural cavity increases R_L, probably due to lung collapse.[10] Direct measurement of sGaw, on the other hand, can be carried out noninvasively and because of its good sensitivity and high reproducibility is most suitable for long-term repetitive studies.

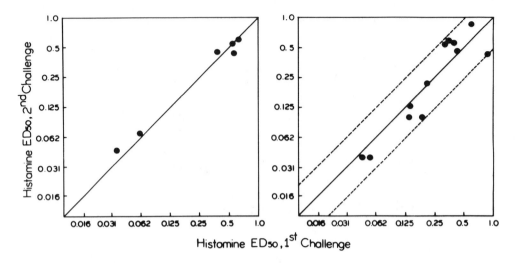

FIGURE 12.   The reproducibility of histamine ED_{50} in 6 guinea pigs after 10 min to 2 h (left), and in 12 guinea pigs after 2 to 4 weeks (right). The results are highly reproducible within 2 h but show an up to twofold variability (shown by broken lines) over a period of 2 to 4 weeks. (Based on data from Agrawal, K. P. and Hyatt, R. E., *J. Appl. Physiol.*, 60, 2089, 1986. With permission.)

B. RATS

Distribution of airway responsiveness in inbred rats was studied by Wang et al.[47] in response to methacholine challenge. Studies were carried out in anesthetized rats. Pleural pressure changes was measured using an esophageal catheter and airflow by a pneumotachograph connected to a plexiglass box fitted over the muzzle. V_T was obtained by integrating the flow signal. R_L was determined by using the isovolume method as shown in Figure 1A. Rats were found to be comparatively insensitive to methacholine and some of them (23 out of 70) did not show even a 50% increase in R_L in response to 30 s inhalation of an aerosol generated from 128 mg/ml methacholine solution. Using the doses of methacholine, producing a 50% increase in R_L over the control value ($ED_{150}R_L$), a log normal frequency distribution of airway responsiveness was observed in 47 rats which responded to 2 to 128 mg/ml methacholine. Assigning an arbitrary $EO_{150} R_L$ value of 256 mg/ml to the nonresponders, these workers reported a 128 times variation in the airway responsiveness of the least and the most sensitive animals.

Short-term reproducibility of airway responsiveness was studied on two to four different days in five reactive and two nonreactive rats, and up to a fivefold variability was observed. Long-term reproducibility was studied after 3 months and the results showed even greater variability. Whether this is due to high day-to-day variability of airway responsiveness in individual rats or to some inaccuracy in the measurement is difficult to say.

These workers did not monitor changes in Cdyn. However, equal falls in Cdyn and G_L were observed in normal rats by Casey and Abboa-Offei[48] in response to antibody against IgE. These workers used a method similar to the one described by Dennis et al.[32] Brunet et al.[36] also observed equivalent changes in Cdyn and R_L in response to serotonin aerosol. Airflow in this study was measured with a pneumotachograph attached to a tracheal cannula, and volume was measured by integrating the flow signal. Cdyn and R_L were computed breath by breath using a Buxco respiratory analyzer.

The method described by Wang et al.[47] is noninvasive and suitable for long-term, repeated measurements. However, determination of Cdyn should also be carried out.

C. DOGS

Early observations in dogs were made by Giles et al.[34] They measured intrapleural pressure with a cannula inserted into the pleural cavity and airflow with a pneumotachograph attached to a tracheal cannula. V_T was obtained by integration of the flow. Cdyn and R_L were determined using an analog computer at end- and midtidal volumes, respectively, as shown in Figure 1A. They observed about a 35% fall in Cdyn and a 110% increase in R_L in response to fixed doses of inhaled histamine. Snapper et al.[25] measured the doses of histamine aerosol in 102 anesthetized, spontaneously breathing mongrel dogs to produce a 35% fall in Cdyn and a 100% increase in R_L. Intrapleural pressure was measured using an esophageal balloon, flow with a pneumotachograph attached to an endotracheal tube, and volume by integration of the flow signal. Cdyn and R_L were determined at midtidal volume using X-Y plots as shown in Figure 1C. The lowest dose of histamine to produce a 35% fall in Cdyn in any dog (0.09 mg/ml) was almost equal to the dose which produced a 100% increase in R_L (0.11 mg/ml). The highest doses were 4.51 and 6.63 mg/ml (50 and 60 times), respectively. These observations show that in dogs, both Cdyn and R_L can be used for measuring airway responsiveness, though the increase in R_L is almost twice the fall in Cdyn at any given dose (a 35% fall in Cdyn is equivalent to a 54% increase in dynamic elasticity).

Snapper et al.[25] also carried out repetitive studies in some of these dogs over a period of up to 20 months and got highly reproducible results. The method is thus suitable for long-term studies.

D. MONKEYS

In monkeys, Kelly et al.,[35] using an esophageal catheter for recording intrapleural pressure changes, an endotracheal tube connected to a pneumotachograph to measure airflow and V_T, and an analog computer as described by Giles et al.,[34] observed that changes occurred in Cdyn as well as in R_L in response to a fixed dose of inhaled histamine, but the increase in R_L was somewhat more pronounced (about 1.6 times) than the fall in Cdyn. Michoud et al.,[49] using the setup shown in Figure 3 and the electrical subtraction method of measuring R_L (Figure 4), found that R_L and Cdyn were equally sensitive parameters for measuring the airway response to histamine, methacholine, and antigen in a mixed population of *Ascaris suum*-sensitive (n = 5) and -insensitive (n = 3) monkeys. However, they preferred to use a 50% increase in R_L for determining the threshold doses of histamine and methacholine. A 60 times variation (0.08 to 5.0 mg/ml) was found for histamine and 50 times (0.02 to 1.0 mg/ml) for methacholine. In a later study using the same method of measurement, Paré and Nicholls[50] observed only an eight times variation (0.44 to 3.3 mg/ml) in the doses of histamine producing a 50% increase in R_L in ten monkeys. However, a 24 times variation (0.47 to 11.3 mg/ml) was found when doses were determined for a 50% fall in Cdyn. Four monkeys were sensitive to *A. suum*, but this did not influence the airway sensitivity to histamine.

Measurements were carried out twice in two monkeys (interval not mentioned) by Michoud et al.[49] Highly reproducible results were obtained. The method does not involve any surgical intervention and is suitable for long-term use.

E. SHEEP

Studies in sheep using different methods of measuring Cdyn and R_L have produced conflicting results. Abraham et al.,[51] using an esophageal balloon for measuring pleural pressure changes and an endotracheal tube connected to a spirometer for measuring V_T and airflow as described by Wanner and Reinhart,[23] observed changes in R_L in response to a fixed dose of carbachol in normal as well as in allergic sheep. On the other hand, Snapper et al.,[26] using a chronically implanted 4 × 3 cm silastic envelope in the pleural cavity for measuring pleural pressure changes and a plethysmograph for measuring V_T and airflow, have reported higher sensitivity of Cdyn than R_L for measuring airway responses to carbachol as well as histamine. However, looking at their data it is evident that a somewhat higher sensitivity of Cdyn (1.6 times) for measuring airway responsiveness to carbachol is simply due to wrong choices of threshold values of fall in Cdyn (35%) and increase in R_L (100%). If doses of carbachol were determined for equivalent changes in Cdyn and R_L, i.e., a 35% fall in Cdyn and a 50 or 55% increase in R_L, the results could have been similar to those of Abraham et al.[51] For histamine, these workers have reported threshold doses only for a 35% fall in Cdyn (0.05 to >50 mg/ml). They observed a 100% or more increase in R_L in only 17 of the 55 sheep. If they had used a 50% increase in R_L, probably the results would have been different. It is therefore difficult to say whether or not Cdyn is a more sensitive parameter to measure airway responses to histamine.

Wanner and Reinhart[23] measured changes in R_L and sG_L in response to methacholine in sensitized and nonsensitized sheep. In sensitized sheep they observed comparatively larger changes in sG_L. Nonsensitized sheep did not respond to methacholine challenge. A similar trend was observed by Wanner et al.[20] while measuring antigen-induced bronchospasm by determining changes in R_L and sG_L. This is because an increase in R_L is partly offset by an increase in FRC. On the other hand, sG_L is independent of lung volume and its determination is more suitable for measuring airway responses. However, the determination of sG_L is a two-step process and not as good as direct determination of sGaw. Measurement of sGaw may therefore be preferable and could be carried out using the same setup by making the animal breathe within the body plethysmograph.

The reproducibility of the fall in Cdyn in response to histamine, either infused through a pulmonary artery or delivered by aerosol, was examined by Hutchison et al.[52] in three sheep on three different days within a week. Each group had two sheep (one was common). Results were quite reproducible for both the routes, but more so with pulmonary artery infusion.

Within-day reproducibility of airway responsiveness was examined for histamine in 18 sheep by Snapper et al.[26] Highly reproducible results were obtained for doses of histamine producing a 35% fall in Cdyn and for doses of carbachol producing either a 35% fall in Cdyn or a 100% increase in R_L.

These results show that chronically instrumented unanesthetized sheep are suitable for long-term studies. However, as the data obtained by using esophageal balloon and endotracheal tube in intact conscious sheep differ markedly, more observations are needed to draw any definite conclusion.

ACKNOWLEDGMENT

I thank Mr. S. K. S. Chauhan for his help in the preparation of this manuscript.

REFERENCES

1. **Macklem, P. T. and Mead, J.,** Resistance of central and peripheral airways measured by a retrograde catheter, *J. Appl. Physiol.,* 22, 395, 1967.
2. **Woolcock, A. J., Vincent, N. J., and Macklem, P. T.,** Frequency dependence of compliance as a test for obstruction in small airways, *J. Clin. Invest.,* 48, 1097, 1969.
3. **Amdur, M. O. and Mead, J.,** Mechanics of respiration in unanesthetized guinea pigs, *Am. J. Physiol.,* 192, 364, 1958.
4. **Neergaard, K. V. and Wirz, K.,** Über eine Methode zur Messung der Lungenelastizität am lebenden Menschen, insbesondere beim Emphysem, *Z. Klin. Med.,* 105, 35, 1927.
5. **Neergaard, K. V. and Wirz, K.,** Die Messung der Strömungswiderstände in den Atemwegen des Menschen, insbesondere bei Asthma und Emphysem, *Z. Klin. Med.,* 105, 51, 1927.
6. **Cook, C. D., Sutherland, J. M., Segal, S., Cherry, R. B., Mead, J., McIlroy, M. B., and Smith, C. A.,** Studies on respiratory physiology in the new born infant. III. Measurements of mechanics of respiration, *J. Clin. Invest.,* 36, 440, 1957.
7. **Mead, J. and Whittenberger, J. L.,** Physical properties of human lungs measured during spontaneous respiration, *J. Appl. Physiol.,* 5, 779, 1953.
8. **Frank, N. R., Mead, J., and Whittenberger, J. L.,** Comparative sensitivity of four methods for measuring changes in respiratory flow resistance in man, *J. Appl. Physiol.,* 31, 934, 1971.
9. **Brody, A. W. and DuBois, A. B.,** Determination of tissue, airway and total resistance to respiration in cats, *J. Appl. Physiol.,* 9, 213, 1956.
10. **Mead, J.,** Control of respiratory frequency, *J. Appl. Physiol.,* 15, 325, 1960.
11. **Hull, W. E. and Long, E. C.,** Respiratory impedence and volume flow at high frequency in dogs, *J. Appl. Physiol.,* 16, 439, 1961.
12. **Ferris, B. G., Jr., Mead, J., Opie, L. H.,** Partitioning of respiratory flow resistance in man, *J. Appl. Physiol.,* 19, 653, 1964.
13. **Fisher, A. B., DuBois, A. B., and Hyde, R. W.,** Evaluation of the forced oscillation technique for the determination of resistance to breathing, *J. Clin. Invest.,* 47, 2045, 1968.
14. **DuBois, A. B., Botelho, S. Y., and Comroe, J. H., Jr.,** A new method for measuring airway resistance in man using a body plethysmograph: values in normal subjects and in patients with respiratory disease, *J. Clin. Invest.,* 35, 327, 1956.
15. **Johanson, W. G. and Pierce, A. K.,** A non-invasive technique for measurement of airway conductance in small animals, *J. Appl. Physiol.,* 30, 146, 1971.
16. **Pennock, B. E., Cox, C. P., Rogers, R. M., Cain, W. A., and Wells, J. H.,** A non-invasive technique for measurement of changes in specific airway resistance, *J. Appl. Physiol.,* 46, 399, 1979.
17. **Agrawal, K. P.,** Specific airway conductance in guinea pigs: normal values and histamine induced fall, *Respir. Physiol.,* 43, 23, 1981.
18. **Drazen, J. M., Loring, S. H., and Venugopalan, C.,** Lung volumes after antigen infusion in the guinea pig in vitro. Effects of vagal section, *J. Appl. Physiol.,* 45, 957, 1978.
19. **Paré, P. D., Michoud, M. C., Boucher, R. C., and Hogg, J. C.,** Pulmonary effects of acute and chronic antigen exposure of immunized guinea pigs, *J. Appl. Physiol.,* 46, 346, 1979.
20. **Wanner, A., Mezey, R. J., Reinhart, M. E., and Eyre, P.,** Antigen-induced bronchospasm in conscious sheep, *J. Appl. Physiol.,* 47, 917, 1979.
21. **Hirshman, C. A., Leon, D. A., and Bergman, N. A.,** The basenji-greyhound dog: antigen-induced changes in lung volumes, *Respir. Physiol.,* 43, 377, 1981.
22. **Briscoe, W. A. and DuBois, A. B.,** The relationship between airway resistance, airway conductance and lung volume in subjects of different age and body size, *J. Clin. Invest.,* 37, 1279, 1958.
23. **Wanner, A. and Reinhart, M. E.,** Respiratory mechanics in conscious sheep: response to methacholine, *J. Appl. Physiol.,* 44, 479, 1978.
24. **Hirshman, C. A., Malley, A., and Downes, H.,** The basenji-greyhound dog model of asthma: reactivity to *Ascaris suum,* citric acid and methacholine, *J. Appl. Physiol.,* 49, 953, 1980.
25. **Snapper, J. R., Drazen, J. M., Loring, S. H., Schneider, W., and Ingram, R. H., Jr.,** Distribution of pulmonary responsiveness to aerosol histamine in dogs, *J. Appl. Physiol.,* 44, 738, 1978.
26. **Snapper, J. R., Lefferts, P. L., Stecenko, A. A., Hinson, J. M.,, and Dyer, E. L.,** Bronchial responsiveness to nonantigenic bronchoconstrictors in awake sheep, *J. Appl. Physiol.,* 61, 752, 1986.
27. **Douglas, J. S., Dennis, M. W., Ridgway, P., and Bouhuys, A.,** Airway dilatation and constriction in spontaneously breathing guinea pigs, *J. Pharmacol. Exp. Ther.,* 180, 98, 1972.
28. **Jaeger, M. J. and Otis, A. B.,** Effect of compressibility of alveolar gas on dynamics and work of breathing, *J. Appl. Physiol.,* 19, 83, 1964.
29. **Agrawal, K. P.,** A non-invasive technique to study anaphylactic reaction and airway reactivity in guinea pigs, *Aspects Allergy Appl. Immunol.,* 8, 37, 1975.

30. **Pare, P. D., Michoud, M. C., and Hogg, J. C.,** Lung mechanics following antigen challenge of *Ascaris suum*-sensitive rhesus monkeys, *J. Appl. Physiol.,* 41, 668, 1976.

31. **Drazen, J. M., Loring, S. H., and Regan, R.,** Validation of an automated determination of pulmonary resistance by electrical subtraction, *J. Appl. Physiol.,* 40, 110, 1976.

32. **Dennis, M. W., Douglas, J. S., Casby, J. U., Stolwijk, J. A. J., and Bouhuys, A.,** On-line analog computer for dynamic lung compliance and pulmonary resistance, *J. Appl. Physiol.,* 26, 248, 1969.

33. **Douglas, J. S., Dennis, M. W., Ridgway, P., and Bouhuys, A.,** Airway constriction in guinea pigs: interaction of histamine and autonomic drugs, *J. Pharmacol. Exp. Ther.,* 184, 169, 1973.

34. **Giles, R. E., Finkel, M. P., and Mazurowski, J.,** Use of an analog on-line computer for the evaluation of pulmonary resistance and dynamic compliance in the anesthetized dog, *Arch. Int. Pharmacodyn. Ther.,* 194, 213, 1971.

35. **Kelly, J. F., Cugell, D. W., Patterson, R., and Harris, K. E.,** Acute airway obstruction in rhesus monkeys induced by pharmacologic and immunologic stimuli, *J. Lab. Clin. Med.,* 83, 738, 1974.

36. **Brunet, G., Piechuta, H., Hamel, R., Holme, G., and Fordhutchinson, A. W.,** Respiratory responses to leukotrienes and biogenic amines in normal and hyperreactive rats, *J. Immunol.,* 131, 434, 1983.

37. **Silbaugh, S. A. and Mauderly, J. L.,** Noninvasive detection of airway constriction in awake guinea pigs, *J. Appl. Physiol.,* 56, 1666, 1984.

38. **DuBois, A. B., Botelho, S. Y., Bedell, G. N., Jr., Marshall, R., and Comroe, J. H., Jr.,** A rapid plethysmographic method for measuring thoracic gas volume: a comparison with nitrogen washout method for measuring functional residual capacity in normal subjects, *J. Clin. Invest.,* 35, 322, 1956.

39. **Agrawal, K. P. and Hyatt, R. E.,** Airway responses to inhaled ouabain and histamine in conscious guinea pigs, *J. Appl. Physiol.,* 60, 2089, 1986.

40. **Lorino, A. M., Mariette, C., Lorino, H., Macquin, I., Rey, P., and Harf, A.,** A microcomputer based system for real-time calculation of airway conductance in awake guinea pigs, *Comput. Methods Programmes Biomed.,* 20, 161, 1985.

41. **Ryan, G., Dolovich, M. B., Obminski, G., Cockcroft, D. W., Juniper, E., Hargreave, F. E., and Newhouse, M. T.,** Standardization of inhalation provocation tests: influence of nebulizer output, particle size, and method of inhalation, *J. Allergy Clin. Immunol.,* 67, 156, 1981.

42. **Stein, M., Schiavi, R. C., Ottenberg, P., and Hamilton, C.,** The mechanical properties of the lungs in experimental asthma in the guinea pig, *J. Allergy,* 32, 8, 1961.

43. **Amdur, M. O.,** The respiratory response of guinea pig to histamine aerosol, *Arch. Environ. Health,* 13, 29, 1966.

44. **Nath, P., Joshi, A. P., and Agrawal, K. P.,** Biochemical correlates of airway hyperreactivity in guinea pigs: role of lysophosphatidylcholine, *J. Allergy Clin. Immunol.,* 72, 351, 1983.

45. **Popa, V., Douglas, J. S., and Bouhuys, A.,** Airway responses to histamine, acetylcholine, and propranolol in anaphylactic hypersensitivity in guinea pigs, *J. Allergy Clin. Immunol.,* 51, 344, 1973.

46. **Douglas, J. S., Pamela, R., and Brink, C.,** Airway responses of the guinea pig *in vivo* and *in vitro, J. Pharmacol. Exp. Ther.,* 116, 1977.

47. **Wang, C. G., Dimaria, G., Bates, H. T., Guttman, R. D., and Martin, J. G.,** Methacholine-induced airway reactivity in inbred rats, *J. Appl. Physiol.,* 61, 2180, 1986.

48. **Casey, F. B. and Abboa-Offei, B. E.,** Pulmonary function changes in normal rats induced by antibody against rat IgE, *Clin. Exp. Immunol.,* 36, 473, 1979.

49. **Michoud, M. C., Pare, P. D., Boucher, R., and Hogg, J. C.,** Airway responses to histamine and methacholine in *Ascaris suum*-allergic rhesus monkeys, *J. Appl. Physiol.,* 45, 846, 1978.

50. **Paré, P. D. and Nicholls, I.,** Bronchial response to histamine after inhaled propranolol and atropine in monkeys, *J. Allergy Clin. Immunol.,* 69, 213, 1982.

51. **Abraham, W. M., Oliver, W., Jr., Matthew, J. W., King, M. M., Wanner, A., and Sackner, M. A.,** Differences in airway reactivity in normal and allergic sheep after exposure to sulfur dioxide, *J. Appl. Physiol.,* 51, 1651, 1981.

52. **Hutchison, A. A., Brigham, K. L., and Snapper, J. R.,** Effect of histamine on lung mechanics in sheep, *Am. Rev. Respir. Dis.,* 126, 1025, 1982.

Chapter 8

CLINICAL METHODS TO EVALUATE AIRWAY REACTIVITY

Russell J. Hopp, Againdra K. Bewtra, and Robert G. Townley

TABLE OF CONTENTS

I. Relationship to Bronchial Asthma 168

II. Indications for Testing 168

III. Measurement of Response 169

IV. Factors Influencing Response 169
    A. Drugs...170
    B. Aerosol Generation...170
    C. Technical Factors..171

V. Expression of Results 171

VI. Reproducibility 172

VII. Pharmacologic Challenges 172
    A. Histamine and Methacholine 172
        1. Preparation...172
        2. Methods 172
    B. Other Pharmacologic Agents 173

VIII. Physiologic Challenges 173
    A. Exercise 174
    B. Cold-Air Hyperventilation...174
    C. Ultrasonic Nebulized Distilled Water Challenge........................175

IX. Allergen Challenge 175
    A. Method...175

Acknowledgments...176

References..176

I. RELATIONSHIP TO BRONCHIAL ASTHMA

Asthma is recognized clinically by reversible airway obstruction and airway hyperresponsiveness. Airway hyperresponsiveness is essential to the definition of asthma, and an understanding of its mechanism is crucial to the elucidation of the pathogenesis of asthma.[1-4] The severity of asthma is correlated with the degree of hyperresponsiveness.[1-4] In asthma, airway hyperresponsiveness appears to arise from both genetic and acquired mechanisms, but increased airway responsiveness can be temporarily associated with exposure to environmental stimuli such as allergens, infection, or ozone.[5]

Bronchial challenges, using both physiologic and pharmacologic methods, have provided an important tool to advance the understanding of airway reactivity and the pathogenesis of bronchial asthma. The purpose of such testing includes diagnosis, occupational screening, research, epidemiology, and evaluation of the efficacy of various pharmacologic agents for the treatment of asthma.[5-7] Precise inhalation methods are essential for the study of airway hyperresponsiveness, regardless of the purpose of such testing.

Although the asthmatic individual shows hyperresponsiveness to a wide variety of physiologic and pharmacologic stimuli, it is quite certain there are important differences in the mechanism whereby these stimuli induced bronchoconstriction. Methacholine or histamine induce direct smooth-muscle constriction; exercise, inhalation of cold dry air, or inhalation of ultrasonically nebulized distilled water (UNDW) appear to do this by more indirect mechanisms, including mast cell mediator release. Furthermore, the response to the pharmacologic stimuli provides a more sensitive parameter than those of the physiologic stimuli. The latter, however, provides a higher degree of specificity. Thus, all current asthmatics respond to methacholine inhalation, whereas only 75 to 80% will respond to the various physiologic stimuli to the point of resulting in a 20% decrease in the 1-s forced expiratory volume (FEV_1).[3,8,9]

The differences between the pharmacologic and physiologic bronchial challenges are both qualitative and quantitative. Tests with exercise, inhaled water, or hyperventilation of cold dry air will not produce a response of 20% fall in the FEV_1 in subjects without asthma even with the maximum stimulus. In contrast, pharmacologic challenges with methacholine or histamine can produce significant airway narrowing in some subjects without asthma.

II. INDICATIONS FOR TESTING

The primary clinical indication for inhalation challenge with methacholine, histamine, UNDW, or cold-air hyperventilation (CAHC) is to identify the presence of bronchial reactivity, an essential component of the asthmatic state.[1,6,7,10-15] Most patients presenting with asthma have classical symptoms, and diagnostic bronchial challenges are not necessary. However, a patient may present with cough or dypsnea as his only symptom and have normal physical findings and spirometry. In these situations a bronchial challenge may be useful as a clinical test. A negative methacholine challenge test rules out current bronchial asthma and would guide the clinician to consider other causes of bronchial disease such as tumor, bronchiectasis, or possibly chronic bronchitis. The indications for antigen challenge and for pharmacologic challenge are listed in Table 1.

Various manufacturing and mining operations, exposure to agricultural environments, and animal handling may be associated with a high rate of occupational asthma. In these situations inhalation challenge may be valuable to determine and identify those workers who are at potential risk for occupational asthma because of preexisting bronchial responsiveness.

Bronchial provocation tests may provide a valuable test of drug efficacy. They are not, however, a substitute for clinical trials.

TABLE 1
Clinical Indications for Inhalation Challenge

Antigen challenge
1.   Clarification of the role of specific allergens in asthma, especially when other diagnostic criteria are negative. It should be recognized that a false-positive reaction is possible, that is, allergic patients may have a bronchial response to antigens that are clinically unrelated to their having asthma. Conversely, antigen challenge may be useful to clarify the nonrelevance of cutaneous or serum tests when the history is equivocal. Provocation with antigen should have clinical relevance, such as determining the need for immunotherapy or specific avoidance.
2.   Evaluation of new drugs for asthma. All new antiasthma medications should be tested against allergen challenges.
3.   Clarification of the mechanism of asthma.
   a.   Antigen challenges have been used extensively to study mediators of allergic asthma. Histamine, leukotriene LTC_4, LTD_4, NCF, and PAF release have been documented after antigen challenge.
   b.   Antigen challenge helps define the immediate and delayed reactions. The immediate reaction begins within minutes, reaches a peak within 10 to 20 min, and is clear within 1.5 to 3 h. The immediate reaction is caused by smooth-muscle constriction as a result of endogenous mediator release. The early response is determined by the level of airway responsiveness to histamine or methacholine, the dose of antigen, and the level of specific IgE antibodies. The late response usually begins between 3 to 4 h, peaks between 8 and 12 h, and may last 24 to 36 h. The late responses are associated with prolonged increases in airway responsiveness to histamine and methacholine. To define, when appropriate, the natural history of antigen sensitivity when there is no immunologic intervention or, conversely, for evaluation of the therapeutic effect of immunotherapy.
4.   For the evaluation of new or unrecognized allergens or provocative agents in pulmonary disease, such as for the assessment of occupational inhalants in susceptible patients.
Methacholine, carbachol, or histamine challenge
1.   To identify the patient with hyperactive airways regardless of cause, as well as to measure the extent of such hyperactivity when appropriate.

III. MEASUREMENT OF RESPONSE

The FEV_1 remains as the most important measurement of airway responsiveness. Its virtues are its simplicity and reproducibility and the fact that its measurement is readily available. It also provides the best differentiation of patients who have asthma and those who do not. Other tests, however, may be used, but it is important that a FEV_1 also be included for comparison.

Other commonly used tests are airway resistance and conductance (Raw and SGaw), and partial expiratory flow volume curves. These measurements provide sensitive measures of response and avoid the full inspiratory maneuver of the FEV_1, which may have a minimal bronchodilator effect. For this reason they are useful for measuring responses to a smaller stimulus. Changes in these parameters can be obtained even when normal individuals are challenged with agents that would not ordinarily produce a PD_{20} FEV_1. They have the disadvantage of being more variable and less reproducible than the FEV_1.

IV. FACTORS INFLUENCING RESPONSE

Factors that can influence the response to bronchial challenge should be avoided, or if unavoidable, taken into consideration in evaluating bronchial challenge results. These include acute viral respiratory infections, bacterial respiratory infections, and pollutants such as NO_2 and SO_2, which are known to increase reactivity. Seasonal exposure to naturally occurring antigen or recent antigen challenge may increase airway hyperresponsiveness. Similarly, power of suggestion can also influence airway reactivity.

TABLE 2
Recommended Ideal Time Interval Between Last
Medication and Bronchial Challenge

Drug	Time interval (hours)
Inhaled bronchodilators	
Isoproterenol	4
Isoetharine	6
Metaproterenol	8
Terbutaline	12
Salbutamol	12
Atropine and its analogs	10
Injected bronchodilators	
Epinephrine	4
Terbutaline	12
Oral Bronchodilators	
Liquid theophyline preparations	12
Short-acting theophyline preparations	18
Aminophylline preparations	18
Intermediate-acting theophyline preparations	24
Long-acting theophyline preparations	48
Cromolyn sodium	48
Long-acting antihistamines	48
Hydroxyzine	96
Terfenadine	72

Note: Patients with an FEV_1 less than 70% of predicted should not
be tested.

A. DRUGS

A variety of drugs that can influence bronchial challenge and recommended withdrawal times prior to challenge are listed in Table 2.

B. AEROSOL GENERATION

In order for airway responsiveness studies to be valid, an aerosol with appropriate and reproducible properties must be delivered to the subject. Important aerosol properties include electric charge, surface area, particle density, composition, volatility, shape, and mass distribution.[16] The DeVilbiss Jet Nebulizer Model 646 is commonly used for methacholine, histamine, and other pharmacologic agents, as well as antigen. The nebulized particle size has a mass median diameter (MMD) of 4.4 μm ± 2.2 μm. The other commonly used nebulizer is the Wright nebulizer, which has a smaller MMD than the DeVilbiss 646. Characteristics of the nebulizers have been reviewed.[16] Similar histamine bronchoconstricting effects and dose-response curves were produced using a DeVilbiss 646 (with dosimeter) and a Wright nebulizer with 2 min of tidal breathing.[17]

Tubing, mouthpieces, and other devices between the aerosol generator and the patient's mouth should remain the same for all measurements because the particle size will vary due to evaporation and impaction of the larger droplets within the tubing.

Ultrasonic nebulization is produced when high-frequency sound waves are focused onto an air-liquid interface. The initial average particle diameter is a function of the crystal frequency used to generate the sound waves. Considerable variation occurs in the effectiveness of different types of ultrasonic nebulizers in inducing bronchoconstriction with UNDW.

C. TECHNICAL FACTORS

The stability of the various concentrations of the inhaled agents in diluent is an important consideration. Methacholine chloride and histamine acid phosphate should be prepared in buffered saline to a pH of 7.4 to avoid the possible potent bronchoconstricting effect of hypotonic solutions. These agents are stable for at least 3 months when stored at 4°C.[7,18] Preservatives such as benzyl alcohol or 0.45 phenol are added to maintain sterility. As an additional precaution, it is recommended that the final solution be passed through a bacterial filter before use. However, other pharmacologic agents such as prostaglandin and leukotriene LTC_4 and LTD_4 are very unstable and therefore should be prepared fresh each day. Platelet activating factor, when used for inhalation studies, should also be made fresh and used within 12 h if stored at 2°C.

The effect of inhalation of normal saline needs to be determined prior to obtaining the dose reponse to any agent. If a fall in FEV_1 of 10 to 20% occurs after inhalation of saline solution, the validity of any subsequent results is questionable, at least for that day. The time between inhalations and the time of spirometry measurement should be constant. The reponses should then be compared to the post-saline measurement. The inhaled agents are delivered in stepwise increasing doses. Concentrations of the bronchoprovocation agent are increased until the FEV_1 has decreased by 20%, the airway conductance or resistance or expiratory flow volume curves have changed by 35 to 40%, or the final dose is reached. The results are expressed as the PD_{20}, FEV_1, or the PD_{35} SGaw and are discussed in Section V. The dose is expressed in breath units for methacholine or histamine. One breath unit is defined as one inhalation of a concentration of 1 mg/ml.[6,7] It is also appropriate to express the dose in milligrams or micromoles and to specify whether the dose is cumulative or noncumulative.

V. EXPRESSION OF RESULTS

The factors which most affect interpretation of tests of airway responsiveness are the dose delivered, how the dose-response curve is plotted, the values used to express its position, the slope and shape of the dose-response curve, and the lung function test used.

The degree of airway responsiveness to methacholine can be expressed as milligrams per milliliter for concentration (noncumulative); micromoles and breath units (cumulative) for individuals with severe, moderate, and mild asthma, as well as for normal subjects; e.g., 1 mg/ml = 0.5 μM = 10 breath units.

Although the PD_{20} FEV_1 is the usual method of expressing results, some subjects without asthma, particularly those with allergic rhinitis, may have a positive reaction, as evidenced by attaining an FEV_1 PD_{20}, and then demonstrating a plateau phenomena.[2,3,19,20] In these subjects, further administration of methacholine or histamine will fail to produce progressive airway narrowing. In contrast, patients with asthma, when administered increasing doses of inhaled histamine or methacholine, have a progressive airway narrowing. Woolcock,[20] and Townley et al.,[2,19] and Reed and Townley[3] have shown that when a FEV_1 PD_{35} is used, one can clearly differentiate between individuals with this plateau phenomena vs. those with asthma. However, as one goes beyond the FEV_1 PD_{35}, a concern for the severity of airway narrowing makes further administration of the bronchoconstrictive agent too uncomfortable or dangerous.[19,20]

An important advantage of determining the area under the dose-response curve is that it allows quantitative measurements in subjects who never achieve a 20% fall in FEV_1 (PD_{20} FEV_1) to either histamine or methacholine.[2,19,20] The determination of an area under the dose-response curve is not necessary for diagnostic studies, but is valuable in epidemiologic and pharmacologic studies.

VI. REPRODUCIBILITY

It is preferable to assess the airway response to mediators at the same time of the day, as circadian variation has been observed with histamine. The 95% confidence limits for the reproducibility of the PC_{20} for methacholine and histamine challenges done on different days with an interval of 1 to 2 weeks was $+/-$ on single twofold concentration.[17] This same degree of reproducibility was shown for both dosimeter and continuous tidal breathing methods.[17]

VII. PHARMACOLOGIC CHALLENGES

A. HISTAMINE AND METHACHOLINE

Of the known pharmacological challenge agents, methacholine and histamine are the most commonly used and have been well standardized. Methacholine is a parasympathomimetic agent which appears to stimulate the muscarinic receptors on bronchial smooth muscles directly, increasing the bronchomotor activity. Methacholine is inhibited by atropine and its analogs.[2,5,21] Histamine induces bronchoconstriction primarily by a direct bronchoconstrictive effect and partly by reflex vagal stimulation.[21]

Methacholine and histamine are both extensively used in research as well as in diagnostic testing. Selection of the agent to be used generally depends upon the investigator's experience and familiarity with the agent. Histamine has a shorter duration of action and may cause headache, flushing, and hoarseness at higher doses.[22,23]

1. Preparation

Patients should have the procedure fully explained. An informed consent should be obtained whenever possible. A physician and emergency equipment must be available at the site of the challenge testing. A general physical examination should be carried out before the challenge and the findings should be recorded.

2. Methods

Methacholine and histamine are available as dry powder. Methacholine has been recently approved by the FDA and made available through Hoffman La Roche Pharmaceutical Co. Its preparation and preservation has been described in Section IV.C.

Two methods of challenge with methacholine and histamine are widely used and both require nebulization of the solution. A DeVilbiss nebulizer 646 is used for Rosenthal-French dosimeter,[7,14] and a Wright nebulizer is used for the continuous aerosol method.[4] Baseline spirometry should be performed and the FEV_1 should be at least 70% of the predicted value.

Serial dilutions of methacholine or histamine are prepared. The standard procedure utilizes the following concentrations and sequence of five inhalations of 0.075, 0.15, 0.31, 0.62, 1.25, 2.5, 5.0, 10 and 25 mg/ml for a total of 225 bu.[6,7] An abbreviated version of the 1975 American Academy of Allergy dose schedule[6] has been suggested.[14] A 2-ml dose of the solution is put into the DeVilbiss no. 646 nebulizer and the plumbing tube is attached to the compressed air reservoir. The aerosol is generated by the compressed air delivered at 20 psi through the nebulizer. The input is controlled by a valve which is triggered by the inspiration and is kept open for 0.6 s. A noseclip is used. The subjects are instructed to inhale slowly from the functional residual capacity (FRC) to total lung capacity (TLC). During the inhalation the vent of the nebulizer should be kept open. Spirometric measurements are taken 3 min after the aerosol inhalation of each dilution. The test is generally terminated if the FEV_1 drops by 20% or more of the control value or if the final dilution is reached. Failure to drop by 20% or more is considered to be a negative challenge. The results are evaluated as discussed in Section VI. The inhalation methodology for the continuous tidal breathing method has been recently reviewed.[24]

Throughout the challenge, spirometric measurements are taken in duplicate. Consistency is defined as a FEV_1 within 5% of the other, and the best of the two values is taken for the challenge evaluation at each step.

If the challenge is to be repeated in the same subject, the same nebulizer should be used each time to avoid the inter-nebulizer variation.[7]

B. OTHER PHARMACOLOGIC AGENTS

The previously discussed bronchial challenge procedures have widespread diagnostic applications. However, research in asthma and bronchial reactivity includes bronchial provocation testing with various other chemicals. Many of these agents are known to be released during mast cell-dependent events and may partially mimic naturally occurring asthma. These agents are likely to be more widely used in the coming years, especially as tools for the investigation of basic mechanisms in asthma.

The technical aspects, as they relate to inhalation challenge tests with these agents, are quite variable when compared to more standardized challenge protocols. It is important for investigators to clearly outline the inhalation technique used to allow for comparison between studies. Dose concentrations and nebulizer outputs should be detailed in published manuscripts. Since the action of these agents is not always well understood, it is not uncommon that inhaled dose and pulmonary function changes are deliberately and appropriately limited.

Prostaglandin D_2 is released in significant amounts after IgE-mediated stimulation of human lung mast cells. A recent report[25] showed that inhaled prostaglandin D_2 has a ten times more potent effect on airways than does histamine. Prostaglandin D_2 had a minimal effect in the normal subjects, while F_2 alpha showed no effect at the doses used.

Leukotrienes C_4, D_4, and E_4 have been shown to have potent bronchoconstrictive properties in humans.[26,27] Although this fact is well recognized, conflicting data have arisen concerning: (1) the site of action of leukotriene,[28] (2) the relative sensitivity of asthmatics and normals to include leukotrienes,[29] and (3) the relative sensitivity of leukotrienes in asthmatics and normals when compared to methacholine.[30]

Platelet activating factor (PAF) has recently been implicated to be an active bronchoconstrictive agent. It also has potent inflammatory generating properties in experimental animals.[31] The effect of inhaled PAF on normal controls has been recently reported.[32] The role of PAF in the induction or accentuation of nonspecific bronchial reactivity requires further investigation.

Adenosine inhalation challenges have gained limited use, predominately in the United Kingdom. Adenosine, and its precursor nucleotide AMP, induces bronchial constriction in asthmatics, but not in normals.[33]

The well-recognized clinical observation that beta-blockers can induce bronchoconstriction in asthmatics has resulted in the use of propranolol as an inhalation challenge procedure. Propranolol sensitivity in asthmatics is less than that seen with histamine[34] and methacholine.[35]

VIII. PHYSIOLOGIC CHALLENGES

As with inhalation studies of methacholine, histamine, and antigen, graded exercise and cold-air hyperventilation (CAHC) can also produce bronchoconstriction in susceptible individuals. These tests are used to assess latent asthma, evaluate the severity of known exercise-induced bronchoconstriction, and to evaluate the effects of medications.[8,13,14] The specificity approaches 100%; however, the sensitivity varies from 50 to 100% depending on the criteria for a positive response. Reproducibility is high if performed more than 2 h apart.[36]

A. EXERCISE

Exercise studies entail free running, treadmill running, and cycloergometer.[37] Free running, though, has many uncontrollable factors which make the test less than optimal.[37] As a result, treadmill running and cycle studies in a controlled environment are more popular.

With exercise challenges, the energy of each subject should be quantitated by a measurement of the work rate[38] needed to increase the oxygen consumption by 30 to 40 ml/min/kg[39,40] or to increase the heart rate by 80 to 90% of maximum heart rate based on the subject's age.[38]

For subjects over 25 years old, a three-step graded increment approach for treadmill testing is advised for safety reasons.[37,38] With subjects younger than 25 years of age, the target heart rate can be reached in the first 1 to 2 min of exercise.[37] The target heart rate should be sustained for 6 to 8 min for a maximum response; longer bouts of exercise will not increase the bronchoconstriction and may even promote bronchodilation.[37,39-42] The mechanics of each challenge have been described elsewhere.[38]

Within the first 4 min of exercise, bronchodilation occurs and is thought to be due to increased sympathetic drive.[37] This is followed by a progressive airway constriction that peaks 3 to 4 min after exercise is completed in children and up to 15 min later in adults.[37,38] Baseline function is attained on an average 20 to 30 min later.[37,38]

As with other bronchoprovocation studies, baseline pulmonary functions are obtained immediately prior to the study, and FEV_1 and PEFR should be at least 65 to 70% of predicted and within 80% of the subject's usual level.[41] The response should be measured every 2 min postexercise up to 10 min and then every 5 min thereafter until baseline is achieved.[41] Disagreement exists regarding what degree of change in the indices represents a positive response.[37-41]

B. COLD-AIR HYPERVENTILATION

For those in whom exercise testing is contraindicated, CAHC may be used to produce similar results; a good correlation exists between the two.[15,38,42]

The setup consists of compressed air entrained through a heat exchanger capable of generating a final temperature at the patient's mouth of at least $-10°C$.[15] It is necessary to measure and control minute ventilation (V_E). End tidal CO_2 need not be measured, but plays an important part as hyperventilation will produce hypocapnia, which itself causes bronchoconstriction.[38]

The inspired and expired air temperature, T_I and T_E, respectively, as well as V_E are measured with V_E and T_I being controlled. The only other important variable is the humidity of the inspired and expired air, WC_I and WC_E, respectively. WC_I can be measured from the compressed air source or produced through a bubble humidifier on the inspired line; WC_E can be assumed to be completely saturated for all practical purposes and obtained from standard saturation-temperature relationships.[43]

To initiate the test, the subject performs a baseline spirometery to determine the FEV_1. V_E is then set at either (1) 20 to 35 times the baseline FEV_1, which is comparable with the V_E attained with moderately strenuous exercise;[15,44] (2) maximal voluntary ventilation (MVV);[60] or (3) a cumulative dose response of 20, 40, 60, 80% of predicted MVV or 7.5, 15, 30, 60 l/min, then MVV.[44,45] Regardless of the method, each is maintained for 3 to 4 min.[15,44,45] Although a single V_E of 20 to 35 times the FEV_1 may produce good results, MVV alone or with a cumulative dose gives more consistent results.[45] A cumulative-dose method also allows better observation of the effect of a drug and decreases the chance of marked bronchoconstriction.[46]

As with exercise tests, the maximal bronchoconstrictive response peaks 4 to 8 min after challenge, starts resolving within the next 5 min, and approaches baseline after 15 to 60 min.[38,44] Here, too, controversy exists as to what is considered a positive response; most agree that a positive response is at least a 10% decrease in FEV_1; for SGaw a positive response is $\geq 30\%$ change.[14,44,45] Measurements are done at either 2 to 3 min intervals, until maximal response is achieved, and then at 5-min intervals until recovery begins.[46,47] The results can be expressed in terms of V_E, the respiratory heat exchange,[38,46] or the maximum drop in FEV_1 obtained.

C. ULTRASONIC NEBULIZED DISTILLED WATER CHALLENGE

Anesthesiologists were first to observe an increase in airway resistance after inhalation of ultrasonic water. Allegra and Bianco[48] used UNDW as a bronchial provocation in 1974. Anderson[49] introduced a dose-response curve and calculated the PD_{20} of UNDW.

The test appears to be very specific, but the sensitivity ranges between 30 to 100%.[20] The correlation between UNDW challenge and methacholine is variable; a better correlation is found between exercise and CAHC.[50]

Various methods of UNDW challenge are being employed and a standardized protocol has yet to be established. The basic principles in doing UNDW challenge include: (1) starting with a low dose; (2) increase the dose gradually; (3) obtain a dose-response curve. UNDW challenge is a safe, specific, moderately sensitive test for bronchial asthma, and it can be used as a valuable research tool in testing the pathophysiology of asthma.

Hypertonic aerosols with osmolarity up to 1280 have been used as a bronchial challenge. The bronchoconstriction induced by inhalation of 3.6% normal saline was equal to that induced by UNDW inhalation.[51]

IX. ALLERGEN CHALLENGE

Antigen provocation was first described by Lowell and Schiller.[52] Although it is widely used by many investigators, its use as a clinical diagnostic tool is restricted because it adds limited information over the skin test. Investigators have found considerable overlap in the antigen provocation response among patients who have atopic asthma and patients who suffer from allergic rhinitis.[1,3,53]

There is a good correlation between skin tests and *in vitro* tests and bronchial provocation. The stronger the skin reaction the greater the chance of positive bronchial provocation.[1,53] A recent report has suggested that an allergen challenge test to determine an early asthmatic response to a particular antigen could be replaced with a skin test and a measure of nonspecific bronchial reactivity.[54]

With few exceptions, a negative antigen provocation test to a certain antigen rules out the possibility that the antigen is responsible for asthma. On the other hand, a positive challenge only indicates sensitivity to the antigen.

Pollens, house dust, mites, molds, and animal danders have been used in antigen provocation tests. Pollens are more likely to cause positive responses than house dust in comparable skin-reactive patients, possibly due to the lack of homogeneity of house dust extracts.

A. METHOD

The aqueous antigenic extracts are diluted with a diluent containing 0.5% sodium chloride, 0.275% sodium bicarbonate, and 0.40% phenol (pH 7.0). Lyophilized extracts are preferable if available. The degradation can be reduced by storage between 4 and $-20°C$ and by addition of a stabilizer such as serum albumin. Limited data indicate that concentrations up to 1:20 can be stored at 4°C for 1 year.[6] Anything more dilute than 1:20 should be utilized within 7 d of preparation. When performing studies of drug efficacy against allergen-induced responses, the extracts should be reconstituted or thawed and diluted shortly before use, preferably on the same day.[6,7,55] It is important that the potency and stability of the antigenic extracts are assured. Antigen should be labeled on a weight per volume basis, but the protein nitrogen units (pnu/ml) and/or μg of protein nitrogen per milliliter determination should also be indicated.[6] One inhalation unit equals one inhalation of 1:5000 W/V or one inhalation of solution with 1 μg protein nitrogen per milliliter or 100 pnu/ml. The general precautions and safety measures for bronchial challenge also apply. Additional precautions pertain to the greater variability, severity, and duration of the response to allergens, especially the late response.[56,57]

A properly performed skin test should be done using both skin prick and intradermal tests. Serially diluted antigen extracts are given from 10^{-5} to 10^{-3} W/V dilution. The diluent control is used as well as histamine. The initial antigen concentration used for the first challenge should be the one which produces a 2+ reaction on intracutaneous injection, i.e., >5 mm wheal (minus diluent control). The antigen should be delivered from a nebulizer connected to a dosimeter as discussed previously.

Pulmonary function studies are performed 10 min following inhalation of 5 breaths of diluent. This diluent value is the control, and if the FEV_1 is not reduced 10% from the baseline, the subject enters the study. The challenge begins with five breaths of the antigen concentration that was required to elicit the 2+ skin test.[6,7] If less than a 15% reduction from the control FEV_1 value occurs 10 min post-antigen, the next dilution is given. If the reduction is 15 to 19%, an additional 5 to 10 min wait is indicated. When approaching the end point which is equal or greater than a 20% fall in FEV_1 from the diluent control, less than five breaths may be given to reduce the possibility of a precipitous fall in the FEV_1.

The cumulative inhalation units of antigen appear logarithmically on the abscissa and the percentage of FEV_1 on the ordinate and the PD_{20} can be calculated in breath units.[6,7] A beta-agonist by inhalation should be given and postbronchodilator spirometry done to be sure that the FEV_1 returns to or near the baseline value. A potential late reaction could be expected to begin within 3 to 8 h. If it is feasible the patient should be studied at hourly intervals, or a peak flow meter can be used and results recorded.[14,54]

If another antigen challenge needs to be done it is wise to wait 1 week or longer. The increase in nonspecific bronchial reactivity may take 1 week or more to return to baseline.[55-57] The subsequent challenge should be started at least two concentrations lower than the previous concentration which induced a significant drop in the FEV_1.

ACKNOWLEDGMENTS

We thank Drs. R. Trivedi, F., Suliaman, and S. Lemire for their contribution, and Rosemary Batts and Nannette Royle for their skillful assistance in preparing this manuscript.

REFERENCES

1. **Townley, R. G., Dennis, M., and Itkin, J. M.,** Comparative action of acetyl-beta-methacholine, histamine and pollen antigens in subjects with hay fever and patients with bronchial asthma, *J. Allergy,* 36, 121, 1965.
2. **Townley, R. G., Bewtra, A. K., Nair, N. H., Brodkey, F. D., Watt, G. D., and Burke, K.M.,** Methacholine inhalation challenge studies, *J. Allergy Clin. Immunol.,* 64(6)2, 569, 1979.
3. **Reed, C. and Townley, R. G.,** Asthma: classification and pathogenesis, in *Allergy: Principles and Practice,* 2nd ed., Middleton, E., Jr., Reed, C. E., and Ellis, E. F., Eds., C. V. Mosby, St. Louis, MO, 1983, 811.
4. **Cockcroft, D. W., Killian, D. N., Mellon, J. J. A., and Hargreave, E. E.,** Bronchial reactivity to inhaled histamine: a method and clinical survey, *Clin. Allergy,* 7, 235, 1977.
5. **Boushey, H. A., Holtzman, M. J., Sheller, J. R., and Nadel, J. A.,** (STATE OF ART) Bronchial hyperreactivity, *Am. Rev. Respir. Dis.,* 121, 389, 1980.

6. **Chai, H., Farr, R. S., Froehlich, L. A., Mathison, D. A., McLean, J. A., Rosenthal, R. R., Sheffer, A. L., II, Spector, S. L., and Townley, R. G.**, Standardization of bronchial inhalation challenge procedures, *J. Allergy Clin. Immunol.*, 56(4), 322, 1975.

7. **Cropp, G. J., Bernstein, I. L., Boushey, H. A., Jr., Hyde, R. W., Rosenthal, R. R., Spector, S. L., and Townley, R. G.**, Guidelines for bronchial inhalation challenges with pharmacologic and antigenic agents, *ATS News*, 11, Spring 1980.

8. **Townley, R. G., Hopp, R., Weiss, S., Lang, W., McCall, M.**, Mechanisms and management of bronchial asthma, in *Clinical Medicine*, ed. Spitell, 1986, 7.

9. **Ramsdale, E. H., Morris, M. M., Roberts, R. S., and Hargreave, F. E.**, Bronchial responsiveness to methacholine in chronic bronchitis: relationship to airflow obstruction and cold air responsiveness, *Thorax*, 39, 912, 1984.

10. **Findlay, S. R. and Lichtenstein, L. M.**, Basophil releasability in patients with asthma, *Am. Rev. Respir. Dis.*, 122, 53, 1980.

11. **Felarca, A. B. and Itkin, I.**, Studies with the quantitative inhalation challenge technique. I. Curve of dose response to acetyl-beta-methacholine in patients with asthma of known and unknown origin, hayfever subjects and non-atopic volunteers, *J. Allergy*, 37, 223, 1966.

12. **Itkin, I. H.**, Bronchial hyperreactivity to mecholyl and histamine in asthma subjects, *J. Allergy*, 40, 245, 1967.

13. **Bewtra, A. K. and Townley, R. G.**, Bronchoprovocative tests — clinical usefulness and limitations, *Arch. Intern. Med.*, 144, 925, 1984.

14. **Rosenthal, R. R.**, Inhalation challenge in asthma, in *Allergy*, Kaplan, A. P., Ed., Churchill Livingstone, New York, 1985, 14.

15. **Deal, E. C., McFadden, E. R., Ingram, R. H., Breslin, F. J., and Jaeger, J. J.**, Airway responsiveness to cold air and hyperpnea in normal subjects and in those with hay fever and asthma, *Am. Rev. Respir. Dis.*, 121, 621, 1980.

16. **Swift, D. L.**, Aerosol generation for inhalation challenge in airway responsiveness, in *Airway Responsiveness: Measurement and Interpretation*, Hargreaves, F. E. and Woolcock, A. J., Eds., Astra Pharmaceutical, Mississauga, Ontario, 1985, 1.

17. **Ryan, G. Dolovich, M. B., Roberts, R. S., Frith, P. A., Juniper, E. F., Hargreave, F. E., and Newhouse, M. T.**, Standardization of inhalation provocation tests: two techniques of aerosol generation and inhalation compared, *Am. Rev. Respir. Dis.*, 123, 195, 1981.

18. **Dolovich, M. B.**, Technical factors influencing response to challenge aerosols in airway responsiveness, in *Airway Responsiveness: Measurement and Interpretation*, Hargreave, F. E. and Woolcock, A. J., Eds., Astra Pharmaceutical, Mississauga, Ontario, 1985, 9.

19. **Townley, R. G., Ryo, U. Y., Kolotkin, B. M., and Kang, B.**, Bronchial sensitivity to methacholine in current and former asthmatic and allergic rhinitis patients and control subjects, *J. Allergy Clin. Immunol.*, 56(6), 429, 1975.

20. **Woolcock, A. J.**, Expression of results of airway hyperresponsiveness in airway responsiveness, in *Airway Responsiveness: Measurement and Interpretation*, Hargreave, F. E. and Woolcock, A. J., Eds., Astra Pharmaceuticals, Mississauga, Ontario, 1985, 80.

21. **Simonsson, B. G., Jacobs, F. M., and Nadel, J. A.**, Role of the autonomic nervous system and the cough reflex in the increased responsiveness of airways in patients with obstructive airway disease, *J. Clin. Invest.*, 46, 1812, 1967.

22. **Hargreave, F. E., Ryan, G., Thomson, N. C., O'Byrne, P. M., Latimer, K., Juniper, E. F., and Dolovich, J.**, Bronchial responsiveness to histamine or methacholine in asthma: measurement and clinical significance, *J. Allergy Clin. Immunol.*, 68(5), 347, 1981.

23. **Kang, B., Townley, R. G., Lee, C. K., and Kolotkin, B. M.**, Bronchial reactivity to histamine before and after sodium cromoglycate in bronchial asthma, *Br. Med. J.*, 1, 867, 1976.

24. **Townley, R. G. and Hopp, R. J.**, Inhalation methods for the study of airway responsiveness, *J. Allergy Clin. Immunol.*, 80, 111, 1987.

25. **Hardy, C. C., Robinson, C., Tattersfield, A. E., and Holgate, S. T.**, The bronchoconstrictor effect of inhaled prostaglandin D_2 in normal and asthmatic men, *NEJM ed.*, 311, 209, 1984.

26. **Holroyde, M. C., Altounyan, R. E. C., Cole, M., Dickson, M., and Elliott, E. V.**, Bronchoconstriction produced in man by leukotriences C and D, *Lancet*, 2, 17, 1981.

27. **Weiss, J. W., Drazen, J. M., Cole, M., McFadden, E. R., Weller, P. S., Corey, E., Lewis, R. A., and Austen, K. F.**, Bronchoconstrictor effects of leukotriene C in humans, *Science*, 216, 196, 1982.

28. **Griffen, M., Weiss, J. W., Leitch, A. F., McFadden, E. R., Corey, E. J., Austen, K. F., and Drazen, J. M.**, Effects of leukotriene D on the airways in asthma, *NEJM ed.*, 308, 436, 1983.

29. **Smith, L. J., Coreenberger, P. A., Patterson, R., Krell, R. D., and Bernstein, P. R.**, The effect of inhaled leukotriene D_4 in humans, *Am. Rev. Respir. Dis.* 131, 368, 1985.

30. **Adelroth, E., Morris, M. M., Hargreave, E. E., and O'Byrne, P. M.,** Airway responsiveness to leukotrienes C_4 and D_4 and to methacholine in patients with asthma and normal controls, *NEJM ed.,* 315, 480, 1986.

31. **Vargaftig, B. B., Lefort, J., Chignard, M., and Benveniste, J.,** Platelet-activating factor induces a platelet-dependent bronchoconstriction unrelated to the formation of prostaglandin derivatives, *Eur. J. Pharmacol.,* 65, 185, 1980.

32. **Cuss, F. M., Dickson, C. M. S., and Barnes, P. J.,** Effects of inhaled platelet activating factor on pulmonary function and bronchial responsiveness in man, *Lancet,* 2, 189, 1986.

33. **Cushley, J. M., Tattersfield, A. E., and Holgate, S. T.,** Adenosine antagonism as an alternative mechanism of action of methylxanthines in asthma, *Agents Actions,* 13 (Suppl.), 109, 1983.

34. **Woolcock, A. J., Cheung, W., and Salome, C.,** Relationship between bronchial responsiveness to propranolol and histamine, *Am. Rev. Respir. Dis.,* 133, A177, 1986.

35. **De Vries, K., Gokemeyer, J. D. M., Koeter, G. H., De Monchy, J. G. R., Van Bork, L. E., Cauffman, H. L., and Meurs, H.,** Cholinergic and adrenergic mechanisms in bronchial reactivity, in *Bronchial Hyperreactivity,* Morley, J., Ed., Academic Press, London, 1982, 107.

36. **Anderson, S. D. and Schoeffel, R. E.,** Standardization of exercise training in the asthmatic patient: a challenge in itself, in *Airway Responsiveness: Measurement and Interpretation,* Hargreave, F. E. and Woolcock, A. J., Eds., Astra Pharmaceuticals, Mississauga, Ontario, 1985, 51.

37. **Godfrey, S.,** Exercise-induced asthma — clinical, physiological, and therapeutic implications, *J. Allergy Clin. Immunol.,* 56, 1, 1975.

38. **Souhrada, J. F. and Kivity, S.,** Exercise testing in *Provocative Challenge Procedures: Bronchial, Oral, Nasal, and Exercise,* Vol. II, Spector, S. L., Ed., CRC Press, Boca Raton, FL, 1983, 75.

39. **Cropp, G. J. A.,** The exercise bronchoprovocation test: standardization of procedures and evaluation of response, *J. Allergy Clin. Immunol.,* 64, 642, 1979.

40. **Eggleston, P. A., Rosenthal, R. R., Anderson, S. D., Anderton, R., Bierman, C. U., Bleeker, E. R., Chai, H., Cropp, G. J. A., Johnson, J. D., Konis, P., Morse, J., Smith, L. J., Summers, R. J., and Trautloin, J. J.,** Guidelines for the methodology of exercise testing of asthmatics, *J. Allergy Clin. Immunol.,* 64, 642, 1979.

41. **Anderson, S. D. and Schoeffel, R. E.,** Standardization of exercise training in the asthmatic patient: a challenge in itself, in *Airway Responsiveness: Measurement and Interpretation,* Hargreave, F. E. and Woolcock, A. J., Eds., Astra Pharmaceutical, Mississauga, Ontario, 1985, 51.

42. **Anderson, S. D.,** Issues in exercise-induced asthma, *J. Allergy Clin. Immunol.,* 76, 763, 1985.

43. **Eschenbacher, W. L. and Sheppard, D.,** Respiratory heat loss is not the sole stimulus for bronchoconstriction induced by isocapnic hyperpnea with dry air, *Am. Rev. Respir. Dis.,* 131, 894, 1985.

44. **Mclaughlin, F. J. and Dozor, A. J.,** Cold air inhalation challenge in the diagnosis of asthma in children, *Pediatrics,* 72, 503, 1983.

45. **Malo, J. L., Cartier, A., and L'Archeveque, J.,** Cold air inhalation has a cumulative bronchospastic effect when inhaled in consecutive doses for progressively increasing degrees of ventilation, *Am. Rev. Respir. Dis.,* 134, 990, 1986.

46. **O'Byrne, P. M.,** Airway challenge using isocapnic hyperventilation, in *Airway Responsiveness: Measurement and Interpretation,* Hargreave, F. E. and Woolcock, A. J., Eds., Astra Pharmaceuticals, Mississauga, Ontario, 1985, 60.

47. **Tessier, P., Cartier, A., L''Archeveque, H., Chezzo, H., Martin, R. R., and Mallo, Jean-Luc,** Within and between day reproducibility of isocapnic cold air challenges in subjects with asthma, *J. Allergy Clin. Immunol.,* 78, 379, 1986.

48. **Allegra, L. and Bianco, S.,** Non-specific broncho-reactivity obtained with an ultrasonic aerosol of distilled water, *Eur. J. Respir. Dis.,* 61 (Suppl. 106), 41, 1980.

49. **Anderson, S.,** Bronchial challenge by ultrasonically nebulized aerosol, *Clin. Rev. Allergy,* 3, 427, 1985.

50. **Bascom, B. and Bleecker, E. R.,** Bronchoconstriction induced by distilled water, *Am. Rev. Respir. Dis.,* 134, 248, 1986.

51. **Schoeffel, R. E., Anderson, S. D., and Altounyan, R. E. C.,** Bronchial hyperreactivity in response to inhalation of ultrasonically nebulized solutions of distilled water and saline, *Br. Med. J.,* 283, 1285, 1981.

52. **Lowell, F. C. and Schiller, I. W.,** Measurement of change in vital capacity as a means of detecting pulmonary reactions to inhaled aerosolized allergenic extracts in asthmatic subjects, *J. Allergy,* 19, 100, 1948.

53. **Bruce, C. A., Rosenthal, R. R., Lichenstein, L. M., and Norman, P. S.,** Quantitative inhalation bronchial challenge in ragweed hayfever patients: a comparison with ragweed-allergic asthmatics, *J. Allergy Clin. Immunol.,* 56, 331, 1975.

54. **Cockcroft, D. W., Murdock, K. Y., Kirby, J., and Hargreave, F.,** Prediction of airway responsiveness to allergen from skin sensitivity to allergen and airway responsiveness to histamine, *Am. Rev. Respir. Dis.,* 135, 264, 1987.

55. **Hargreave, F. E. and Fink, J. N.,** The role of bronchoprovocation, *J. Allergy Clin. Immunol.,* 78(2), 517, 1986.

56. **Hargreave, F. E. and Dolovich, J.,** Bronchial responsiveness and late asthmatic response, in *Asthma: Physiology, Immunopharmacology and Treatment,* Kay, A. B., Lichtenstein, L. M., and Austen, K. F., Eds., Academic Press, London, 1984, 263.

57. **Hargreave, F. E., Frith, P. A., Dolovich, M., Cartier, A., Ryan, G., Juniper, E. F., Dolovich, J., and Newhouse, M. T.,** Allergen-induced airway responses and relationships with nonspecific reactivity, in *Airway Reactivity: Mechanisms and Clinical Relevance,* Hargreave, F. E., Ed., Astra Pharmaceuticals, Mississauga, Ontario, 1980, 145.

Chapter 9

PULMONARY REFLEX EFFECTS ON AIRWAY SMOOTH MUSCLE AND VENTILATION

Dale R. Bergren

TABLE OF CONTENTS

I.   Introduction 182

II.   Significance of Pulmonary Afferent Receptors on Pulmonary Function 182
       A.   The Hering-Breuer Stretch Reflex 182
       B.   Reflex Bronchomotor Tone 183

III.   Pulmonary Receptors with Afferent Fibers within the Vagi 186
       A.   Slowly Adapting or Pulmonary Stretch Receptors (PSRs) 186
              1.   Location 186
              2.   Stimuli 187
                     a.   Activity During Eupneic Breathing 187
                     b.   Mechanical 187
                     c.   Chemical 191
              3.   Reflex Actions of PSRs 192
       B.   Rapidly Adapting Receptors (Irritant Receptors) 194
              1.   Location 194
              2.   Stimuli 195
                     a.   Activity During Eupneic Breathing 195
                     b.   Mechanical 195
                     c.   Chemical 199
              3.   Reflex Effects of Rapidly Adapting Receptors 205
       C.   Pulmonary and Bronchial C-Fiber Endings 206
              1.   Location 206
              2.   Stimuli 207
                     a.   Activity During Eupneic Breathing 207
                     b.   Mechanical 207
                     c.   Pathological Stimulants of C-Fiber Endings 210
                     d.   Chemical 211
              3.   Reflex Resulting from C-Fiber Ending Stimulation 212
                     a.   Capsaicin and the Chemoreflex 212

IV.   Studies Concerning the Integration of Pulmonary Reflexes 213
       A.   Drug Inhibition of Pulmonary Reflexes 213
       B.   Central Integration of Pulmonary Receptors 214
       C.   Action of Local Anesthetic on Pulmonary Receptor Activity 215

V.   Conclusion 216

References 216

I. INTRODUCTION

Reflex control of airway smooth muscle originating from the lungs occurs not only during stressful conditions, such as in the defense of the lungs, but also during normal conditions as well. For example, pulmonary receptors whose afferent fibers travel through the vagal nerves influence patterns of ventilation, airway resistance, and pulmonary compliance during eupneic breathing. Then during stressful conditions the reflex actions of these pulmonary receptors may go on to influence not only pulmonary functions by altering ventilation patterns, increasing airway smooth-muscle tone, decreasing lung compliance, and increasing secretions within the airways, but also cardiovascular functions by inducing tachycardia or bradycardia, vasodilation, and hypotension as seen during anaphylaxis. The purpose of this review is to discuss recent studies concerning reflex actions originating from the lungs which affect its ventilation, resistance, and compliance. Earlier studies will be employed to establish a basis for various discussions. An all-inclusive review, however, is not the purpose of this chapter, as there has been a number of recent and comprehensive reviews available presented by a number of prominent investigators.[1-10] Omission of studies from this review which have already been reviewed elsewhere is not intended to minimize the importance of those studies.

II. SIGNIFICANCE OF PULMONARY AFFERENT RECEPTORS ON PULMONARY FUNCTION

Reflexes originating within the lungs which influence ventilation include the Hering-Breuer stretch and deflation reflex, reflexes which either increase or decrease bronchomotor tone, reflexes which shorten or prolong either inspiratory or expiratory time, and other reflexes such as coughing, gasps, and sighs. The strength, magnitude, or significance of these pulmonary reflexes depend upon the species being studied, the individual, and the state of consciousness or level of anesthesia of that individual.

A. THE HERING-BREUER STRETCH REFLEX

The Hering-Breuer stretch reflex is more easily demonstrated in some species as compared to others.[11,12] In rabbits, the inflation reflex has been reported to be quite strong.[12,13] Tidal volume has been reported to increase 65% after bilateral vagotomy.[13] Dogs are a species in which this reflex can be observed even in an unsedated state.[14-16] Distraction or other factors limit this reflex in the conscious dog.[15] In humans, the strength of the Hering-Breuer stretch reflex has been thought to be extremely weak or even absent.[11,12,17-20] The Hering-Breuer inflation reflex is difficult to demonstrate in conscious human subjects, although the reflex has been demonstrated in anesthetized human subjects.[12,19,21] With the development of heart-lung transplants more has been learned concerning this reflex in human beings. The breathing patterns of eight patients having undergone heart-lung transplantation, eight patients having undergone heart transplantation, and eight subjects having no surgery were compared.[22] No differences in the breathing patterns could be demonstrated among the three groups. Even occasional augmented breaths and sighs occurred in the patients who had undergone heart-lung transplantation. The observations from this study suggest that the Hering-Breuer stretch reflex is negligible in conscious man as was previously thought. Furthermore, because augmented breaths and sighs were also present in the group having received heart-lung transplantation, other pulmonary receptors, such as the rapidly adapting receptor, thought essential in initiating these augmented breaths and sighs which periodically occur during normal breathing patterns to restore normal lung compliance, may not be. The time interval between the surgery and the study was reported to be from 1 month to 2 years. Could reinnervation of the lungs account for these findings? The authors reasoned that this likelihood was remote. Although the cough reflex was not tested, elevated resting heart rates suggested reinnervation of at least the heart had not occurred.

The reestablishment of the Hering-Breuer stretch reflex has been demonstrated 12 to 14 weeks after lung denervation in beagle dogs.[23] In a later study these investigators recorded nerve activity from the vagus nerve in dogs which had undergone lung denervation 19 months earlier.[24] Activity of pumonary stretch receptors (PSRs) was demonstrable in these dogs. In addition, stroking the lung surface stimulated these receptors in the reinnervated lung.

Recent studies in human subjects demonstrate the existence of the Hering-Breuer stretch reflex under certain resting conditions, however. In 11 laryngectomized subjects, lung inflations were performed through a tracheal stoma.[20] No reproducible apnea occurred when the subjects were conscious. However, during deep, nonrapid eye-movement sleep, apnea did occur after lung inflation. The duration of the apneic period was directly proportional to the volume of the lung inflation. These results imply that the length of the apnea is a function of PSR activity. Apnea following lung inflation has also been demonstrated by other investigators in anesthetized human subjects.[19,21] Therefore, in humans consciousness overrides the Hering-Breuer stretch reflex.

B. REFLEX BRONCHOMOTOR TONE

The contribution of pulmonary receptors to basal bronchomotor tone or to the reflex component of bronchoconstriction during anaphylaxis depends not only upon the species being studied, but also upon the individual and current conditions of the individual, be it either animal or man.[25] Worthy of exploration, however, is whether or not pulmonary reflexes make "significant" alterations in bronchomotor tone despite the difficulty in its quantification.

Although highly resistant to the effects of putative mediators of pulmonary anaphylaxis as compared to other species, rats are used in the study of airway mechanics and its reflex control. In three strains of rats, Albino, Brown Norwegian, and Wistar, neither baseline resistance nor dynamic compliance values were affected after bilateral vagotomy.[26,27] However, the dose-response curves of resistance and dynamic compliance to carbachol were shifted to the right after bilateral vagotomy.[26] This suggests that the airway responsiveness to carbachol is affected at some point in the reflex arc in rats.

The importance of pulmonary receptors in determining the base level of ventilation in newborn rats was more demonstrable. Vagotomy decreased ventilation by some 38%, while tidal volume increased three times, inspiratory time increased two times, and expiratory time increased six times in neonatal rats.[28] Isoflurane administration produced effects similar to that of vagotomy. Therefore, isoflurane must be a potent inhibitor of PSR activity in the rat. Thus far, limited information exists on the characteristics of pulmonary afferents in this species. Tsubone[29] has described stretch receptors, deflation receptors, and "irritant"-like receptors in the rat. Sapru et al.,[30] recording from thin vagal filaments in five rats, reports D Met-pro^5-enkephalinamide and halothane stimulate pulmonary J receptors. The use of phenyl diguanide and the absence of rapidly adapting responses of these receptors to lung inflation were used to identify the receptors as type J receptors. Neither location nor conduction velocity were reported. No one has systematically characterized the effect of chemical stimuli on pulmonary receptors in the rat.

Vagal influence on lung mechanics is demonstrable in guinea pigs. In spontaneously breathing guinea pigs bilateral vagotomy reduced the effect of intravenously injected histamine by 33% on pulmonary conductance, but did not block the effect of histamine upon pulmonary compliance. In paralyzed and artificially ventilated guinea pigs, vagotomy reduced the effect of histamine 75% upon conductance and 50% upon compliance.[31] In a similar study of guinea pigs Drazen and Austen[32] reported that histamine as well as bradykinin and prostaglandin $F_{2\alpha}$ ($PGF_{2\alpha}$) had reflex action. The magnitude of the reflex component of histamine challenge was very similar to that reported by Mills and Widdicombe[31] for both resistance and compliance. Histamine may even act as a neurotransmitter in the central nervous system to induce reflex bronchoconstriction.[33] Slow-reacting substance of anaphylaxis and the early effects of $PGF_{2\alpha}$ had no demonstrable reflex action. Late affects of $PGF_{2\alpha}$ were reduced approximately 60% after atropine administration for both compliance and resistance. Bradykinin had obvious reflex actions only at 3.0 μg/kg, but not at either higher or lower doses. Atropine reduced the effect of bradykinin upon compliance 50% and resistance 80%.

In rabbits, bilateral vagotomy decreased lung resistance by 18% in one study[34] and by some 16 to 37% in another, depending on the anesthetic used,[13] demonstrating baseline vagal tone in this species. Rabbits also have a demonstrable reflex component of bronchoconstriction.[34,35] Stimuli which induce reflex bronchoconstriction in the rabbit include histamine, phenyl diguanide, antigen, cold air, and sulfur dioxide.[34-39] The response to cold air increased in these sensitized rabbits compared to nonsensitized rabbits.[36,39] Vagally mediated bronchoconstriction to SO_2 exposure is demonstrable only acutely,[37,38] while prolonged exposure to SO_2 exposure increases lung resistance through an inflammatory process and lacks a vagal component.[34] The inflammatory effect of SO_2 with prolonged exposure is supported by the observations that the reactions to both phenyl diguanide and cold-air exposure, which are reflex in nature, are suppressed after SO_2 exposure.[34] The observed effects of SO_2 are not only affected by the duration of its exposure, but also on whether or not anesthetics are also used and which agents are used. Exposure to SO_2 increased ventilatory volume and decreased respiratory frequency when urethane was used as the anesthetic, while the ventilatory responses of SO_2 exposure were attenuated when sodium pentobarbital was the anesthetic.[13] These results were not observed in newborn rabbits, as even the apneic response to lung inflation could not be abolished. With SO_2 administration base level compliance in adult rabbits increased approximately 40% after either sulfur dioxide administration or bilateral vagotomy with either urethane or pentobarbital administered as the anesthetic. When a barbiturate was used as an anesthetic, resistance decreased after either sulfur dioxide administration or bilateral vagotomy. Although these results are difficult to interpret, the increase in compliance after bilateral vagotomy may reflect the contribution of efferent activity to the smooth muscle. These authors thought this to be an unlikely explanation, however. Furthermore, changes in end-expiratory volume were also thought to be unlikely. Therefore, explanation for the increase in compliance after SO_2 administration remains obscure.

In anesthetized but spontaneously breathing cats, vagal afferents contribute considerably to base level bronchomotor tone.[40] Unilateral vagotomy reduced pulmonary resistance 29%. Section of the contralateral vagal nerve only weekly added to the effect because the total reduction in resistance thereafter was only 31%. Atropine also reduced the effects of histamine injection by about 30% upon compliance and by about a factor of 1 log-dose upon resistance. Procaine administered bilaterally to the vagi resulted in a similar decrease in resistance to that of bilateral vagotomy. The effect of procaine was attributed to abolishing the conduction of action potentials of C-fibers carried through the vagal nerves.

Dogs have also been used in a number of studies for the purpose of demonstrating reflex bronchoconstriction. Indeed, studies which first demonstrated reflex bronchoconstriction used dogs as the model.[41,42] Substances which induce reflex bronchoconstriction in the dog include histamine,[41-46] acetylcholine,[44,45] bradykinin,[47] serotonin,[44] capsaicin,[48] various prostaglandins,[49] hypotonic saline, and distilled water.[50]

There are conflicts as to whether or not there exists a reflex component for certain mediators of the list above. A number of inestigators have demonstrated minor or no vagal reflex action of histamine upon bronchomotor tone in dogs.[43,51-55] For example, histamine challenge, limited to a single bronchi via a fiber-optic bronchoscope, increased resistance in collateral areas of the lungs. Vagotomy, however, failed to alter resistance through these collateral channels.[51] The reasons for the disparities remain difficult to explain, although axon reflexes originating from C-fiber endings may possibly explain some of these disparities.

In the Basenji-greyhound dogs the reflex component to antigen challenge has been estimated to be about one third of the total bronchoconstriction.[56,57] Administration of volatile anesthetics reduced the reflex component of bronchomotor tone by one half in this species as compared to that observed when thiopental was used as the anesthetic agent.[57] In addition, atropine also blocked approximately half (54%) of the resistance increase which develops in this breed of dog when challenged with aerosol of hypotonic saline.[50]

An earlier study in beagle dogs compared the effect of pentobarbital anesthesia with that of chloralose anesthesia on the reflex component of bronchoconstriction induced by histamine.[45] In that study vagotomy reduced the resulting bronchoconstriction induced by histamine by a factor of six when chloralose was used as an anesthetic. No reflex component of bronchoconstriction could be demonstrated in these dogs when pentobarbitone was used as the anesthetic agent. Furthermore, particle size of the histamine aerosol also greatly affected resulting resistance. Aerosols averaging 0.5 μM produced relatively small increases in resistance, while aerosols averaging 10 μM produced much larger increases in resistance. There results suggest that histamine is a more potent constrictor of the upper rather then than the lower airways. This finding is also in agreement with Dixon et al.[58] A combination of the factors above could account for some of the discrepancies reported in the literature concerning the reflex action of various mediators.

Some assessment has been made on the strength of pulmonary reflexes in the human being. Reflexes elicited from within the human trachea by distilled water administration include apnea, expiration, spasmatic breathing and panting, slow breathing, cough, and rapid shallow breathing.[59] Cough and slow breathing were the most susceptible to anesthetic blockade, while apnea was the least. To determine the reflex contribution of receptors to basal tone in the upper airway, lidocaine was topically applied to the pharynx.[60] Airway resistance to inspiratory flow decreased 63% and resistance to expiratory flow decreased 40% as the result of the lidocaine administration. These observations were made during conditions of sleep and conscious, quiet breathing. Therefore, activity or receptors in the pharyngeal airways in humans enhance the patency of the airway lumen. Airflow itself may be a stimulus under normal conditions which serves to dilate the airways.

During more stressful conditions the reflex action of histamine aerosol challenge to the airways of asthmatic subjects was studied through the administration of aerosols of atropine prior to the histamine challenge. The attenuation afforded by the atropine administration ranged from 2- to 36-fold in these patients.[61] Ipratropriun has also been shown to be effective in attenuating the effects of both methacholine and PGD_2 in asthmatic subjects, but not $PGF_{2\alpha}$.[62] In another study atropine reduced the effect of histamine upon specific airway conductance (sGaw) by approximately 100% in asthmatic subjects and 50% in nonasthmatic subjects.[63] On the other hand, other investigators found no reflex component of bronchoconstriction to histamine in humans.[64] Possible explanations for the inconsistency of the observed results may include the dosage used and the size of the aerosol particles.

Reflex bronchodilation apparently occurs in humans as well. Glanville et al.[65] studied the effect of lung inflation on induced bronchoconstriction in normal subjects and subjects having had heart-lung transplantation. Lung inflation reversed the bronchoconstriction only in the normal subjects, suggesting that the reflex bronchodilation was mediated by PSRs.

Therefore, many studies demonstrate, but not without contention, significant reflex contributions from pulmonary receptors to bronchomotor tone during "normal" conditions and to bronchoconstriction during conditions of stress in a number of species studied thus far, including man.

III. PULMONARY RECEPTORS WITH AFFERENT FIBERS WITHIN THE VAGI

Presently there are but three major accepted categories of pulmonary afferent receptors within the vagi believed to exist in the lungs. Three categories of receptors must therefore explain the origins of many pulmonary reflexes.[66] These three categories are PSRs, also called slowly adapting receptors, rapidly adapting receptors (RARs), or the so-called "irritant" receptor and C-fiber endings. Subclassifications of C-fiber endings now exist: either pulmonary C-fiber endings (type J receptors)[67] or bronchial C-fiber endings.[68] Both are named after the system of blood supply within which these receptors are located.

Subclassification have been suggested for PSR as well,[69] those being low- (tonic) and high- (phasic) threshold receptors. Location of the PSRs may also contribute to differing reflex effects.[70,71] Other investigators disagree as there appears to be too much of a continuum of PSRs between the extremes to justify upholding the separation of this type of receptor into subclassification.[72,73] This topic will be discussed further later in this review.

Subclassification has even been suggested for the RAR.[6,35,74-77] Laryngeal and perhaps tracheal RARs have been proposed to mediate reflexes differing from those of the RARs found in the lower airways.[10]

The notion that only three categories of pulmonary afferents has been closely guarded. However, the existence of other types of receptors cannot be absolutely ruled out at this time. For example, recently, purely deflationary receptors have been described in the rat.[29,78] Deflationary receptors have been described in the past as well in rabbits and guinea pigs,[79-82] but up until the present time they have been continually placed in the categories of other existing receptor types, such as the "irritant" or RARs. However, the existence of purely deflationary receptors should be reconsidered, at least in some species.

A. SLOWLY ADAPTING OR PULMONARY STRETCH RECEPTORS (PSRs)
1. Location

Slowly adapting PSRs are thought to be anatomically associated with airway smooth muscle and possibly with surrounding collagen fibers as well. Removing the tracheal mucosa does not inactivate tracheal PSRs.[83] Krauhs[84] describes what are believed to be PSRs which were located with the trachealis muscle layer of dogs. These receptors appear to be mechanoreceptors having a number of unmyelinated endings. Some portions of these endings may terminate in the extracellular spaces and may have association with collagen in the area of the basal lamina. In the trachea, PSRs may be located only in the membranous posterior wall.[83]

The distribution of the PSRs within the tracheal-bronchial tree has been the subject of a number of studies. PSRs are located from the extrathoracic airways,[85] even within the larynx, down to the terminal bronchioles,[86] and possibly within the alveolar duct. The area of actual anatomical concentration has been more controversial, but may be partially explainable through species variation.

In cats, earlier studies found the majority of receptors to be located in the central airways distal to the trachea,[87] while recently Paintal and Ravi[88] and Ravi[89] report that 84% of the PSRs studied were found in the lung parenchyma in this species. The majority of those receptors in the latter study were concentrated in the diaphragmatic lobe. The use of veratrine injection into the pulmonary circulation, punctate stimulation, and local mechanical stimulations provided evidence of their peripheral location. The studies of Armstrong and Luck[90] also report more peripheral PSR locations in this species. In dogs, Miserocchi et al.[86,91] found nearly half and Bartoli et al.[92] found over half of the PSRs studied to be located in the extrapulmonary airways. In functional studies using high-frequency oscillation, Wozniak et al.[93] report in dogs that of 56 PSRs studied, 7 were extratracheal, 24 were intrathoracic tracheal, and 26 were intrapulmonary in their location.

The distribution of PSRs in the airways has been studied in several other species besides dogs and cats. In rabbits, the distribution of PSRs is seemingly equally divided between central and peripheral airways in one study,[71] while in another report[94] the central airways contained the majority of the PSRs that were studied. In the opossum the distribution of 93 PSRs studied favors a peripheral location, 22% located in the trachea and 77% located more distally.[95]

The location of PSRs may be important to its reflex nature. The PSRs in the large airways may sense airflow,[8] either inspiratory or expiratory,[96] while PSRs located more distally may sense changes in tension of the surrounding tissue. These properties may lead to different reflex actions of "two" types of PSRs and may influence ventilation at different times during the breathing cycle. PSR activity during the inspiratory phase appear to influence inspiratory time (T_I). PSR activity during the expiratory phase of the respiratory cycle appears to influence expiratory time (T_E). Generally, only PSRs within the central airways have expiratory activity. During high-frequency ventilation (HFV)[93] and end-expiration loading,[97] activity of centrally located or tonically active PSRs is influenced more so than of periphereal located or phasic PSRs. This then favors reflex action of centrally located rather than peripherally located PSRs during these circumstances.

Some evidence of location and differing chemical sensitivity of PSRs has been established. In studies conducted by Kohl et al,[71] the location of the PSRs was determined and then the response of the receptors to inflation and to ammonia challenge was compared with the anatomical location of the PSR considered. Ammonia inhalation increased activity more with PSRs with peripheral than within central locations. The same pattern of response was observed with lung inflation. Therefore, if approximately equal numbers of PSRs are distributed in the central as compared to the peripheral airways, as has been observed in some species, then peripheral PSRs may have the greater reflex input to some stimuli.

2. Stimuli

a. Activity During Eupneic Breathing

PSR activity during eupneic breathing varies greatly with individual receptors. Activity may range from 1 or 2 impulses per breath to 50 or even more impulses per breath (Figure 1). As lung volume nears total lung capacity PSR activity may become as high as 300 impulses per second, and at this high frequency a few PSRs even cease firing until lower lung volumes are again attained.[98]

b. Mechanical

Touch or mechanical pressure stimulates PSRs, but these receptors are not exquisitely sensitive to such stimuli.[87] However, probing of the lung parenchyma is useful to estimate PSR location.[24,99] Although mechanical stimulus of PSRs may not be as impressive as it is for RARs, cardiac rhythm can be detected in the activity of some PSRs as well as it can for RARs. During 10- and 30-cm H_2O constant pressure inflations of the lungs, a cardiogenic component of PSR activity could be discerned from the data presented by Ogilvie.[72] This pulsation waveform was more apparent at 30- vs. 10-cm H_2O inflation pressure. Therefore, pulse pressure does affect PSR activity. Cardiac modulation of PSRs has also been observed by others.[98,100,101]

As lung volume or transpulmonary pressure increases, so does the activity of intrapulmonary PSRs. One will find that PSRs will mirror insufflation pressure (Figure 1), be it induced mechanically or chemically.[12,70,72,102] During artificial ventilation at constant tidal volume the number of action potentials of PSRs is remarkably consistent (Figure 1A and 1C). This is also true of ventilatory maneuvers such as stepwise hyperinflation of the lungs or constant-pressure hyperinflation of the lungs (Figure 1A). Despite the consistency found within a single receptor to mechanical stimuli, there is a great range in both the sensitivity

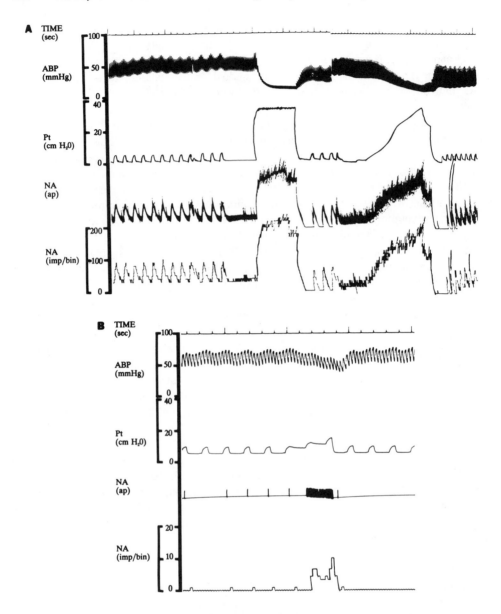

FIGURE 1.   Ventilatory characteristics of intrapulmonary pulmonary stretch receptors (PSR) of the anesthetized and artificially ventilated guinea pig. As in all subsequent figures, from top to bottom are time, arterial blood pressure, insufflation pressure, and nerve activity of single units of the vagal nerve. (A) Constant pressure and constant-rate inflations of the lung. (B) High-threshold PSR contrasting the activity range of this category of pulmonary receptor.

and threshold level of PSRs (Figure 1B). Threshold levels of 21 PSRs in dogs were reported by Barnas et al.[103] and ranged from less than 2.2 cm H_2O for 7 PSRs, 2.2 to 5.0 for 2 PSRs, 5.0 to 10.2 for 8 PSRs, and greater than 10.2 for 12 PSRs. One study of 12 PSRs in dogs reports an average threshold pressure inducing PSR activity to be 5.8 ± 1.5 cm H_2O.[104] As the threshold of these PSRs increased, so did the reported adaptation index. Some PSRs are tonically active at functional residual capacity, (FRC), while others are not. In reiteration, the activity may reflect the anatomical location of the PSRs.

During constant-volume hyperinflation of the lungs, some PSRs will partially adapt to the stimulus over time. In a recent review, maintained lung inflation has even been said to

189

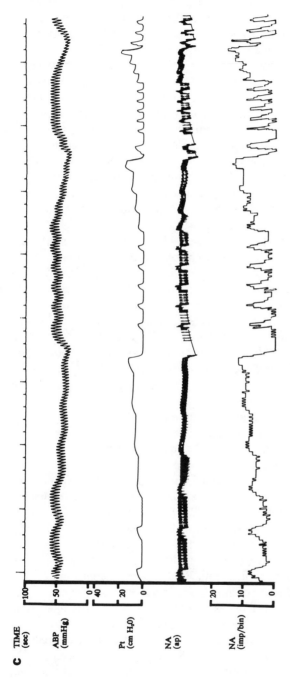

FIGURE 1C. The effect of rate on PSR activity during stepwise lung inflation induced by clamping the expiratory line of the ventilator. The ventilator was set at rates of approximately 25, 40, and 80 cycles per minute.

produce a "rapid decline" in PSR activity.[9] The slowly adapting receptor has become a popular term to describe this category of receptor. A portion, or perhaps a large portion, of the adaptation during constant-volume inflation of the lungs, at least for some of these PSRs, may be due to changes in tension of the tissue that surrounds the receptor (visceolastic properties). Davenport et al.[105] studied the adaptation of PSRs in the trachea of dogs. Adaptation occurred over the 30-min period of constant inflation, with the greatest change being within the first 3 min. However, these investigators concluded that the adaptation was the result of the viscoelastic properties of the tracheal tissue rather than of changes in PSR signal propagation. Transpulmonary pressure rather than volume appears to be the better estimator of the stimulus at the receptor site.[73,94,102,106,107] This would be especially applicable for PSRs found in the periphery of the lung as this area is more distensible than the central airways. Constant-pressure inflations of the lungs are more likely to correct for changes in airway tension due to the viscoelastic properties of the surrounding tissue rather than constant-volume inflations of the lungs, because circumference tension may accurately approximate the sensing characteristics of PSRs. In determining adaption indices of PSRs, Davis et al.[102] selected periods during the maintained inflation when both volume and pressure were nearly constant. In their study, 34 of 49 PSRs had an adaptation index of less than 10%. Therefore, constant-pressure ventilatory maneuvers would better assess the adaptation characteristics of the PSR.

Bartlett and St. John[108] have studied 84 PSRs and their adaptation rates in six different mammalian species. The adaptation rate was studied with constant-pressure inflations of 2, 5, and 10 cm H_2O. The adaptation index (initial — final spike frequency/initial $\times$ 100) ranged from 15 and 16 in the dog and guinea pig, respectively, to 27 in the hamster. No significant species variations could be determined for the adaptation index or the half time to full adaptation. The duration of the inflation was not clear, although an example presented in one figure was at least 7 s. In the studies of Ogilvie et al.,[72] static inflations of 5 s in duration showed no clear changes in the interspike interval of 81 of 83 tracheal PSRs studied in dogs. The adaptation index reported for these PSRs studied ranged from 7.4 to 29.2% (mean = 16.2). Of 15 PSRs studied by Kappagoda et al.[99] in dogs, all had an adaptation index of less than 20%.

Although adaptation of the PSR does occur, constant-pressure inflation is rarely held for more than a moment physiologically during normal conditions. Furthermore, during HFV, PSRs apparently do not adapt to this stimulus, although RARs apparently do.[109] Therefore, is PSR adaptation of physiological significance? One must also wonder how much adaptation of PSRs can be sensed by the central nervous system for two reasons. Firstly, the period of time at which constant volumes are held above FRC of the lung is normally short as compared to the adaptation rate of PSRs. Secondly, the reduction in PSR activity (or adaptation rate) is generally a small percentage of the overall activity. A number of investigators have also observed PSR activity to be influenced by the rate of lung inflation.[73,102,106,110] Although rate of inflation (increases in airflow) increases the activity of the PSR, the effect is not as remarkable as it is with RARs. Upon examination of data presented by Pack et al.,[73] increasing the rate of inflation affects PSR activity in an additive manner at best, but not in an exponential manner as it does with RARs.[111] The increase in PSR activity due to increased flow rates could possibly be explained through increased shear wall stress due to increasing turbulence within the airways in higher flow rates as predicted by Reynold's number. This would be especially true for the PSRs which are located in the more central airways and those located at airway bifurcations. Therefore, though rate sensitivity has been reported for PSRs by a number of investigators, the magnitude of the change in receptor activity is smaller than the magnitude of the change in airflow. If the PSR is affected by rates of inflation, changes in the rate of inflation should also change the magnitude of their reflex effects.

What effect does HFV have on activity of PSRs? Barnas et al.[103] observed that during HFV of 15 Hz in dogs, activity of PSRs showed no tendency to adapt in that the discharge frequency during the first 3 s of the HFV was was no different from the last 3 s. Duration of the HFV ranged from 8.5 to 29.5 s. Similar findings were observed by Rewa et al.[112] at various frequencies. No adaptation was observed when HFV was maintained for 3 min at frequencies of 8, 16, 28 Hz. High-frequency oscillatory ventilation in this study increased PSR activity at 28 Hz vs. 8 Hz when oscillatory volume and mean airway pressures were held constant.[112] However, if the average PSR frequency is divided by the oscillation frequency, then PSR activity per breath becomes 5.5, 2.8, and 1.9 at 8.16, and 28 Hz, respectively. Changes in tidal volume did not increase PSR activity when ventilation frequency and mean airway pressure were held constant. Changes in mean airway pressure increased PSR activity when breathing frequency and tidal volume were held constant. Increases in thoracic gas volume may explain the increased PSR activity. PSRs may have dynamic properties as these authors conclude; however, if PSR activity per cycle is analyzed it appears that there is a decrease in PSR activity as breathing frequency increases during HFV. Homma et al.[109] report nearly steady activity of PSRs with triangular-wave high-frequency inflation (HFI) of 10 to 50 Hz.

What evidence exists which supports different categories of PSRs? Because of the differences in the viscoelastic properties of the central vs. the peripheral airways, PSRs in the central airways tend to have a lower threshold of activation to increasing lung volume and are also more likely to have tonic activity. PSRs in the more distal airways tend to have a higher threshold of activation to increasing lung volume and are more likely to display phasic activity during the ventilation cycle. Therefore, PSRs have been categorized as low- and high-threshold receptors as proposed by Paintal[113] and type I or type II receptors are proposed by Miserocchi and Sant' Ambrogio.[69] Type I receptors are lower threshold and show a plateau in activity as a function of increasing airway pressure (saturated above 10 cm H_2O). Orientation of their receptive ending within the airway smooth muscle is proposed to be one of parallel organization.[86] These receptors also tend to be active throughout the respiratory cycle and have been called tonic PSRs. PSRs which behave in this manner are most likely to be located in the central airways. Type II receptors are higher threshold and show no plateau in activity as airway pressures increase above 10 cm H_2O. Orientation of their receptive endings within the airway smooth muscle is proposed to be one of series organization.[86] These receptors tend to be active during inspiration and silent during expiration; therefore, these receptors have been called phasic PSRs. The PSRs are most likely to be located more peripherally in the lungs. Ravi[89] has also categorized PSRs as either high or low threshold in cats and has also demonstrated the anatomical basis for the categorization. Low- and high-threshold pulmonary receptors have also been demonstrated recently in turtles.[114] In agreement with the studies of Ravi,[89] the majority of receptors in this study were also of the high-threshold type. The concept of subcategories of PSRs has been disputed by Pack et al.[72,73] and others. These receptors admittedly exist, but a continuum of receptor responses can be shown between these two extremes. These investigators have come to the same conclusion by studying numerous PSRs from a single airway.[72] No evidence supported two distinct subtypes of PSRs from studies using a range of static inflation and deflation maneuvers.

c. Chemical

The chemical stimulation of the PSR has been difficult to demonstrate. Agents which apparently stimulate PSRs directly include ammonia[71] and veratrine,[25,115] while local anesthetics,[116-118] SO_2 in rabbits only,[38] and volatile anesthetics such as ether, halothane, and acrylamide[119,120] depress or acutely abolish PSR activity. The effect of SO_2 apparently depresses PSR activity selectively because the cough reflex, assumed to be mediated by

RARs, remained functional after SO_2 administration.[121] Other agents such as histamine and acetylcholine appear to stimulate PSR activity secondarily through smooth-muscle contraction.[87,101,110,122,123]

Whether CO_2 acts directly or indirectly on PSRs has been controversial. Extratracheal pulmonary receptors apparently are not affected by either changes in either CO_2 levels or pH.[85] A number of studies have shown that PSR activity is inversely related to airway CO_2.[124-126] However, since CO_2 increases tone of airway smooth muscle, the PSR activity will also be indirectly affected.[12,106,122,124] Supportive of this assumption is that only PSR threshold activity is affected by CO_2 rather than PSR sensitivity to lung volume as has been discussed by Pack.[7] Other investigators report that CO_2 and perhaps increased hydrogen ion concentrations may stimulate PSR activity.[127]

If PSRs are indeed contained within the airway smooth muscle, then local P_aCO_2 rather than P_ACO_2 may be more influential upon PSR activity. It is thought that hydrogen ions may affect PSR activity as carbonic anhydrase administration reduces the effect of CO_2 on PSR activity. Mitchell and Vidruk[128] found no consistent effect of P_aCO_2 on PSR activity in 28 intrapulmonary PSRs of mongrel dogs, a finding consistent with earlier studies[85,124] even though increasing P_aCO_2 reduced the relationship between airway pressure and phrenic nerve activity. Therefore, alteration of this relationship must be of central rather than pulmonary origin.

3. Reflex Actions of PSRs

The category of receptor which mediates the Hering-Breuer stretch reflex is undoubtedly the PSR. Increasing PSR activity corresponding to increasing lung volumes contributes to "switching off" inspiration.[129,130] Elimination of PSR input to the central nervous system through vagotomy or through SO_2 administration in rabbits increases tidal volume, inspiratory time T_I, and blocks the apnea induced by lung inflation.[13,37,38,130]

The PSR is the only category of pulmonary receptor thus far which has been shown to produce reflex bronchodilation.[53,130-132] The probability of this effect has been well accepted. Receptors of the nonadrenergic, noncholinergic nervous system may cause reflex dilation as well;[133] however, this system may not be operative in the upper airways of the cat.[134] Lung inflation reflexly decreases the smooth-muscle tone in isolated segments of the trachea.[131,135] Stimulation of PSRs during HFV also induces reflex bronchodilation.[136] Furthermore, increased activity from tracheal and bronchial stretch receptors induced by lung inflation decreases the activity of the genioglossus muscle and delay its phasic onset of activation.[135,137,138] Sorkness and Vidruk[131] demonstrated that isocapneic changes in ventilation altered the smooth-muscle tone of the trachea in dogs. Interestingly, when frequency and tidal volume were altered reciprocally, holding alveolar ventilation constant, no change occurred in tracheal pressure. However, if either parameter was changed independently, the tracheal pressure also changed. These effects were blocked with vagotomy, which suggests the reflex action was due to activity originating from PSRs.

Does reflex bronchodilation occur in humans? In a group of seven "normal" subjects and of seven heart-lung transplant recipients, Glanville et al.[65] demonstrated that either slow or rapid lung inflation to total lung capacity lowered bronchomotor tone, but only in the seven normal subjects. Therefore, some category of receptor even in human beings apparently mediates reflex bronchodilation. Increasing the rate of inflation did not change the observed results as compared to slow inflation rates. This suggests that under these conditions RARs did not influence airway tone.

The use of HFV as a research tool has led to further understanding of the pulmonary reflexes originating from not only PSRs, but from RARs as well. HFV causes apnea in dogs ventilated at 15 Hz with constant mean lung volumes and constant end-expiratory CO_2 levels.[103] Neuronal recordings from pulmonary afferents during HFV showed that activity of most PSRs increases during its application, while activity of RARs did not increase during HFV as long as mean lung volume remained above FRC. Results similar to those of Barnas are reported by Homma et al.[109,139] using a triangular pulse wave rather than a sinusoidal wave. Both HFI and high-frequency deflation (HFD) were tested. Peak airway pressures in the first study were 7.3 ± 0.8 cm H_2O, while those of the second were reported to be 10 cm H_2O. Peak pressures of 10 cm H_2O would be expected to stimulate a number of RARs even at ventilatory rates within the physiological range. However, the number of spikes ''locked'' to each HFI pulse decreased for RARs and remained constant for PSRs as the frequency of the HFI increased from 10 to 50 Hz.[109] HFI prolonged T_E at higher frequencies and shortened T_E at lower frequencies, which probably reflects PSR activity. HFD shortened T_E. During near single-fiber recording, HFI stimulated both PSRs and RARs, but HFD stimulated RARs only. RARs may therefore decrease T_E, at least during HFD. It is uncertain whether or not changes in FRC may have influenced the results of this study.

C-fiber endings are assumed not to be stimulated by HFV unless lung volumes became very high. However, no study has recorded C-fiber ending activity during HFV. Therefore, the reflex effects due to HFV which were observed above FRC are assumed to be mainly mediated by PSR stimulation. These reflexes included apnea or prolonged T_E and bronchodilation. Furthermore, T_E duration is thought to be a direct function of PSR activity.[109,139-141] Bilateral vagotomy in a number of species or SO_2 administration in rabbits prevents both the apnea or prolonged T_E due to the HFV, demonstrating that these affects were indeed due to reflex actions.[109,139,141] Quantitatively, Zuperku et al.[142] report that for each increase in 1 cm H_2O of airway pressure, T_E increases 400%. Barnas et al.[103] observed an approximate increase of three impulses per second in PSR activity for each 1 cm H_2O increase in static airway pressure.

To demonstrate that the mechanism of activation for both PSRs and RARs includes HFV and not just changes in FRC, the activity of PSRs and RARs were compared during conditions of spontaneous breathing, static lung inflations to levels equal to the increase in FRC induced by HFV, and during HFV itself at 29 Hz.[93] Because the distending pressure during HFV dissipates as a function of the airway generation, these investigators also localized the receptors of their study. PSR response to HFV decreased as the receptors were more peripheral in their location. PSR activity increased with static inflation of the lungs which reflects the change in pressure induced by HFV. However, the activity of the PSRs increased considerably more during the application of HFV. The increase in PSR activity during HFV vs. static inflation was increased 3.7 times for extratracheal PSRs, 3.2 times for PSRs in the upper intrathoracic trachea, 2.5 times for PSRs in the lower intrathoracic trachea, and 2.1 times for intrapulmonary PSRs. Therefore, the effect of HFV upon PSR activity diminishes as a function of the airway generation. RARs did not respond to the static inflation because of its low volume, but did respond to HFV. The effect of location and HFV upon RAR activity was not analyzed in this study. Therefore, the stimulation of both receptor types was due primarily to HFV and secondarily to increased FRC.

T_E has been shown to increase during conditions other than HFV. Davenport and Wozniak[97] increased the expiratory load, which increased the discharge of PSRs during the expiratory phase of ventilation in rabbits, and found T_E to increase. At equivalent levels of end expiratory volume (V_E), resistive loading increased T_E more than did elastic loading. This relationship between V_E and T_E was also abolished with the administration of SO_2, implicating the activity of PSRs in the reflex. Furthermore, unilateral vagotomy reduced the resulting increase in T_E associated with increased expiratory load administration. These authors believe the length of T_E is a function of the temporal (number of impulses from a fiber as a function of time) and spacial (number of active fibers at one time) conditions.

PSRs also influence expiratory muscle activity. In opossums, continuous positive airway pressure (CPAP of 6 to 8 cm H_2O) increased activity of abdominal muscles to enhance expiratory effort.[100] During the application of CPAP the vagi were bilaterally cooled in steps of 2° at 5-min intervals beginning at 14°C. Abdominal muscle activity ceased at temperatures ranging from 12 to 7.6°C (9.6°C average). Concurrently, both spacial and temporal activity of the diaphragm (EMG) increased. As the vagi were further cooled by an average of 4 more degrees, diaphragm EMG further increased. Pulmonary afferent recordings demonstrated that PSR activity increased with CPAP while RAR activity increased initially, but then adapted to this stimulus. A minority of PSRs which originally had tonic expiratory activity during CPAP ceased tonic expiratory activity to CPAP after 5 min. During cooling of the vagi, temperatures of 12 to 7°C attenuated PSR activity more than it did RAR activity. Although C-fiber endings were not recorded in this study, C-fiber endings are presumed to be less affected at these temperatures than either PSRs or RARs whose fibers are myelinated.[143] This increased activity of the diaphragm could originate from either RARs or C-fiber endings in addition to PSR inhibition. Studies in rabbits also demonstrate the diaphragmatic activity increased with HFV and was further enhanced with SO_2 administration.[141]

PSRs and RARs have myelinated fibers, and the overlap of the conduction velocities is great as determined in the dog[66] and in the guinea pig.[144] However, reflexes generated from PSRs appear to be affected in graded cooling studies before those of RARs.[100,141] Furthermore, through cross-correlation studies, the lag time between PSR activity and peak airway pressure was significantly shorter than RARs.[109] This lag time is a function of conduction velocity. These results suggest the conduction velocities or the time to peak generator potential of PSRs are faster than those of RARs. Therefore, augmented inspiratory activity can be attributed in part to the removal of PSR input at 7°C. This enhancement of inspiratory effort could also be due to unantagonized inspiratory reflexes originating from RARs at a temperature of 7°C, as RARs may still have limited function at this temperature. In the study by Farber,[100] further inspiratory augmentation was observed at an average temperature decrease of 4°C beyond the temperature where the effect was observed initially. Inspiratory augmentation could be mediated only through unmyelinated afferent fibers at lower temperatures once RAR receptor activity ceases. This may be another reflex action of C-fiber endings.[145] Since it is likely that increased airway tone would be observed as PSR activity becomes much reduced at approximately 9.6°C, this alone could be an explanation. RARs may not reflexly increase airway tone. As RARs appear to be functional at temperatures lower than those of PSRs, the further increase in airway tone observed at 5 to 6°C may correspond to elimination of this second group of myelinated afferent neurons, namely the RARs, leaving C-fiber endings totally unantagonized which undoubtedly contributes to airway tone.

PSRs apparently reflexly affect functions outside the lungs in addition to their respiratory reflexes. Low lung volumes appear to cause tachycardia,[104,146] while higher lung volumes may cause bradycardia.[147] However, the Hering-Breuer stretch reflex has a lower threshold. Therefore, there may be little physiological significance of such a reflex. Lung inflation also produces varying effects on various vascular beds. These results are discussed in detail by De Burgh Daly.[148]

B. RAPIDLY ADAPTING RECEPTORS (IRRITANT RECEPTORS)
1. Location
The RARs are presumed to be located within the airway epithelium. Supportive evidence for this presumption remains circumstantial.[117,149,150] Histological studies have shown certain endings ramify to the airway lumen with unmyelinated dendrites traveling between epithelial cells.[151-154] Indirect proof of the RAR association with the epithelium has been reported by Mortola et al.[155] and Sant' Ambrogio et al.[149] The response to mechanical probing of RARs may be eliminated by the removal of the epithelial layer. However, its fiber will still respond to lung inflation maneuvers. Therefore, the RAR may be a complex of terminals, some

associated with the epithelium and others with deeper layers, perhaps collagen or even smooth muscle.

Analysis of RAR distribution within the airways has been reported by several groups of investigators. In dogs, Mortola et al.[155] reported studying 196 RARs, of which 14% were associated with the trachea, 19% in the bronchus, 25% in the lobar bronchi, and 42% in the bronchioles. The highest concentration of RARs per square centimeter occurred in the lobar bronchi. Widdicombe's[101] earlier studies in the cat are supportive of these findings. More recently, Jonzon et al.[156] reported that of 31 RARs studied in dogs, approximately half were in the main or lobar bronchi, while the others were more distally located. In one study of 42 RARs recorded from the left cervical vagus nerve in dogs, we found 15% in the extrapulmonary airway, 8% in the upper lobe, 39% in the middle lobe, 32% in the lower lobe, and 6% were located in the contralateral lung.[157]

The distribution of RARs in the airways of guinea pigs appears to be very similar to the distribution of RARs reported in the dog. We have found that in the guinea pig 9% of the receptors studied were associated with the trachea, 33% with the carina and hilar region, 39% with the lower peripheral lung, and 18% with the upper peripheral lung in one study,[144] and a very similar distribution in another.[158] RARs may also be concentrated at airway bifurcations.[101,149,155,159] It is likely that the RARs exist from the larynx[160] down to distal airways in which PSRs have already been shown to exist.

In the trachea, RARs are located in both the regions of the cartilage and the trachealis muscle, which is unlike the distribution of PSRs.[149] PSRs have been demonstrated to be associated with the membranous posterior wall of the trachea only.[83] This has lead Wozniak et al.[93] to propose two different groups of RARs. RARs associated with the trachealis muscle may be primarily mechanoreceptors responding to various ventilatory maneuvers, while RARs associated with the cartilaginous regions of the trachea may respond more to irritants.

2. Stimuli

a. Activity During Eupneic Breathing

RARs activity during eupneic breathing shows individual variation among individual receptors, but not nearly like that observed with PSRs. Generally, activity of the RARs during eupneic breathing is irregular and sparse. In rabbits, of 24 RARs, 10 had virtually no eupneic activity, while 14 had basal activity ranging from 0.2 to 6.3 impulses per second.[159] The basal activity of RAR in rabbits,[159] dogs,[161] and guinea pigs[144] has been reported to be quite low, being 0.8, 0.3, and 0.2 impulses per second, respectively. Mills et al.[76] report that RAR activity increases during prolonged experimentation, presumably as lung compliance decreases. This is phenomena that we also observe in guinea pigs. In addition, RAR discharge in rabbits was observed to increase when both vagi rather than one had been severed.[162]

b. Mechanical

RARs respond vigorously to pressure or touch of their receptive endings,[76,77] much more so than PSRs. One may use this method of RAR stimulation to define the area of the lungs which house the field of the RAR. In larger animals this may be accomplished through the use of a fiber-optic bronchoscope. An example of probing the receptive field of an RAR and its resulting response is shown in Figure 2A.

RARs respond to rapid changes in lung volume, be it either inflation or deflation (Figure 2B and 2C).[109,111,139,144,159] RARs tend to have higher thresholds of activation when compared to PSRs. Generally, this threshold begins at approximately two times the normal tidal volume. Kaufman et al.[104] report an average threshold level of 13.5 ± 2.2 cm H_2O for RAR activation during an inflation rate of 1.5 to 2.0 cm H_2O per second beginning at 2.5 cm H_2O and ending at 30.0 cm H_2O. Not only the volume change, but the rate of change (dP/dt) influences the degree of RAR stimulation (Figure 2C, and Figure 3). If one analyzes the response of

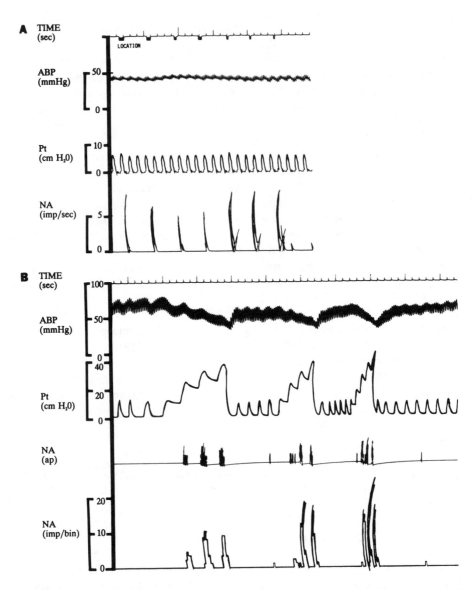

FIGURE 2.   Mechanical and ventilatory characteristics of intrapulmonary rapidly adapting receptors (RAR) in guinea pigs. (A) Location of RARs after thoracotomy. The probe was a small cotton pledget soaked in 0.9% NaCl. (B) The effect of rate on RAR activity during stepwise lung inflation. The ventilator was set at rates of approximately 20, 40, and 80 cycles per minute.

RARs to a stepwise inflation of the lung by occluding the expiratory line of the ventilator, activity of the RAR occurs primarily when the volume of the lungs is changing. However, the functional relationship "fits" best when changes in transpulmonary pressure are used rather than changes in lung volume. Therefore, changes in transpulmonary pressure may be the more accurate representation of the stimuli of the RAR rather than changes in lung volume. The rate of volume change often lowers the threshold of the receptors and it is also possible to change volume slowly enough so as not to stimulate some RARs even up to volumes near total lung capacity (TLC) (Figure 2C). If one examines the pattern of discharge of the RARs during the corresponding changes in insufflation pressure, the greatest activity of these receptors corresponds to the period in time in which insufflation pressure is changing the most.[111,163] Thereafter, even though airway pressures are held high, but remain constant,

197

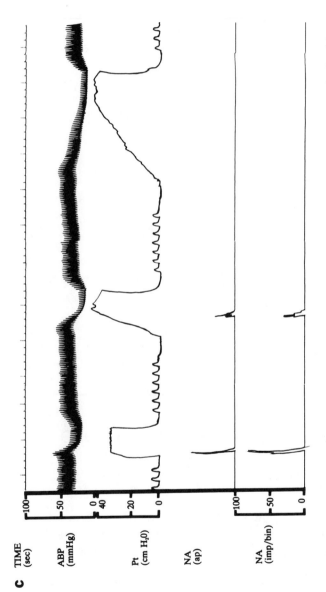

FIGURE 2C. The effect of flow rate on RAR activity during ramp inflations. This receptor had obvious rate-related activity.

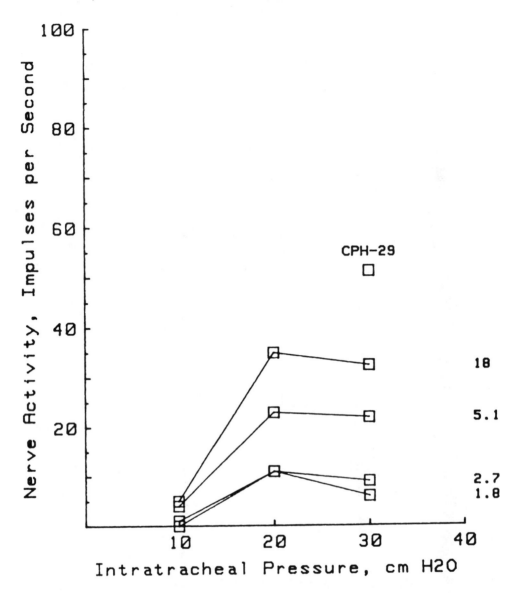

FIGURE 3.   The effect of rate on one RAR in a guinea pig. Ramp inflations are 1.8, 2.7, 5.1, and 18 cc/s and constant pressure inflation is 29 cm H$_2$O. RAR activity increases as a function of rate of airflow.

RAR activity will adjust dramatically to a lower and sporadic level of activity or may even stop firing altogether. On further analysis of the data of Pack and Delaney,[111] modeling of the data reveals that the response of the RAR to changes in airflow rate fits an exponential function or a power function.

To be classified as a RAR, Widdecombe established a criteria that 70% of the action potential recorded from fibers innervating an RAR must occur within 2 s of the beginning of a maintained constant-pressure inflation of the lungs.[101,164] This criteria remains the standard for identification of these receptor types. In studies of RARs in dogs, Pack and Delaney[111] report an average adaptation index of 94.1% for the 37 receptors studied. Barnas et al.[103] report 86.8% for 6 receptors, Sampson and Vidruk[161] report 93.1% for 35 receptors, and Kappagoda et al.[99] report 82.6% for 11 receptors.

c. Chemical

Because the sensory endings of RARs apparently project to the airway lumen, it has been logical to assume that this strategic location supports the assumption that the RARs are important receptors in mediating pulmonary defense mechanisms. RARs are thought to be activated by noxious gases, chemicals, congestion, emboli, pneumothorax, and even mediators of anaphylaxis of allergic reactions.[76,165] Thus, the original terminology of RAR was replaced by Widdicombe with the term of "irritant" receptors, which gained popularity and wide acceptance in both the basic and the clinical sciences.[66] Many defense reflexes began to be associated with this category of receptor. Initial studies clearly demonstrated that increased activity of the RARs occurs concurrently with the challenge of numerous putative mediators of anaphylaxis, irritant gases, and foreign chemicals. Activity of RARs increases with the administration of histamine,[58,76,144,161,166-168] bradykinin,[47,169] $PGF_{2\alpha}$,[158,166,167,169,170] serotonin,[58] substance P,[171] and adenosine.[172,173] The list of gases which stimulate RARs include ammonia, chlorine, cigarette smoke,[144,174,175] and volatile anesthetics such as ether and halothane.[144,174,176] Foreign chemicals which have been reported to increase RAR activity includes phenyl diguanide[77,159] and capsaicin, but indirectly in the cat[159] and the guinea pig,[306a] and veratridine.[8,115]

The stimulation of the RAR by these putative mediators and foreign chemicals, but necessarily not by the gases, are usually accompanied by increases in airway resistance or intra-airway pressure. In dogs, Sampson and Vidruk[167] found that histamine stimulated 88% of the RARs studied. This stimulation was accompanied by increases in insufflation pressure. With the administration of 5 to 10 µg/kg of isoproterenol prior to the histamine challenge, the increase in insufflation pressure to the histamine challenge was reduced 81%, but RAR activity was reduced only 26%. Sampson and Vidruk[161] further tested the correlation of RAR irritability and insufflation pressure by administering equimolar doses of histamine and acetylcholine as an aerosol to the lungs of dogs. They found histamine to have more of an effect on the RARs than did acetylcholine, while acetylcholine had more potent action in increasing intra-airway pressure than did histamine. Other studies have supported a direct mechanism of histamine.[31,77,175] Perhaps an alternative explanation may be that histamine may have greater action on central airways,[45,58] while cholinergic agents such as acetylcholine or methacholine may have greater action on peripheral airways.[177] In addition, Shioya et al.[178] demonstrated that methacholine is a potent bronchoconstrictor in the first six generations of the airways, but progressively increases in its effects in the lower generations. If a RAR being studied was located in the central airways, then histamine may appear to have the greater direct action on the receptor. Similar effects may be observed if the aerosol favored either central airway or peripheral airway deposition.[179] In addition, Kariya et al.[180] determined that methacholine had greater potency upon the lung parenchyma as measured by monitoring resistance during slow ventilation with a large tidal volume as compared to the potency of methacholine upon the central airways by monitoring resistance during fast ventilation with a small tidal volume.

The association of RAR or "irritant" receptor activation and its mediation of reflex bronchoconstriction by mediators such as histamine has been thought to occur not only in animals, but in man as well.[181] However, the probability that RARs mediate defense reflexes across species lines becomes unlikely as RARs were characterized in species other than the dog and the rabbit. However, even in the dog, stimulation of RARs by either histamine or $PGF_{2\alpha}$ appeared to be related to ventilation mechanics.[166] RARs in the cat have not been shown to be activated by histamine unless accompanied by changes in lung mechanics.[159] Similarly, RARs of guinea pigs[80,144,158] increase activity as the result of histamine challenge. However, as in the cat, this activity shows great correlation with the accompanying increase in insufflation pressure.[158] This activation of RARs in the guinea pig by histamine is dependent upon changes in insufflation pressure which reflects changes in either compliance or resistance or both. The viscoelastic properties of the tissues which support or house the nerve endings would necessarily have to become "stiffer" in order to activate these receptor endings. In the guinea pig, if increased smooth-muscle tone is prevented from developing by the administration of a beta 2 adrenergic receptor agonist such as epinephrine, isoproterenol, or terbutaline, then RAR activation can be attenuated as well (Figure 4).[144] The activation of RARs by leukotriene C_4 (LTC_4) and bradykinin also appears to be an indirect one in the guinea pig.[182,183] Furthermore, either salicylic acid or acetylsalicylic acid antagonized increases in both RAR activity and insufflation pressure induced by either LTC_4 or bradykinin challenge.[182] Therefore, in guinea pigs the smooth-muscle activation by either LTC_4 or bradykinin appears to be a product of arachidonic acid metabolism. The activation of the RAR then appears to be due either to a product of arachidonic acid metabolism or smooth-muscle contraction as the result of its release.

Of the putative mediators studied thus far, $PGF_{2\alpha}$ has probable direct action on RAR activity in the guinea pig[158] and possibly in the dog.[184] A point must be made, however, that activation of a receptor by a putative mediator of anaphylaxis even by direct means does not predispose that receptor to then mediate reflex bronchoconstriction. Such a supposition then leads to a puzzling contradiction when faced with situations where chemicals or gases such as ether, which do not necessarily develop subsequent bronchoconstriction, stimulate RARs very strongly, at least in guinea pigs. Furthermore, stimulation by either aerosol challenge or by intravenous injection of a mediator undoubtedly causes the release of other agents which may be the actual stimulating agent. For example, adenosine may affect certain pulmonary receptors.[172,173] However, adenosine has been shown also to stimulate histamine release from human mast cells.[185] There yet may be a mediator released which stimulates RARs directly. Antigen aerosol in dogs (*Ascaris suum*) stimulated RARs[157,186] and also in guinea pigs sensitized to ovalbumin (Figure 5). The activity of this particular RAR appears to be far beyond the corresponding mechanical changes of the airways. As noted in Figure 5, not all RARs respond in this manner. The activity of some receptors in response to antigen challenge is obviously the result of changes in airway mechanics. Investigators in the laboratory of Coleridge, Sampson, and Widdencombe have all commented on the great variability of RARs not only in response to chemicals, but in basal activity as well. Those in the past who have suggested subcategories of this receptor may yet see this reconsidered.

Ozone exposure has been suspected to contribute to obstructive pulmonary disease, especially in asthmatic patients. Bronchial hyperirritability occurs in man after exposure to ozone.[187] In that study, histamine aerosol of the same concentrations increased airway resistance significantly more after ozone exposure than before ozone exposure. Furthermore, atropine pretreatment blocked the increase in airway resistance produced by histamine. Therefore, a cholinergic pathway was suspected to mediate the reflex component of bronchoconstriction. These investigators suggested that ozone may sensitize bronchial irritant or RARs to mediators such as histamine. In dogs,[188-190] exposure to ozone increased the bronchomotor response to aerosol challenge of histamine and of $PGF_{2\alpha}$. This response was also blocked by atropine pretreatment or by cooling the vagal nerves.

Since dogs and humans treated with ozone become hypersensitive to either histamine or $PGF_{2\alpha}$ and because RARs are suspected to be stimulated by these agents to cause reflex bronchoconstriction, we studied the effect of ozone on the response of RARs to histamine or $PGF_{2\alpha}$ aerosol challenge.[191] The experiments were done in a blind manner in that the dogs were treated with ozone or compressed air in another laboratory. The dogs were challenged with histamine or $PGF_{2\alpha}$ aerosol 24 h later while recording from fibers of RARs. The airway response to aerosol challenge of histamine of $PGF_{2\alpha}$ was either greater or unchanged from that in the sham-treated dog (Figure 6). However, the response of the RARs to the aerosol challenge of histamine or $PGF_{2\alpha}$ in the dogs treated with ozone was less then those of the sham-treated dogs.

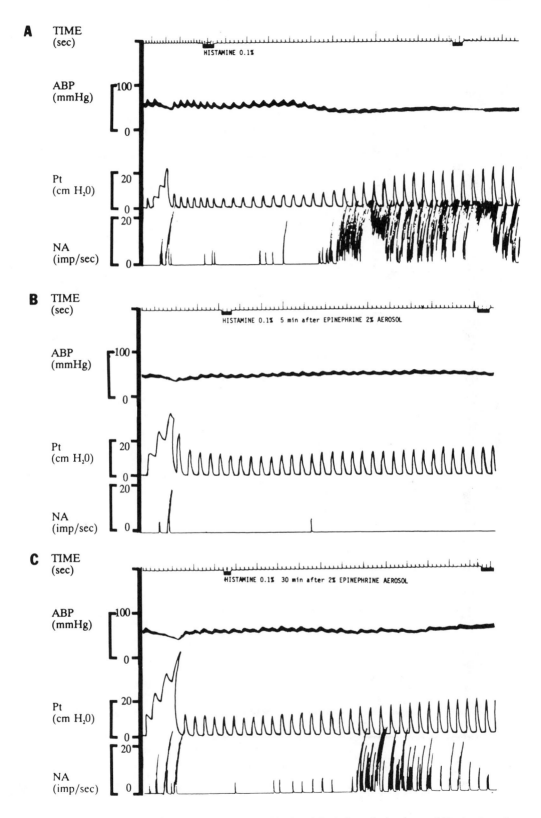

FIGURE 4.   Histamine aerosol challenge of 0.01% and RAR activity before, 5 min after, and 30 min after prior epinephrine aerosol administration of 2.0% (30 s). RAR activity appears dependent upon changes in pulmonary mechanics.

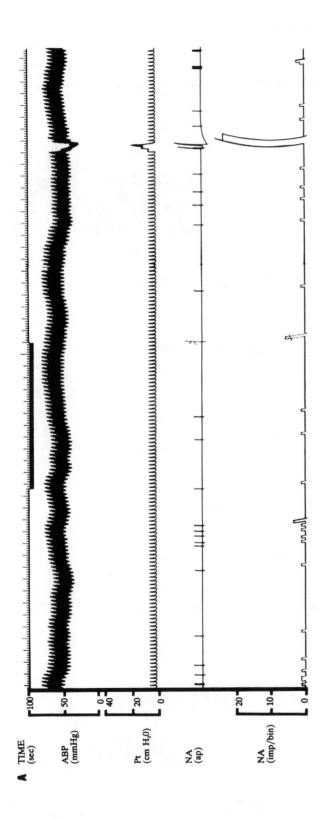

203

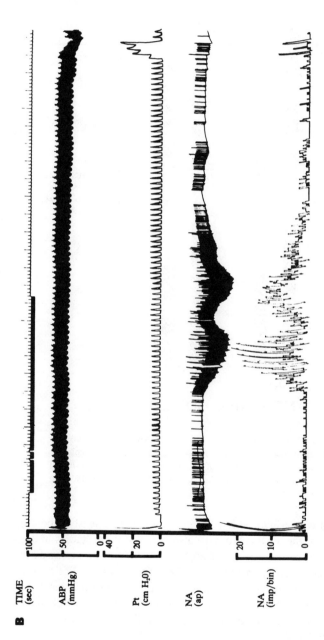

FIGURE 5A and B. Comparison of the effect of aerosol administration of distilled water (A) and ovalbumin (B) upon RAR activity in an OA-sensitized guinea pig; OA% is as indicated by event markers. Not all RARs react to OA in such a manner. Other RARs are activated in relationship to changes in intratracheal pressure (Pt).

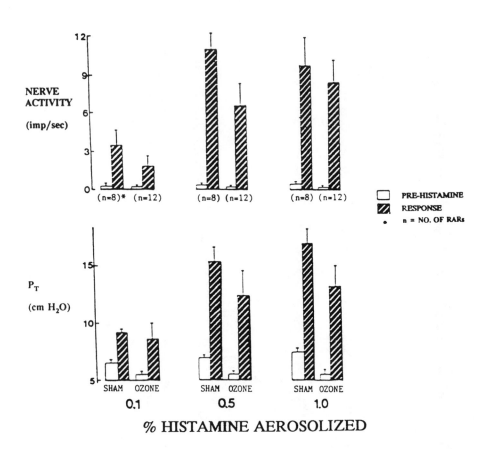

A. SUMMARY OF AIRWAY AND RAR RESPONSES TO HISTAMINE

(Mean ± SE)

FIGURE 6.   The effect of ozone on Pt and RAR nerve activity in dogs. Open columns are base level. First hatched columns represent compressed air-treated (2 h) dogs and second hatch columns represent ozone-treated dogs (0.1%, 2 h). The reactivity of the airways and RARs were studied 24 h after exposure in response to histamine aerosol challenge (A) or $PGF_{2\alpha}$ aerosol challenge (B). In neither case was RAR activity increased.

   Therefore, the mechanism of ozone-induced hyperirritability is not, at least in the dog, the result of increased sensitivity of the RARs. We have also repeated these studies in dogs while studying the effects of ozone on the activity of 24 PSRs. Ozone again increased the action of histamine and $PGF_{2\alpha}$ on insufflation pressure. The response of the PSRs in the dogs exposed to ozone was depressed when challenged with histamine aerosol compared to the sham-treated dogs (Figure 6A). However, the reverse was true for aerosol challenge with $PGF_{2\alpha}$. For two doses of $PGF_{2\alpha}$ tested, the discharge of PSRs was greater in dogs treated with ozone as compared to the sham-treated dogs (Figure 6B). If the activity of PSRs is not universally depressed by ozone treatment, then it is unlikely that the hyperirritability of the airways after ozone exposure is due to the elimination of the bronchodilatory affects of PSRs. To understand the reflex mechanism of ozone one must also know what effect ozone has upon C-fiber endings. Such experiments have not yet been performed.

B. SUMMARY OF AIRWAY AND RAR RESPONSES
   TO PROSTAGLANDIN F$_{2\alpha}$

(Mean ± SE)

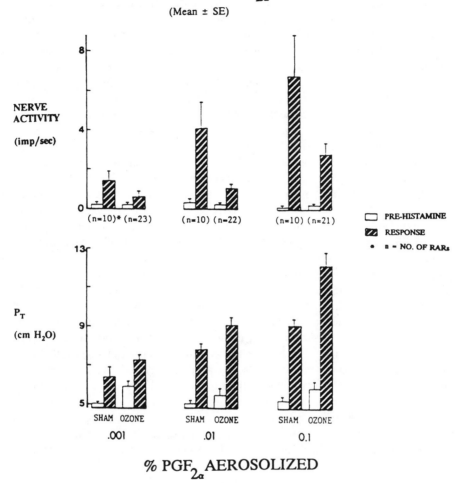

FIGURE 6B.

3. Reflex Effects of Rapidly Adapting Receptors

What are the other possible functions that may be attributed to the RARs? One possible function of these receptors is that RARs may be important in relaying the state of compliance of the lungs to the medulla or even higher centers, such as the pneumotaxic centers.[76,77,156,162,192] A decrease in pulmonary compliance induced by removing positive end expiratory pressure in dogs being ventilated with an open chest proved to be a strong stimulus for RARs in dogs[156] and also in cats and rabbits.[192] This type of stimulus has little or no affect on changing the activity of PSRs or C-fiber endings. In guinea pigs, deflation of the lungs is a strong stimulus for RARs[80,144] and an ineffective stimulus to most PSRs.[306a] However, in dogs, some PSRs may be tonically activated by such a ventilatory maneuver.[9] C-fiber endings are reported to be relatively insensitive to deflation.[2,159,193]

Deflation or decreases in compliance, which seem to activate RARs selectively, may then initiate the gasp reflex or the periodic sighs which are seen during normal ventilation patterns.[120,141,194-198] Inspiratory activity below FRC cannot be explained by absence of PSR activity alone (disinhibition). Phrenic activity in rabbits at subatmospheric intratracheal pressure is greater with the vagi intact as compared to activity after vagotomy.[199] Furthermore, as the vagi are cooled to 30, 8, and 0°C, tonic inspiratory activity is reduced as the temperature is lowered in response to the administration of subatmospheric intratracheal pressure. Since smaller temperature changes from 8 to 0°C were not studied, this affect cannot be definitively attributed to either RARs or C-fiber endings alone. The increased inspiratory activity from these pulmonary receptors would induce lung inflation. The inflation of the lungs during these conditions would restore compliance by expanding peripheral airways, open closed airways or collapsed alveoli, and increase the efficiency of the surfactant system.

HFV studies support the possibility that RAR stimulation increases inspiratory activity. In dogs, HFV above FRC under certain conditions has no effect on RARs.[103,112] However, RARs have been reported to increase their activity to HFV[93] and especially when the pattern of ventilation was triangular in nature.[109,139] When the lung volume was below FRC during HFV, RAR activity was increased[103] as it was with HFD.[109,139] The mechanism of this activation of the RARs was thought to be due to airway deformation.[103] In another study, HFV was observed to increase diaphragmatic activity in rabbits.[141] The oscillatory pressure used in this study was both positive and negative. Although the increased diaphragmatic activity could have been caused by either RAR or C-fiber activity, perhaps both, RARs seem to be the more likely candidate with the knowledge available at present. No studies of HFV have been performed while recording from unmyelinated pulmonary receptors.

In rabbits, treatment with SO_2, which eliminates activity of PSRs to the central nervous system, T_I and diaphragmatic activity has been shown to increase, while T_E decreases with deflation.[37,38,102,200] Furthermore, in rabbits during HFV, phrenic nerve activity (or EMG) decreased prior to SO_2 administration, but increased after SO_2 administration.[141] Therefore, RARs may function to increase T_I in addition to inducing augmented inspiration such as sighs or gasps.[162,201] This is supportive of earlier studies which report that T_I increases as the result of RAR activation.[202,203] However, there are studies which suggest that this may not be the case. In human patients with lung transplantation, periodic sighs are demonstrable despite the apparent lack of nervous connections to the central nervous system.[22] Elimination of PSR activity could possibly explain both the observed increase in T_I and phrenic activity. In summary, because RAR stimulation by bronchoactive chemicals appears for the most part to be related to airway smooth-muscle tone, the direct cause-effect relationship of RAR activation by mediators of anaphylaxis and reflex bronchoconstriction appears to be weak. Therefore, RARs may not function to cause reflex-increased smooth-muscle tone, but may activate augmented lung inflation to large lung volumes. Through this mechanical means the diameter of small airways may be increased by stretching airway smooth muscle, thereby decreasing airway resistance. Compliance of the lung may also be restored by overcoming the critical closing pressure of affected airways or alveoli and redistributing the surfactants, thereby increasing the effective volume of the lungs. Reflex actions other than these remain obscure with respect to the RAR. Therefore, RARs may not induce increases in bronchomotor tone, but may actually decrease airway resistance through inducing certain ventilatory maneuvers.

C. PULMONARY AND BRONCHIAL C-FIBER ENDINGS
1. Location
The blood supply to the C-fiber endings has been used to categorize this receptor type into two subcategories: pulmonary and bronchial C-fiber endings. Type J receptors, originally described[204] and termed by Paintal,[67,204,205] are those C-fiber endings which are closely associated with the region of the alveolus and the alveolar or "pulmonary" capillary blood supply. Therefore, the term "pulmonary C-fiber endings" is used to describe these receptors.[67] Histological investigations of C-fiber endings in the mouse in this region shows unmyelinated fibers of a sensory appearance (presence of neurotubules and mitochondria) associated with the alveolar type I cell and the alveolar duct.[206] A group of C-fiber endings,

however, have been demonstrated to have a shorter latency to provocative chemicals such as capsaicin injected through the bronchial vs. the pulmonary circulation,[68] hence the term "bronchial C-fiber ending". The receptive endings of this category of C-fibers could possibly reach the lumen of the conducting airways. Nerve fiber endings have been observed in the bronchial walls and epithelium.[154,207]

Identification of pulmonary or bronchial C-fiber endings by drug injections alone may be misleading. Determination of the location of some C-fiber endings through pulmonary or bronchial circulation by drug injection has proved to be difficult, as anastomosis exists between these two circulatory routes.[57,104,208] This could lead to incorrect conclusions of the type of C-fiber endings being studied. Therefore, caution must be used in categorizing these receptor types by drug injection and by determination of its conduction velocity alone. For example, C-fibers were studied in rabbits, and phenyl diguanide was injected via the pulmonary or bronchial circulation. The latency of stimulation of the receptor was used to test their location. Of the 15 fibers tested, apparently 4 were pulmonary C-fiber endings, 6 were bronchial, and the remaining 6 were accessible with equal latency through either intravenous or carotid artery injection.[40] A similar observation was made by Trenchard et al.[288] in the rabbit. Of 20 nonmyelinated pulmonary receptors, 3 were named "pulmonary-bronchial" receptors.

Fiber-optic bronchoscopy can be used in larger animals to determine C-fiber location, but this is not an alternative procedure for locating C-fiber endings in small animals. Coleridge and Coleridge[68,218] have reported locating the receptor site by probing the lungs after the experiment and advise such substantiation of the location of the C-fiber endings. An example of the response of C-fiber endings to pressure is demonstrated in a study by Paintal.[67]

In summarizing their location, C-fiber endings are probably present throughout the tracheal-bronchial tree (bronchial C-fiber endings), as well as within or around the alveolus itself (pulmonary C-fiber endings). Indeed, Armstrong and Luck[159] report no area of specific C-fiber ending concentration within the tracheal bronchial tree. Boushey et al.[209] demonstrated C-fibers in the afferent pathway of the superior laryngeal nerve. Physiological evidence of this through cold-air challenge has been reported by Jammes et al.[210] There are those who believe that C-fiber endings may have some association with neuroepithelial bodies of the airways.[211,212] The possibility of this association needs further study.

2. Stimuli
a. Activity During Eupneic Breathing

Base level activity for C-fiber endings during breathing has been reported to be about 0.2 impulses per second for pulmonary C-fiber endings and about 2 impulses per second for bronchial C-fiber endings in dogs[143] in one study and approximately 1.4 and 2.4 impulses per second in another study for nine C-fiber endings each.[99] The pattern of C-fiber activity during eupneic breathing is typically low and can be either seemingly quite independent of any ventilatory correlation with either regular or irregular activity, especially that of bronchial C-fibers. Bronchial C-fibers display irregular but sustained activity during maintained lung inflation as well.[104] On the other hand, the activity of some C-fibers may appear to have ventilatory modulation and may be activity originating from pulmonary C-fibers. However, pulsatile pressures have been reported not to stimulate type J receptors,[67] which is not the case for PSRs and RARs.

b. Mechanical

Mechanical stimulation by constant pressure or stepwise inflation of the lungs of either category of C-fiber ending is weak compared to either of the other two categories of pulmonary receptors (Figure 7).[67,104,159,213,214] For example, stepwise inflation of the lungs to TLC may elicit but a few action potentials from either pulmonary or bronchial C-fiber

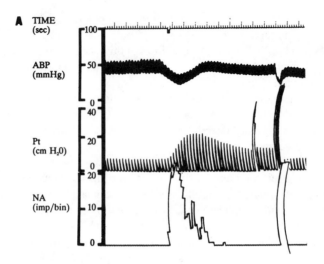

FIGURE 7. Comparison of the effect of capsaicin 10 μg/kg in two different guinea pigs, while recording from a RAR (A) and from a C-fiber ending (B). The subclassification of the C-fiber ending was not determined. Its conduction velocity was 1.2 m/s.

endings.[68,159,214,215] There is an apparent difference in sensitivity of the subcategories of C-fiber endings to mechanical stimulation. Pulmonary C-fiber endings are more sensitive to changes in intrapulmonary pressure.[104] The average pressure found to activate 13 pulmonary C-fiber endings was found to be about 16 cm H_2O, while that of bronchial C-fiber endings was 27 cm H_2O.[104] Of the 10 bronchial C-fiber endings, 2 had threshold pressures of 46 cm H_2O to induce receptor activation. Some bronchial C-fiber endings may not respond to lung inflation.[68] The observation indirectly confirms the existence of the two different anatomical locations of C-fiber endings. The lung parenchyma where pulmonary C-fiber endings are located would be under greater elastic stress when the lungs are being inflated than bronchial C-fiber endings which are located in larger airways.

Deflation appears to be a weak stimulus for C-fiber endings. Coleridge et al.[215] and Coleridge and Coleridge[3,68] report that in dogs neither pulmonary nor bronchial C-fiber endings are stimulated by the collapse of the lungs in dogs with an open chest or when a negative pressure (i.e., forced deflation) is applied to the tracheal cannula. Armstrong and Luck[159] also report deflation of the lungs to have no affect on C-fiber activity in cats. However, others have reported that deflation does stimulate at least some C-fiber endings.[205,214,216] Hyperdeflation of the lungs, which results in mechanical deformation of the bronchial walls, has been reported to stimulate bronchial C-fiber endings in cats.[216]

Although only several studies report the effect of rates of inflation on PSR and RAR activity, no systematic report exists on the dynamic nature of C-fiber endings. Kaufman et al.[104] have recorded from C-fiber endings during a slow inflation of 1.5 to 2.0 cm H_2O per second to 30 cm H_2O and a constant-pressure inflation at 30 cm H_2O in dogs. Both pulmonary and bronchial C-fiber endings apparently have adaptive characteristics to constant-pressure inflation of the lungs. The range of adaptation is quite large. Of 13 pulmonary C-fiber endings, 6 stopped firing within 1 min while the remaining 7 fired throughout a 15-min inflation period, but with some adaptation reported. Of 10 bronchial C-fiber endings, 4 stopped firing within 1 min of the application of 30 cm H_2O constant-pressure inflation, 2 did not reach threshold pressure levels, and the remaining 4 either had some adaptation or fired irregularly throughout the 15-min period. Both categories of C-fiber endings were essentially inactive at maintained pressures of 2.5 cm H_2O.

Temperature may also influence the activity of C-fiber endings, especially those located

209

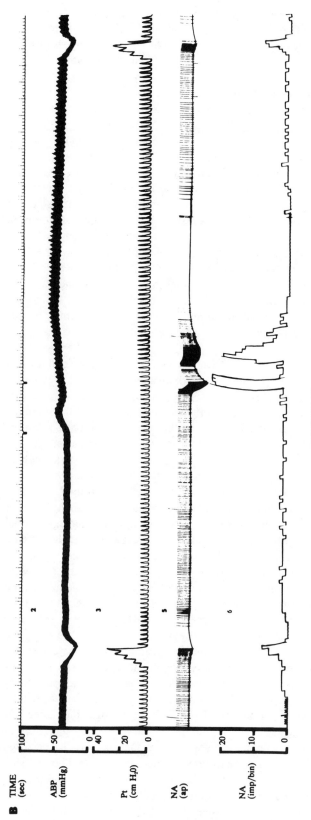

FIGURE 7B.

in the larynx. Sectioning of the superior laryngeal nerve or administration of procaine reduced the increase in airway resistance due to the breathing of cold air.[210] Perhaps future studies will demonstrate that C-fiber endings become hyperirritable to cold air in hypersensitive airways as the effect of cold air are enhanced in the airways of sensitized rabbits.[39]

c. Pathological Stimulants of C-Fiber Endings

Pathologically, pulmonary congestion or edema has long been thought to stimulate pulmonary C-fiber endings (type J receptors).[67,68,113,204,205,213,217,218] Originally, the low activity of the type J receptor to these stimuli led Paintal to believe the response was not impressive and that congestion and edema were weak stimuli of type J receptors. Paintal later stated that edema and congestion were powerful and specific stimuli of C-fiber endings. In addition, due to the shear numbers of C-fiber endings carried by the vagus, relatively small increases in individual receptor activity may be more influential within the central nervous system than is intuitively apparent. More recent support for this proposal has been presented by Roberts et al.[219] Perivascular cuffing produced by saline infusion of 20% of body weight in dogs stimulated both bronchial and pulmonary C-fiber endings and RARs. PSRs were stimulated, but only during the expiratory phase of ventilation. However, when blood was withdrawn to decrease the microvascular pressure to near the baseline level, the activity of both the RARs and PSRs returned to their previous baseline activity. Pulmonary C-fiber ending activity was reduced somewhat, but it remained elevated above the previous baseline level. Bronchial C-fiber ending activity remained elevated only in cases where pulmonary edema was severe.

In contrast to the study of Roberts et al.,[219] Kappagoda et al.[99] report in dogs that sustained increases of pulmonary venous pressure of approximately 10 mmHg increased the activity of PSRs, RARs, and bronchial C-fiber endings, while pulmonary C-fiber endings did not significantly increase in their activity to this stimulus. Upon removal of the stimulus, i.e., release of the pressure from mitral valve obstruction, the activity of all types receptors returned to base level. The greatest changes in activity occurred with the RARs. The differences observed between the studies of Roberts et al.[219] and those of Kappagoda et al.[99] are that the increase in the pulmonary vascular pressure was controlled to a moderate elevation (maximum 10 mmHg increase) and for a limited period of time (15 min) in the later study.

The differences observed in C-fiber characteristics may be explained through the differing experimental methods used. In other studies increases of 20 mmHg or greater in left atrial pressure were used while studying pulmonary receptors,[218-220] vs. the 10 mmHg increase used by Kappagoda et al.[99] In addition, not all pulmonary C-fiber endings were stimulated by pulmonary congestion in the studies of Coleridge and Coleridge.[218] In the studies of Kappagoda et al.[99] the mean increase in activity of the pulmonary C-fiber ending was not statistically elevated, but in the discussion it is stated that six of nine pulmonary C-fiber endings "responded to an increase in left atrial pressure of 10 mmHg". These investigators then comment that their results are compatible with those of Coleridge and Coleridge.[218]

Wead et al.[221] have presented evidence that pulmonary edema may not be a stimulus for C-fiber endings. With lung inflation to 30 cm H_2O, capsaicin, and alloxan injections did elicit the chemoreflex of bradycardia, hypotension, and apnea, elevated pulmonary vascular pressures alone did not. In these experiments the left lung was separately perfused and ventilated. The normal cardiac output and ventilation went to the right lung after left-lung isolation. This may have changed sensory input to the central nervous system, such as heightened PSR activity and RAR activation. However, since the chemoreflex occurred under certain conditions and not others makes the differences among various studies difficult to reconcile. These results support earlier findings of Lloyd.[222]

The reflex effects of such stimulation of the C-fiber endings have been extensively reviewed[2] and are believed to be dyspnea, with apnea,[233] tachypnea,[193,223] constriction of the airway,[216,224] bradycardia,[68,225,226] systemic hypotension,[98,225,226] and mucus secretion.[227] The reflexes evoked by C-fiber stimulation have been called the chemoreflex by a number of investigators.[179,215] This chemoreflex is demonstrable very early in life. This reflex, which includes apnea, shallow breaths, and obstructive inspiratory effects, has been demonstrated even in preterm infants.[228]

d. Chemical

C-Fiber endings are stimulated by a number of endogenous mediators released during anaphylaxis and allergic reactions. Those mediators shown thus far to stimulate the C-fiber endings include histamine,[68,159,166,169,229] $PGF_{2\alpha}$,[166] PGE,[49] bradykinin,[47,229-232] serotonin,[3] substance P,[171] adenosine,[172] and possible enkephalins.[30] Extracts of IgE antigen challenge of human mast cells resulted in increased C-fiber activity as recorded intracellularly from rabbit nodose ganglion cells.[223] Although the identity of the mediator is not precisely known, these investigators believe the agent not to be histamine, but is lipid in character and may be a prostaglandin such as PGD_2.

Exogenous chemicals which stimulate C-fiber endings include capsaicin[215,234] and phenyl diguanide,[3] sodium dithionite for pulmonary C-fiber endings,[208] and possibly kainate.[235] Halothane, ether, chloroform, SO_2, tetraethylammonium (TEA), and ammonia[25,49,67,90,176,205,236] are among the gases known to stimulate C-fiber endings. Cigarette smoke also causes apnea, bradycardia, and hypotension in dogs which is abolished during vagal cooling studies only at temperatures which also block C-fiber transmission.[237] Bronchospasm induced by cold-air challenge may also be mediated by C-fiber endings.[39,238]

Respiratory gases may also affect C-fiber ending activity. Delpierre et al.[216,239] observed in cats that during conditions of various levels of hypercapnia in the presence of hyperoxia, C-fiber activity of bronchopulmonary C-fibers increased from approximately 1 to 2 impulses per second. The C-fiber activity responded to increasing concentrations of inspired CO_2 by "on" and "off" periods of stimulation, therefore detecting dynamic changes in CO_2 concentrations. These investigators concluded that airway CO_2 may be the "most common stimulus" of bronchopulmonary C-fiber endings. In these studies hypoxia was observed to have no effect on these bronchopulmonary C-fiber endings.

Trenchard[127] injected acetic acid, lactic acid, and sodium dithionite into the right atrium to increase concentrations of CO_2 and/or hydrogen ions in order to obtain evidence that pulmonary nonmyelinated vagal afferent endings are sensitive to increased concentrations of either CO_2 or hydrogen ions. The administration of these chemicals increased breathing frequency and FRC, while decreasing expiratory time (T_E) and tidal volume (V_T). Such effects were blocked by vagotomy. However, in another study, administration of CO_2 to the inspired gas ($PCO_2 = 46$ mmHg) produced no change in the activity of either pulmonary of bronchial C-fiber endings.[125] Activity of both receptors decreased when PCO_2 was decreased ($PCO_2 = 19$ mmHg), but was not changed from baseline activity at a PCO_2 of 2 mmHg.

There exists different sensitivities of the two subcategories of C-fiber endings to the various mediators tested. Bronchial C-fiber endings have the greater sensitivity to nearly all naturally occurring mediators. This difference in the sensitivities of the bronchial and pulmonary C-fiber endings has been assumed to be a function of the direct action of the chemical upon the receptor. If airway deformation also affects C-fiber ending activity, then a portion of the excitation of bronchial C-fiber endings to these mediators may be due to mechanical rather than chemical activation. Despite this argument, the fact remains that neither C-fiber ending category is particularly sensitive to various ventilatory maneuvers compared to the two other categories of pulmonary receptors. Therefore, the mechanical aspect of the stimulation of either receptor type may be of little significance until the lungs have become greatly inflated or there is great narrowing or deformation of the airways due to bronchoconstriction.

3. Reflex Resulting from C-Fiber Ending Stimulation

The reflex actions of C-fiber ending stimulation have been extensively and recently reviewed by Coleridge and Coleridge.[2] The major defensive reflexes originating from C-fiber ending stimulation include apnea followed by rapid and shallow breathing,[25,48,176,213,215,223,226,240,241] bronchoconstriction,[216] increased tracheal secretions[227] and systemic hypotension,[98,225,241,242] and bradycardia as has been mentioned.[225,241] Further evidence that C-fiber stimulation reflexly inhibits respiration has been reported by Haxhiu et al.[234] Capsaicin challenge in dogs via right-atrium injection resulted in reduction or absence of upper airway dilating and chest wall and abdominal muscles activity. The upper-airway constrictor muscles and internal intercostal muscles remained active, however. Hypercapnia, hypoxia, or positive end-expiratory pressures did not change the observed response of these muscles, although bilateral vagotomy reversed the observed responses. There has been some disagreement as to whether the rapid-shallow breathing pattern is one that is the direct result of the C-fiber activation or due to the apnea which proceeded it (i.e., elevated P_aCO_2). Coast and Cassidy[243] infused various doses of capsaicin into vascularly isolated dog lungs while measuring diaphragm EMGs. Cessation of diaphragmatic contractions were observed, but no evidence was obtained to support the finding that stimulation of pulmonary C-fiber endings reflexly caused rapid and shallow ventilation.

C-Fiber endings apparently contribute to basal bronchomotor tone. Roberts et al.[145,224] and Pisarri et al.[244] found bronchomotor tone to increase in dogs whose vagal nerves were bilaterally cooled to temperatures ranging from 7 to 2°C. Jonzon et al.[143] demonstrated that only unmyelinated fibers remain active at these temperatures, although they are reduced in their activity. However, one of the first indications that C-fiber endings may contribute to bronchomotor tone even during unstressed ventilation was reported by Jammes and Mei.[40] They found that blocking the C-waves of vagal transmission by procaine decreased bronchomotor tone.

Roberts et al.[145] monitored isolated tracheal smooth-muscle segments supplied by motor innervation from the superior laryngeal nerve *in vivo* while hyperinflating the lungs. When the vagal nerves were at 37°C this maneuver resulted in relaxation of the tracheal smooth muscle. When the vagi were cooled and beginning at temperatures of 8°C the segments contracted in response to lung hyperinflation. This effect failed to occur after the temperature of the vagus nerve fell below 2°C. Furthermore, bilateral vagotomy abolished both relaxation and constriction in response to lung inflations. It was suggested by these investigators that C-fiber endings mediate Head's paradoxical reflex and induce reflex bronchoconstriction via lung inflation.

Therefore, C-fiber endings contribute to bronchomotor tone and ventilatory control through their basal activities during eupnea. Increased C-fiber activity beyond that of eupneic breathing induced either by large inflations of the lungs, increased P_ACO_2, or even by chemical stimulation would therefore enhance or accentuate their affects on bronchomotor tone and ventilation.

a. Capsaicin and the Chemoreflex

Capsaicin has been used as a research tool to induce the chemoreflex in a number of species including dogs,[48,68,215,245] cats,[216,226,240] guinea pigs,[246-249] rats,[249,250] and even man.[251-255] Capsaicin is thought to act selectively on C-fiber endings and as a result of its administration should reflect the reflex nature of C-fiber ending stimulation.

In dogs, capsaicin has no apparent direct action on airway smooth muscle.[3] Capsaicin challenge in dogs results in bronchoconstriction,[123,216,245] apnea followed by rapid and shallow breathing.[223] C-Fiber endings also influence functions outside the lungs including bradycardia[218,225] and hypotension.[98,225] Vascular beds which vasodilate in response to pulmonary C-fiber stimulation include skeletal muscle vessels,[225] coronary vessels,[256,257] and diaphragmatic vessels.[243] The purpose of this reflex is uncertain. Since pulmonary congestion and edema stimulate pulmonary C-fibers, then this reflex may serve to shift vascular volumes to the systemic from the pulmonary circulation.

In guinea pigs similar effects can be observed with capsaicin challenge as compared to the dog.[246,247,249] However, reflex actions of capsaicin have been difficult to demonstrate. Complete bilateral vagotomy does not attenuate the action of capsaicin in this species.[246,247,249] Capsaicin may have direct action on airway smooth muscle in the guinea pig. Another possible explanation for the lack of demonstrable vagal reflexes is that other afferent and efferent routes travel through spinal pathways and the stellate ganglion.[234,258-263] However, capsaicin may also produce some of its actions through an axon reflex.

A number of investigators have proposed that C-fiber endings may participate in an axon reflex,[248,264-268] and possibly even in man.[269] Capsaicin may stimulate C-fiber endings which then may cause the release of tachykinins such as substance P from collateral nerve endings. Calcitonin gene regulatory peptide (CGRP)[171,267,269-273] has been shown to coexist in the C-fiber terminals with substance P. Once released, these tachikinins may cause the observed effects directly or even indirectly through release of other mediators through mast cell degranulation.[265]

Subcutaneous administration of capsaicin not only depletes stores of substance P, but also decreases the number of sensory or C-fiber endings in neonatal rats.[259,274-277] Thereafter the effects of capsaicin challenge are prevented as well as the effects of certain other substances, such as cigarette smoke.[268] Therefore, C-fiber endings in the lungs act not only through vagal and spinal reflex arcs, but through local axon reflex arcs as well.

IV. STUDIES CONCERNING THE INTEGRATION OF PULMONARY REFLEXES

A. DRUG INHIBITION OF PULMONARY REFLEXES

The comparative use of local anesthetics, muscarinic antagonists, and sodium cromoglycate (SCG) has contributed to the knowledge of mechanisms of reflexes involving bronchoconstriction and cough. It is now apparent that the reflexes of bronchoconstriction and cough can involve separate mechanisms. In asthmatic subjects atropine administration attenuated both the increase in airway resistance and the cough caused by aerosol challenge of distilled water,[278] demonstrating that both involve reflex pathways. Lidocaine blocked the cough, but not the increase in airway resistance. Furthermore, SCG blocked the bronchoconstriction, but not the cough. However, these investigators thought the action of SCG may not involve inhibition of airway afferent nerves.

In another study of asthmatic patients, nebulized distilled water was confirmed to cause both cough and bronchoconstriction as measured by decreases in forced expiratory volume (FEV$_1$). Both atropine and SCG blocked the resulting bronchoconstriction, but not the cough. Both atropine and SCG have been reported to decrease airway resistance in other studies as well.[279] The action of SCG in this study was reported to be immediate. This suggested to these investigators that SCG did act through neuronal mechanisms.

RARs, particularly those located in the larynx, may participate in the cough reflex.[6,209,280] Others believe that C-fiber endings may also initiate the cough reflex when stimulated.[280,281] Capsaicin treatment can block the cough reflex to certain stimuli as well as the avoidance behavior to that stimuli.[268] Since capsaicin is thought to act selectively upon C-fiber endings, Forsberg and Karlsson[281] suggest that cough is dependent upon C-fiber endings stimulation. However, capsaicin may affect A-delta fibers if only indirectly as well so as to alter the function of RARs.

Because the administration of SCG attenuates bronchoconstriction, but not the cough induced by capsaicin challenge, it would seem that SCG inhibits the action of C-fiber endings.[282] SCG has been reported to attenuate the response of C-fiber endings to histamine in dogs. However, other investigators[283] were unable to confirm these results. SCG was also reported to decrease the reponsiveness of RARs to histamine challenge in dogs.[284,285] In natively allergic dogs, SCG decreased the airway response and activity of 25 RARs to aerosol challenge of ascaris antigen.[157] However, SCG attenuated neither the airway response nor the activity of 27 RARs to histamine aerosol challenge. Therefore, although SCG may inhibit certain neuronal mechanisms, particularly those of C-fiber endings, confirmatory evidence supporting such a mechanism remains equivocal.

The airways of asthmatic individuals[286] and the airways of laboratory animals whose airways have been sensitized to foreign proteins[39,50,158] are demonstrably hyperirritable to numerous provocative agents. A significant portion of the bronchoconstriction can be shown to have a reflex component. It has not been demonstrated that C-fiber endings become hyperirritable under such circumstances. For example, cold air-induced and histamine-induced bronchoconstriction is greater in sensitized rabbits vs. untreated rabbits.[39] Both vagotomy and SCG block this reaction. If SCG has action on pulmonary reflexes it would most likely be via C-fiber endings.

B. CENTRAL INTEGRATION OF PULMONARY RECEPTORS

Although little is known concerning the integrative processing of all pulmonary afferent fibers within the central nervous system, some information is available. Perhaps the earliest indication that enhancement or elimination of certain categories of pulmonary receptors changes airway smooth-muscle tone and ventilation comes from the classic study done by Head.[287] Upon rewarming the vagi from a temperature of near 0°C, the original inhibitory inflation reflex to lung inflation was replaced instead by an enhanced inspiratory effort. This effect appears to be due not only to suppression of PSR activity during the inflation at these temperatures, but to unopposed activity of pulmonary C-fiber endings as proposed by Roberts et al.[145] Therefore, during normal conditions the reflex action of the myelinated PSRs dominate those of unmyelinated receptors during maneuvers involving lung inflation despite the difference in numbers of the categories of pulmonary receptors. However, Koller and Kohl[288] report that under certain conditions the Hering-Breuer stretch reflex may be overridden by other pulmonary reflexes. During anaphylaxis or attacks of bronchial asthma tachypnea dominates, resulting from a "deflation" or "nociceptive" reflex. These investigators believe lung deflation or collapse receptors (RARs) are responsible for this reflex. However, in light of recent studies, C-fiber endings should also be considered because more than just mechanical factors are involved.

How certain categories of pulmonary receptors influence reflex effects of other categories of receptors such as that stated above remains uncertain to a large extent. Little information concerning the central integration of pulmonary receptor activity is available. The afferent fibers of the pulmonary receptors studied thus far appear to project to different areas of the central nervous system. PSRs have been demonstrated to project monosynaptically to I_B and perhaps P cells of the nucleus tractus solitarius neurons in the medulla.[289-294] PSRs terminate to these neurons largely in the ventral, ventrolateral, lateral, and interstitial nuclei of the tractus solitarius as buttons with hundreds of terminals per axon (650 to 1180) over distance of 1.7 to 2.1 mm.[295,296] RARs also project to the nucleus of the tractus solitarius.[297-300] However, RARs project to different regions of the nucleus tractus solitarius than do PSRs, being primarily to the dorsal and dorsolateral subnuclei and secondarily to the intermediate nuclei.[297-299] This is in contrast to the primary area of termination of PSRs. RARs also terminate as buttons averaging 500 to 1050 per axon over a distance of 4 mm rostrocaudally.[298] Both RARs and PSRs appear to have further rostral projections,[295-298] but these tracts have as of yet not been traced. This may be true in that destruction of the ventrolateral nucleus tractus solitarius does not alter T_I of the Hering-Breuer reflex in the cat.[301] However, the intermediate area of the ventral medulla may affect phrenic activity via RARs.[302] No such studies have provided information as to the projection sites of C-fiber endings.

What influence does shear numbers of pulmonary receptors have on the strength of a reflex? Without doubt, C-fibers are by far the most numerous pulmonary fibers carred in the vagi. Furthermore, Jammes et al.[210] state "non-myelinated afferent fibers constitute the most important sensory component in the vagus nerve". Estimates have placed the total number of vagal fibers to be 5000, and of those, 4000 are C-fiber endings.[303] Of the myelinated fibers the ratio of RARs to PSRs ranges between 0.11 in cats, 0.18 in dogs, 0.22 in opossums, and 0.44 in rabbits.[95] It may be that this difference in the ratio between various species could explain some of the observed differences in reflexes to various stimuli.

Numbers may be deceiving, however, in estimating the strength of respiratory reflexes. In the example of Head's paradoxical reflex, PSR activity dominates reflexes of lung inflation at moderate rates and volumes at least in normal individuals. However, a biphasic response to lung inflation has been reported by Roberts et al.[145] in dogs. Initially, activity of PSR dominated the inflation reflex, inducing bronchodilation. Vagal cooling below 7°C eliminated the bronchodilation effect of inflation. Bronchoconstriction remained until vagal temperatures fell below 2°C. These results imply the PSRs were responsible for the initial relaxation and pulmonary C-fiber endings for the subsequent contraction. What role would rapidly adapting receptors play in these circumstances? Because pulmonary C-fiber activity probably does not increase significantly with constantly maintained inflation, is the adaptation of PSRs enough to account for the biphasic response of smooth-muscle tone? If PSR adaptation is insufficient to account for this change could RAR activity influence airway tone? RARs would be active primarily during the pressure change to the level of maintained inflation. Relatively little activity of RARs would occur beyond the point where pressure ceases to change. It is difficult to conclude that RARs could be responsible for bronchoconstriction in the case of lung hyperinflation. Therefore, could RARs facilitate the bronchodilation reflex of PSRs during conditions of rapid inflation of the lungs to large volumes? This would make physiological sense. During increase rates of inspiratory airflow, which is a major stimulus of RAR, enhanced airway dilation could better accommodate the larger volume of air traveling through the airways.

In spontaneously breathing animals or humans, the gasp reflex may override the inflation reflex under certain conditions. In this situation the RAR presumably mediates this augmented breathing maneuver. In most species RARs are far fewer in number than the PSRs, which mediate the Hering-Breuer inhibition reflex. The limit of the augmented inspiration may then be the limit of elastance of the lungs and chest at TLC nears. The RAR discharge ceases or "adapts" near TLC as the lungs are no longer rapidly changing volume, while the PSRs continue heightened or sustained activity. Expiration then ensues as PSR activity dominates vagal traffic. At this time the Hering-Breuer stretch reflex initiates.

C. ACTION OF LOCAL ANESTHETIC ON PULMONARY RECEPTOR ACTIVITY

Can local anesthetics be useful in separating reflexes of different categories of pulmonary receptors? Aerosol challenge of local anesthetics is a method used to block pulmonary reflexes in addition to cutting, differential cooling, or anodal hyperpolarization of the vagi. In rabbits, Jain et al.[118] reported that bupivacaine inhibited the cough reflex, the Hering-Breuer inflation reflex, and the deflation reflex. However, the ventilatory response to phenyl diguanide was not blocked. This implies that fibers of PSRs and RARs were blocked, while those of C-fiber endings were not. In cats, bupivacaine reduced or completely blocked PSR and RAR activity to mechanical stimuli, but bupivacaine failed to block C-fiber endings. These results would support the earlier studies of Fahim and Jain.[117]

In dogs, bupivacaine decreased or abolished respiratory reflexes of cough, apnea, and the Hering-Breuer inflation reflex.[116] The increased resistance induced by histamine aerosol challenge was also reduced by 71%. These results imply that fibers of perhaps all three categories of pulmonary receptors were blocked or at least attenuated in the dog, as histamine is a potent stimulant of C-fiber endings in this species. Hamilton et al.[179] were unable to demonstrate significant reflex effects of bupivacaine aerosols in dogs when aerosols of 1 to 1.7 μm in diameter were used. However, larger diametered aerosols of 4.8 μm of bupivacaine blocked the cough reflex, the Hering-Breuer stretch reflex, and the pulmonary chemoreflex to capsaicin challenge. Furthermore, intravenous administration of bupivacaine failed to block any of these three reflexes from the lungs. Perhaps the larger-diametered aerosol particles allowed higher concentrations of the bupivacaine to anesthetize receptive endings throughout the airway. This may explain the conflicting results observed when compared with other studies. Camporesi et al.[304] studied the differential effects of lidocaine, bupivacaine, and tetracaine on the activity of PSRs and RARs. Higher concentrations and longer periods of time were required to anesthetize PSRs. These authors conclude that it is possible to block the activity of one type of pulmonary receptor over another.

Aerosol administration of local anesthetics as well as agents such as SCG and cholinergic blocking agents is a method which can be used in human subjects to study pulmonary reflexes as well. In normal subjects, aerosol challenge of distilled water caused both cough and bronchoconstriction.[59,305] Atropine and SCG administration blocked this bronchoconstriction, but not the cough, while just the opposite effects were observed with lidocaine administration. These results suggest the bronchoconstriction and cough reflexes are mediated via different reflex mechanisms. In another study, ipratropium decreased specific airway conductance in asthmatic subjects, but not in normal subjects.[306] Bupivacaine blocked the cough reflex to citric acid aerosol challenge in both groups of subjects, while sodium cromolyn did not. Unlike the results found in dogs, bupivacaine did not block the effects of histamine on specific conductance, nor was the effect of $PGF_{2\alpha}$ blocked. Ipratropriun attenuated the effect of only histamine. Although highly speculative, the dissimilarities between the studies in dogs and those in human subjects may be explained in that the efferent pathway in the human subjects may have remained patent. This possibility was not tested. However, another possible explanation is that humans and dogs are different with respect to the action of bupivacaine in the airways and their receptors.

V. CONCLUSION

Each category of pulmonary receptor therefore has particular functions, not only during stressful conditions, but during eupnea as well. The pathological reflexes should reflect an increase in the intensity of the physiological reflexes. Furthermore, unless modulation of pulmonary reflexes occurs within the central nervous system, these reflexes projecting from a particular category of receptor should demonstrate consistency regardless of the nature of the stimulus. Much is still to be learned concerning the stimuli, pattern of discharge and reflexes of each category of receptor, and what changes occur in airway disease or damaged airways. Most certainly, understanding processes of modulation and central integration of these processes is just beginning.

REFERENCES

1. **Barnes, P. J., Chung, K. F., and Page, C. P.,** Inflammatory mediators and asthma, *Pharmacol. Rev.,* 40(1), 49, 1988.

2. **Coleridge, H. M. and Coleridge, J. C. G.,** Reflexes evoked from tracheobronchial tree and lungs, in *Handbook of Physiology, The Respiratory System, Control of Breathing,* Sect. 3, Vol. II, Part 1, Cherniack, N. S. and Widdicombe, J. G., Eds., American Physiological Society, Bethesda, MD, 1986, 395.

3. **Coleridge, J. C. G. and Coleridge, H. M.,** Afferent vagal C fibre innervation of the lungs and airways and its functional significance, *Rev. Physiol. Biochem. Pharamcol.,* 99, 1, 1984.

4. **Hahn, H.-L.,** Role of the parasympathetic nervous system and of cholinergic mechanisms in bronchial hyperreactivity, *Bull. Eur. Physiopathol. Respir.,* 22 (Suppl. 7), 112, 1986.

5. **Jammes, Y.,** Tonic sensory pathways of the respiratory system, *Eur. Respir. J.,* 1, 176, 1988.

6. **Karlsson, J.-A., Sant' Ambrogio, G., and Widdicombe, J.,** Afferent neural pathways in cough and reflex bronchoconstriction, *J. Appl. Physiol.,* 65(3), 1007, 1988.

7. **Pack, A. I.,** Sensory inputs to the medulla, *Annu. Rev. Physiol.,* 43, 73, 1981.

8. **Sant'Ambrogio, G.,** Information arising from the treacheobronchial tree of mammals, *Physiol. Rev.,* 62, 531, 1982.

9. **Sant'Ambrogio, G.,** Nervous receptors of the tracheobronchial tree, *Annu. Rev. Physiol.,* 49, 611, 1987.

10. **Widdicombe, J. G.,** Sensory innervation of the lungs and airways, *Prog. Brain Res.,* 67, 49, 1986.

11. **Cross, B. A., Guz, A., Jain, S. K., Archer, S., Stevens, J., and Reynolds, F.,** The effect of anesthesia of the airway in dog and man: a study of respiratory reflexes, sensations and lung mechanics, *Clin. Sci. Mol. Med.,* 50, 439, 1976.

12. **Widdicombe, J. G.,** Respiration reflexes in man and other mammalian species, *Clin. Sci.,* 21, 163, 1961.

13. **Mortola, J. P., Fisher, J. T., and Sant'Ambrogio, G.,** Vagal control of the breathing pattern and respiratory mechanics in the adult and newborn rabbit, *Pfluegers Arch.,* 401, 281, 1984.

14. **Clifford, P., Litzow, J. T., von Colditz, J. H., and Coon, R. L.,** Effect of chronic pulmonary denervation on ventilatory responses to exercise, *J. Appl. Physiol.,* 61(1), 603, 1986.

15. **Nadel, J. A., Phillipson, E. A., Fishman, N. H., and Hickey, R. F.,** Regulation of respiration by bronchopulmonary receptors in conscious dogs, *Acta Neurobiol. Exp.,* 33, 33, 1973.

16. **Phillipson, E. A., Hickey, R. F., Bainton, C. R., and Nadel, J. A.,** Effect of vagal blockade on regulation of breathing in conscious dogs, *J. Appl. Physiol.* 29, 475, 1970.

17. **Chaudhary, B. A. and Spier, W. A.,** Effect of lidocaine anesthesia on pattern of ventilation and pulmonary function test, *South. Med. J.,* 72, 1246, 1979.

18. **Christiansen, J. and Haldane, J. S.,** The influence of distention of the lungs on human respiration, *J. Physiol. (London),* 48, 272, 1914.

19. **Guz, A., Noble, M. I. M., Trenchard, D., Cochrane, H. L., and Makey, A. R.,** Studies on the vagus nerves in man: their role in respiration and circulatory control, *Clin. Sci.,* 27, 293, 1964.

20. **Hamilton, R. D., Winning, A. J., Horner, R. L., and Guz, A.,** The effect of lung inflation on breathing in man during wakefulness and sleep, *Respir. Physiol.,* 73, 145, 1988.

21. **Gautier, H., Bonora, M., and Gaudy, J. H.,** Breuer-Hering inflation reflex and breathing pattern in anesthetized humans and cats, *J. Appl Physiol.,* 51, 1162, 1981.

22. **Shea, S. A., Horner, R. L., Banner, N. R., McKenzie, E., Heaton, R., Yacoub, M. H., and Guz, A.,** The effect of human heart-lung transplantation upon breathing at rest and during sleep, *Respir. Physiol.,* 72, 131, 1988.

23. **Clifford, P. S., Bell, L. B., Hopp, F. A., and Coon, R. L.,** The Breuer-Hering reflex (BHR) reappears 12—14 weeks after surgical lung denervation in beagle dogs, *J. Appl. Physiol.,* 54, 1451, 1983.

24. **Clifford, P. S., Bell, L. B., Hopp, F. A., and Coon, R. L.,** Reinnervation of pulmonary stretch receptors, *J. Appl. Physiol.,* 62(5), 1912, 1987.

25. **Dawes, G. S. and Comroe, J. H.,** Chemoreflexes from the heart and lungs, *Physiol. Rev.,* 34, 167, 1954.

26. **Badier, M., Soler, M., Mallea, M., Delprerre, S., and Orehek, J.,** Cholinergic responsiveness of respiratory and vascular tissue in two different rat strains, *J. Appl. Physiol.,* 64(1), 323, 1988.

27. **Caldeira, M. P. R., Saldiva, P. H. N., and Zin, W. A.,** Vagal influences on respiratory mechanics, pressures and control in rats, *Respir. Physiol.,* 73, 43, 1988.

28. **Ledorko, L., Kelly, E. N., and England, S. J.,** Importance of vagal afferent in determining ventilation in newborn rats, *J. Appl. Physiol.,* 65(3), 1033, 1988.

29. **Tsubone, H.,** Characteristics of vagal afferent activity in rats: three types of pulmonary receptors responding to collapse inflation, and deflation of the lung, *Exp. Neurol.,* 92, 541, 1986.

30. **Sapru, H. N., Willette, R. N., and Krieger, A. J.,** Stimulation of pulmonary J receptors by an enkephalin-analog, *J. Pharmacol. Exp. Ther.,* 217, 228, 1981.

31. **Mills, J. E. and Widdicombe, J. G.,** Role of the vagus nerves in anaphylaxis and histamine-induced bronchoconstrictions in guinea-pigs, *Br. J. Pharmacol.,* 39, 724, 1970.

32. **Drazen, J. M. and Austen, K. F.,** Atropine modification of the pulmonary effects of chemical mediators in the guinea pig, *J. Appl. Physiol.,* 38, 834, 1975.

33. **Mauser, P. J., Edelman, N. H., and Chapman, R W.,** Central nervous system control of airway tone in guinea pigs: the role of histamine, *J. Appl Physiol.,* 65, 2024, 1988.

34. **Barthelemy, P., Badier, M., and Jammes, Y.,** Interaction between SO_2 and cold-induced bronchospasm in anesthetized rabbits, *Respir. Physiol.,* 71, 1, 1988.

35. **Karczewski, W. and Widdicombe, J. G.,** The effect of vagotomy, vagal cooling and efferent vagal stimulation on breathing and lung mechanics of rabbits, *J. Physiol. (London),* 201, 259, 1969.

36. **Badier, M., Barthelemy, P., Soler, M., and Jammes, Y.,** *In vivo* and *in vitro* studies on cold-induced airway response in normal and sensitized rabbits, *Respir. Physiol. (London),* 73, 1, 1988.

37. **Davies, A., Dixon, M., Callanan, D., Huszczuk, A., Widdicombe, J. G., and Wise, J. C. M.,** Lung reflexes in rabbits during pulmonary stretch receptor block by sulphur dioxide, *Respir. Phsyiol.,* 34, 83, 1978.

38. **Davies, A., Dixon, M., Widdicombe, J. G., and Wise, J. C. M.,** Lung stretch receptor paralysis by sulphur dioxide, *J. Physiol. (London),* 275, 13P, 1978.

39. **Jammes, Y., Barthelemy, P., Fornaris, M., and Grimaud, C. H.,** Cold-induced bronchospasm in normal and sentitized rabbits, *Respir. Physiol.,* 63, 347, 1986.

40. **Jammes, Y. and Mei, N.,** Assessment of the pulmonary origin of bronchoconstrictor vagal tone, *J. Physiol. (London),* 291, 305, 1979.

41. **DeKock, M. A., Nadel, J. A., Zwi, S., Colebatch, H. J. H., and Olsen, C. R.,** New method for perfusing bronchial arteries: histamine bronchoconstriction and apnea, *J. Appl. Physiol.,* 21, 185, 1966.

42. **Gold, W. M., Kessler, G.-F., and Yu, D. Y. C.,** Role of vagus nerves in experimental asthma in allergic dogs, *J. Appl Physiol.,* 33, 719, 1972.

43. **Bleecker, E. R., Cotton, D. J., Fischer, S. P., Graf, P. D., Gold, W. M., and Nadel, J. A.,** The mechanism of rapid shallow breathing after inhaled histamine aerosol in exercising dogs, *Am. Rev. Respir. Dis.,* 114, 909, 1976.

44. **Delpierre, S., Orehek, J., Beaupre, A., Velardocchio, J. M., Fornaris, M., and Grimaud, C.,** Comparative relfex action of histamine, acetylcholine and serotonin on dog airways, *Bull. Eur. Physiopathol. Respir.,* 19, 489, 1983.

45. **Jackson, D. M. and Richards, I. M.,** The effects of pentobarbitone and chloralose anesthesia on the vagal component of bronchoconstriction produced by histamine aerosol in the anesthetized dog, *Br. J. Pharmacol.,* 61, 251, 1977.

46. **Richards, I. M. and Jackson, D. M.,** An investigation of histamine aerosol induced reflex bronchoconstriction in the anaesthetized dog, *Br. J. Pharmacol.,* 61, 251, 1977.

47. **Kaufman, M. P., Coleridge, H. M., Coleridge, J. C. G., and Baker, D. G.,** Bradykinin stimulates afferent vagal C-fibers in intrapulmonary airways of dogs, *J. Appl. Physiol.: Respir. Environ. Exercise Physiol.,* 48, 511, 1980.

48. **Coleridge, H. M., Coleridge, J. C. G., and Kidd, C.,** Role of the pulmonary arterial baroreceptors in the effects produced by capsaicin in the dog, *J. Physiol. (London),* 170, 272, 1964.

49. **Roberts, A. M., Schultz, H. D., Green, J. F., Armstrong, D. J., Kaufman, M. P., Coleridge, H. M., and Coleridge, J. C. G.,** Reflex tracheal contraction evoked in dogs by bronchodilator prostaglandins E_2 and I_2, *J. Appl. Physiol.,* 58, 1823, 1985.

50. **Osborne, M. L., Evans, T. W., Sommerhoff, C. P., Chung, K. F., Hirshman, C. A., Boushey, H. A., and Nadel, J. A.,** Hypotonic and isotonic aerosols increase bronchial reactivity in Basenji-Greyhound dogs, *Am. Rev. Respir. Dis.,* 135, 345, 1987.

51. **Kaplan, J., Smaldone, G. C., Menkes, H. A., Swift, D. L., and Traystman, R. J.,** Response of collateral channels to histamine: lack of vagal effect, *J. Appl. Physiol.,* 51(5), 1314, 1981.

52. **Krell, J., Chakrin, L. W., and Wardell, J. R.,** The effect of cholinergic agents on a canine model of allergic asthma, *J. Allergy Clin. Immunol.,* 58, 19, 1976.

53. **Loofbourrow, G. N., Wood, W. B., and Baird, I. L.,** Tracheal constriction in the dog, *Am. J. Physiol.,* 191, 411, 1957.

54. **Loring, S. H., Drazen, J. M., and Ingram, R. H., Jr.,** Canine pulmonary response to aerosol histamine: direct versus vagal effects, *J. Appl. Physiol. Respir. Environ. Exercise Physiol.,* 42(6), 946, 1977.

55. **Snapper, J. R., Drazen, J. M., Loring, S. H., Braasch, P. S., and Ingram, R. H., Jr.,** Vagal effects on histamine, carbachol, and prostaglandin $F_{2\alpha}$ responsiveness in the dog, *J. Appl. Physiol.: Respir. Environ. Exercise Physiol.,* 47, 13, 1979.

56. **Hirshman, C. A. and Downes, H.,** Basenji-Greyhound dog model of asthma: influence of atropine on antigen-induced bronchoconstriction, *J. Appl. Physiol.,* 50, 761, 1981.

57. **Hirschman, C. A., Edelstein, G., Peetz, S., Wayne, R., and Downes, H.,** Mechanism of action of inhalational anesthesia on airways, *Anesthesiology,* 56, 107, 1982.

58. **Dixon, M., Jackson, D. M., and Richards, I. M.,** The effects of histamine, acetylcholine and 5-hydroxytryptamine on lung mechanics and irritant receptors in the dog, *J. Physiol. (London),* 287, 393, 1979.

59. **Nishino, T., Hiraga, K., Mizuguchi, T., and Honda, Y.,** Respiratory reflex responses to stimulation of tracheal mucosa in influrane-anesthetized humans, *J. Appl. Physiol.,* 65(3), 1069, 1988.

60. **DeWeese, E. L. and Sullivan, T. Y.,** Effect of upper airway anesthesia on pharyngeal patency during sleep, *J. Appl. Physiol.,* 64(4), 1346, 1988.

61. **Sheppard, D., Epstein, J., Skoogh, B. E., Bethel, R. A., Nadel, J. A., and Boushey, H. A.,** Variable inhibition of histamine-induced bronchoconstriction by atropine in subject with asthma, *J. Allergy Clin. Immunol.,* 73(1), 82, 1984.

62. **Beasley, R., Varley, J., Robinson, C., and Holgate, S. T.,** Cholinergic-mediated bronchoconstriction induced by prostaglandin D_2, its initial metabolite 9_a11B-PGF_2 and $PGF_{2\alpha}$ in asthma, *Am. Rev. Respir. Dis.,* 136, 1140, 1987.

63. **Eiser, N. M. and Guz, A.,** Effect of atropine on experimentally-induced airway obstruction in man, *Bull. Eur. Physiopathol. Respir.,* 18, 449, 1982.

64. **Casterline, C. L., Evans, R., III, and Ward, G. W., Jr.,** The effects of atropine and albuterol aerosols on the human bronchial response to histamine, *J. Allergy Clin. Immunol.,* 58, 607, 1976.

65. **Glanville, A. R., Yeand, R. A., Theodore, J., and Robin, E. D.,** Effect of single respiratory maneuvers on specific airway conductance in heart-lung transplant recipients, *Clin. Sci.,* 74, 311, 1988.

66. **Sampson, S. R.,** Sensory neurophysiology of airways, *Am. Rev. Respir. Dis.,* 115(6), 107, 1977.

67. **Paintal, A. S.,** Mechanism of stimulation of type J pulmonary receptors, *J. Physiol. (London),* 203, 511, 1969.

68. **Coleridge, H. M. and Coleridge, J. C. G.,** Impulse activity in afferent vagal C-fibers with endings in the intrapulmonary airways of dogs, *Respir. Physiol.,* 29, 125, 1977.

69. **Miserocchi, G. and Sant'Ambrogio, G.,** Responses of pulmonary stretch receptors to static pressure inflations, *Respir. Physiol.,* 21, 77, 1974.

70. **Davenport, P. W., Lee, L.-Y., Lee, K., Yu, L. K., Miller, R., and Frazier, D. T.,** Effect of bronchoconstriction on the firing behavior of pulmonary stretch receptors, *Respir. Physiol.,* 46, 295, 1981.

71. **Kohl, J., Koller, E. A., Kuoni, J., and Morky, L.,** Location-dependent characteristics of pulmonary stretch receptor activity in the rabbit, *Pfluegers Arch.,* 406, 303, 1986.

72. **Ogilvie, M. D., Bogen, D. K., Galante, R. J., and Pack, A. I.,** Response of stretch receptors to static inflations and deflations in an isolated tracheal segment, *Respir. Physiol.,* 75, 289, 1989.

73. **Pack, A., Ogilvie, D. M., Davies, R. O., and Galante, R. H.,** Responses of pulmonary stretch receptors during ramp inflations of the lung, *J. Appl. Physiol.,* 61(1), 344, 1986.

74. **Fillenz, M. and Widdicombe, J. G.,** Receptors of the lungs and airways, in *Handbook of Sensory Physiology. Enteroceptors,* Vol. III, Part 1, Neil, E., Ed., Springer-Verlag, New York, 1972, 81.

75. **Larsell, O. and Burget, G. E.,** The effect of mechanical and chemical stimulation of the tracheo-bronchial mucous membrane, *Am. J. Physiol.,* 70, 311, 1924.

76. **Mills, J. E., Sellick, H., and Widdicombe, J. G.,** Activity of lung irritant receptors in pulmonary microembolism, anaphylaxis and drug-induced bronchoconstrictions, *J. Physiol. (London),* 203, 337, 1969.

77. **Mills, J. E., Sellick, H., and Widdicombe, J. G.,** Epithelial irritant receptors in the lungs, in *Ciba Found. Symp. Breathing: Hering-Breuer Centenary Symposium,* Porter, R., Ed., Churchill Livingstone, London, 1970, 77.

78. **Wei, J. Y. and Shen, E. H.,** Vagal expiratory afferent discharges during spontaneous breathing, *Brain Res.,* 335, 213, 1985.

79. **Buff, R. and Koller, E. A.,** Studies on mechanisms underlying the reflex hyperpnoea induced by inhalation of chemical irritants, *Respir. Physiol.,* 21, 371, 1974.

80. **Koller, E. A. and Ferrer, P.,** Discharge patterns of the lung stretch receptors and activation of deflation fibers in anaphylactic bronchial asthma, *Respir. Physiol.,* 17, 113, 1973.

81. **Koller, E. A. and Ferrer, P.,** Studies on the role of the lung deflation reflex, *Respir. Physiol.,* 10, 172, 1970.

82. **Luck, J. C.,** Afferent vagal fibres with an expiratory discharge in the rabbit, *J. Physiol. (London),* 211, 63, 1970.

83. **Bartlett, Jr., D., Jeffery, P., Sant'Ambrogio, G., and Wise, J. C. M.,** Location of stretch receptors in the trachea and bronchi of the dog, *J. Physiol. (London),* 258, 409, 1976.

84. **Krauhs, J. M.,** Morphology of presumptive slowly adapting receptors in dog trachea, *Anat. Res.,* 210, 73, 1984.

85. **Nilsestuen, J. O., Coon, R. L., Woods, M., and Kampine, J. P.,** Location of lung receptors mediating the breathing frequency response to pulmonary CO_2, *Respir. Physiol.,* 45, 343, 1981.

86. **Miserocchi, G. and Sant'Ambrogio, G.,** Distribution of pulmonary stretch receptors in the intrapulmonary airways of the dog, *Respir. Phsyiol.,* 21, 71, 1974.

87. **Widdicombe, J. G.,** The site of pulmonary stretch receptors in the cat, *J. Physiol. (London),* 125, 336, 1954.

88. **Paintal, A. S. and Ravi, K.,** The relative location of low- and higher-threshold pulmonary stretch receptors, *J. Physiol. (London),* 307 (Abstr.), 50P, 1980.

89. **Ravi, K.,** Distribution and location of slowly adapting pulmonary stretch receptors in the airway of cats, *J. Auton. Nerv. Sys.,* 15(3), 205, 1986.

90. **Armstrong, D. J. and Luck, J. C.,** Accessibility of pulmonary stretch receptors from the pulmonary and bronchial circulations, *J. Appl. Physiol.,* 36, 706, 1974.

91. **Miserocchi, G., Mortola, J., and Sant'Ambrogio, G.,** Localization of pulmonary stretch receptors in the airways of dogs, *J. Physiol. (London),* 235, 775, 1973.

92. **Bartoli, A., Cross, G. A., Guz, A., Huszczuk, A., and Jefferies, R.,** The effect of varying tidal volume on the associated phrenic motoneurone output: studies of vagal and chemical feedback, *Respir. Physiol.,* 25, 135, 1975.

93. **Wozniak, J. A., Davenport, P. W., and Kosch, P. C.,** Responses of pulmonary vagal mechanoreceptors to high-frequency oscillatory ventilation, *J. Appl. Physiol.,* 65(2), 633, 1988.

94. **Roumy, M. and Leitner, L.-M.,** Localization of stretch and deflation receptors in the airways of the rabbit, *J. Physiol. (Paris),* 76, 67, 1980.

95. **Farber, J. P., Fisher, J. T., and Sant'Ambrogio, G.,** Distribution and discharge properties of airway receptor in the opossum, didelphis marsupials, *Am. J. Physiol.,* 245, R209, 1983.

96. **Sant'Ambrogio, G. and Mortola, P.,** Behavior of slowly adapting stretch receptors in the extrathoracic trachea of the dog, *Respir. Physiol.,* 31, 377, 1977.

97. **Davenport, P. W. and Wozniak, J. A.,** Effect of expiratory loading on expiratory duration and pulmonary stretch receptor discharge, *J. Appl. Physiol.,* 61(5), 1857, 1986.

98. **Adrian, E. D.,** Afferent impulses in the vagus and their effect on respiration, *J. Physiol. (London),* 79, 332, 1933.

99. **Kappagoda, C. R., Man, G. C. W., and Teo, K. K.,** Behaviour of canine pulmonary vagal efferent receptors during sustained acute pulmonary venous pressure elevation, *J. Physiol. (London),* 394, 249, 1987.

100. **Farber, J. P.,** Pulmonary receptor discharge and expiratory muscle activity, *Respir. Physiol.,* 47, 219, 1982.

101. **Widdicombe, J. G.,** Receptors in the trachea and bronchi of the cat, *J. Physiol. (London),* 123, 71, 1954.

102. **Davis, H. L., Fowler, W. S., and Lambert, E. H.,** Effect of the volume and rate of inflation and deflation on transpulmonary pressure and response of pulmonary stretch receptors, *Am. J. Physiol.,* 187, 558, 1956.

103. **Barnas, G. M., Banzett, R. B., Reid, M. B., and Lehr, J.,** Pulmonary afferent activity during high-frequency ventilation at constant mean lung volume, *J. Appl. Physiol.,* 61(1), 192, 1986.

104. **Kaufman, M. P., Iwamoto, G. A., Ashton, J. H., and Cassidy, S. S.,** Responses to inflation of vagal afferents with endings in the lungs of dogs, *Circ. Res.,* 51, 525, 1982.

105. **Davenport, P. W., Sant'Ambrogio, F. B., and Sant'Ambrogio, G.,** Adaptation of tracheal stretch receptors, *Respir. Physiol.,* 44, 339, 1981.

106. **Bradley, G. W. and Scheurmier, N.,** The transduction properties of tracheal stretch receptors *in vitro,* *Respir. Physiol.,* 31, 365, 1977.

107. **Sant'Ambrogio, F. B., Sant'Ambrogio, G., Mathew, O. P., and Tsubone, H.,** Contraction of trachealis muscle and activity of tracheal smooth receptors, *Respir. Physiol.,* 71, 343, 1988.

108. **Bartlett, D., Jr. and St. John, W. M.,** Adaptation of pulmonary stretch receptors in different mammalian species, *Respir. Physiol.,* 37, 303, 1979.

109. **Homma, I., Isobe, A., Onimaru, H., and Oouchi, M.,** Slowly adapting and rapidly adapting pulmonary receptor responses to high-frequency inflation in rabbits, in *Neurobiology of the Control of Breathing,* von Euler, C. and Lagererantz, H., Eds., Raven Press, New York, 1986, 269.

110. **Bartlett, D., Jr., Sant'Ambrogio, G., and Wise, J. C. M.,** Transduction properties of tracheal stretch receptors, *J. Physiol. (London),* 258, 421, 1976.

111. **Pack, A. I. and DeLaney, R. G.,** Response of pulmonary rapidly adapting receptors during lung inflation, *J. Appl. Physiol.: Respir. Environ. Exercise Physiol.,* 55, 955, 1983.

112. **Rewa, G., Kappagoda, C. T., Man, S. F. P., and Man, G. C.,** The effect of high frequency oscillatory ventilation on pulmonary stretch receptors in the dog, *Clin. Invest. Med.,* 9, 167, 1986.

113. **Paintal, A. S.,** Vagal sensory receptors and their reflex effects, *Physiol. Rev.,* 53(1), 159, 1973.

114. **McLean, H. A., Mitchell, G. S., and Milsom, W. K.,** Effects of prolonged inflation on pulmonary stretch receptor discharge in turtles, *Respir. Physiol.,* 75, 75, 1989.

115. **Sant'Ambrogio, F. B. and Sant'Ambrogio, G.,** Circulatory accessibility of nervous receptors localized in the tracheobronchial tree, *Respir. Physiol.,* 49, 49, 1982.

116. **Dain, D S., Boushey, H. A., and Gold, W. M.,** Inhibition of respiratory reflexes by local anesthetic aerosols in dogs and rabbits, *J. Appl. Physiol.,* 38(6), 1045, 1975.

117. **Fahim, M. and Jain, S. K.,** The effect of bupivacaine aerosol on the activity of pulmonary stretch and "irritant" receptors, *J. Physiol. (London),* 288, 367, 1979.

118. **Jain, S. K., Trenchard, D., Reynolds, F., Noble, M. I. M., and Guz, A.,** The effect of local anaesthesia of the airway on respiratory reflexes in the rabbit, *Clin. Sci.,* 44, 519, 1973.

119. **Hersch, M. I., Satchell, P. M., Sullivan, C. E., and McLeod, J. G.,** Abnormal pulmonary slowly adapting receptors in canine acrylamide neuropathy, *J. Appl. Physiol.,* 60(2), 376, 1986.

120. **Hersch, M. I., Satchell, P. M., Sullivan, C. E., and McLeod, J. G.,** Abnormal cough reflexes in acrylamide neuropathy, *Proc. Aust. Physiol. Pharmacol.,* 16, 182P, 1985.

121. **Sant'Ambrogio, G., Sant' Abrogio, F. B., and Davies, A.,** Airway receptors in cough, *Bull. Eur. Physiopathol. Respir.,* 20, 42, 1984.

122. **Davenport, P. W., Lee, L.-Y., Lee, K., Yu, L. K., Miller, R., and Frazier, D. T.,** Effect of bronchoconstriction on the firing behavior of pulmonary stretch receptors, *Respir. Physiol.,* 46, 295, 1981.

123. **Widdicombe, J. G.,** The activity of pulmonary stretch receptors during bronchoconstriction, pulmonary edema, atelectasis and breathing against a resistance, *J. Physiol. (London),* 159, 436, 1961.

124. **Bartlett, D., Jr. and Sant' Ambrogio, G.,** Effects of local and systemic hypercapnia on the discharge of stretch receptors in the airways of the dog, *Respir. Physiol.,* 26, 91, 1976.

125. **Coleridge, H. M., Coleridge, J. C. G., and Banzett, R. B.,** Effect of CO_2 on afferent vagal endings in the canine lung, *Respir. Physiol.,* 34, 135, 1978.

126. **Sant' Ambrogio, G., Miserocchi, G., and Mortola, J.,** Transient responses of pulmonary stretch receptors in the dog to inhalation of carbon dioxide, *Respir. Physiol.,* 22, 191, 1974.

127. **Trenchard, D.,** $CO_2/H+$ receptor in the lungs of anesthetized rabbits, *Respir. Physiol.,* 63, 227, 1986.

128. **Mitchell, G. S. and Vidruk, E. H.,** Effects of hypercapnia on phrenic and stretch receptor responses to lung inflation, *Respir. Physiol.,* 68, 319, 1987.

129. **Agostoni, E., Citterio, G., and Piccoli, S.,** Reflex partitioning of inputs from stretch receptors of bronchi and thoracic trachea, *Respir. Physiol.,* 60, 311, 1985.

130. **Widdicombe, J. G. and Nadel, J. A.,** Reflex effects of lung inflation on tracheal volume, *J. Appl. Physiol.,* 18, 681, 1963.

131. **Sorkness, R. and Vidruk, E.,** Reflex effects of isocapnic changes in ventilation on tracheal tone in awake dogs, *Respir. Physiol.,* 69, 161, 1987.

132. **Stein, J. E. and Widdicombe, J. G.,** Interaction of reflexes from chemo- and pulmonary stretch receptors in control of airway calibre, *J. Physiol. (London),* 216, 33, 1971.

133. **Ko, W.-C. and Lai, Y.-L.,** The tracheal nonadrenergic noncholinergic inhibitory system during antigen challenge, *Respir. Physiol.,* 74, 129, 1988.

134. **Don, H., Baker, D. G., and Richardson, C. A.,** Absence of nonadrenergic noncholinergic relaxation in the cat cervical trachea, *J. Appl. Physiol.,* 65, 2524, 1988.

135. **Agostoni, E., Cavagna, A. M., and Citterio, G.,** Effects of stretch receptors of bronchi or trachea on genioglossus muscle, *Respir. Physiol.,* 67, 335, 1987.

136. **Camproesi, E. M., Salzano, J. V., and Martel, D.,** Airway smooth muscle tone during high frequency ventilation, *Fed. Proc. Fed. Am. Soc. Exp. Biol.,* 41, 1358, 1982.

137. **Brouillette, R. T. and Thach, B. T.,** Control of genioglossus muscle inspiratory activity, *J. Appl. Physiol.,* 49, 801, 1980.

138. **van Lunteren, E., Strohl, K. P., Parker, D. M., Bruce, E. N., van de Graaf, W. B., and Cherniack, N. S.,** Phasic volume-related feedback on upper airway muscle activity, *J. Appl. Physiol.,* 56, 730, 1984.

139. **Homma, I., Isobe, A., Iwase, M., Onimaru, H., and Sibuya, M.,** Cross-correlation between vagal afferent impulses from pulmonary mechanoreceptors and high-frequency inflation (HFI) and deflation (HFD) in rabbits, *Neurosci. Lett.,* 75, 299, 1987.

140. **Davenport, P. W., Freed, A. N., and Rex, K. A.,** The effect of sulfur dioxide on the response of rabbits to expiratory loads, *Respir. Physiol.,* 56, 359, 1984.

141. **Kohl, J. and Koller, F. A.,** Blockade of pulmonary stretch receptors reinforces diaphragmatic activity during high-frequency oscillatory (HFOV) ventilation, *Pfluegers Arch.,* 411, 42, 1988.

142. **Zuperku, E. J., Hopp, F. A., and Kampine, J. P.,** Central integration of pulmonary stretch receptor input in the control of expiration, *J. Appl. Physiol.,* 52, 1296, 1982.

143. **Jonzon, A., Pisarri, T. E., Roberts, A. M., Coleridge, J. C. G., and Coleridge, H. M.,** Attenuation of pulmonary afferent input by vagal cooling in dogs, *Respir. Physiol.,* 72, 19, 1988.

144. **Bergen, D. R. and Sampson, S. R.,** Characterization of intrapulmonary, rapidly adapting receptors of guinea pigs, *Respir. Physiol.,* 47, 83, 1982.

145. **Roberts, A. M., Coleridge, H. M., and Coleridge, J. C. G.,** Reciprocal action of pulmonary vagal afferents on tracheal smooth muscle tension on dogs, *Respir. Physiol.,* 72, 35, 1988.

146. **Coon, R. L., Zuperku, E. H., and Kampine, J. P.,** Respiratory arrhythmias and airway CO_2, lung receptors, and central inspiratory activity, *J. Appl. Physiol.,* 60, 1713, 1986.

147. **Cassidy, S. S., Eschembacher, W. L., and Johnson, R. L., Jr.,** Reflex cardiovascular depression during unilateral lung hyperinflation in the dog, *J. Clin. Invest.,* 64, 620, 1979.

148. **Daly, M. De Burgh,** Interactions between respiration and circulation, in *Handbook of Physiology, The Respiratory System,* Vol. II, Cherniack, N. S. and Widdicombe, J. G., Eds., American Physiological Society, Washington, D.C., 1986, 529.

149. **Sant' Ambrogio, G., Remmers, J. E., DeGroot, W. J., Callas, G., and Mortola, J.,** Localization of rapidly-adapting receptors in the trachea and main stem bronchus of the dog, *Respir. Physiol.,* 33, 359, 1978.

150. **Widdicombe, J. G.**, Studies on afferent airway innervation, *Am. Rev. Respir. Dis.*, 115(6), 90, 1977.

151. **Das, R. M., Jeffery, P. J., and Widdicombe, J. G.**, The epithelial innervation of the lower respiratory tract of the cat, *J. Anat.*, 126, 123, 1978.

152. **Das, R. M., Jeffery, P. K., and Widdicombe, J. G.**, The structure and function of intra-epithelial nerve fiber of the respiratory tract in the cats, *J. Anat.*, 126(1), 123, 1978.

153. **Jeffery, P. K. and Reid, L.**, Intra-epithelial nerves in normal rat airways: a quantitative electron microscopic study, *J. Anat.*, 114, 34, 1973.

154. **Rhodin, J. A. G.**, Ultrastructure and function of the human tracheal mucosa, *Am. Rev. Respir. Dis.*, 93, 1, 1966.

155. **Mortola, J., Sant' Ambrogio, G., and Clement, M. G.**, Localization of irritant receptors in the airways of the dog, *Respir. Physiol.*, 24, 107, 1975.

156. **Jonzon, A., Pisarri, T. E., Coleridge, J. C. G., and Coleridge, H. M.**, Rapidly adapting receptor activity in dogs is inversely related to lung compliance, *J. Appl. Physiol.*, 61(5), 1980, 1986.

157. **Bergen, D. R., Myers, D. L., and Mohrman, M.**, Activity of rapidly-adapting receptors to histamine and antigen challenge before and after sodium cromoglycate, *Arch. Int. Pharmacodyn. Ther.*, 273, 88, 1985.

158. **Bergren, D. R., Gustafson, J. M., and Myers, D. L.**, Effect of prostaglandin $F_{2\alpha}$ on pulmonary rapidly-adapting receptors in the guinea pig, *Prostaglandins*, 27, 391, 1984.

159. **Armstrong, D. J. and Luck, J. C.**, A comparative study of irritant and type J receptors in the cat, *Respir. Physiol.*, 21, 47, 1974.

160. **Lowry, R. H., Wood, A. W. M., and Higgenbotham, T. W.**, Effects of pH and osmolarity on aerosol-induced cough in normal volunteers, *Clin. Sci.*, 74, 373, 1988.

161. **Sampson, S. R. and Vidruk, E. H.**, Properties of "irritant" receptors in canine lungs, *Respir. Physiol.*, 25, 9, 1975.

162. **Sellick, H. and Widdicombe, J. G.**, Vagal deflation and inflation reflexes mediated by lung irritant receptors, *Q. J. Exp. Physiol.*, 55, 153, 1970.

163. **Gustafson, J. and Bergren, D. R.**, Pulmonary rapidly-adapting receptors in the guinea pig depend on the rate of step-hyperinflation, *Fed. Proc., Fed. Am. Soc. Exp. Biol.*, 41(4), 987, 1982.

164. **Widdicombe, J. G.**, Respiratory reflexes, in *Handbook of Physiology*, Sect. III. Vol. I, Fenn, W. O. and Rahn, H., Eds., Williams & Wilkins, American Physiological Society, Baltimore, 1964, 583.

165. **Sellick, H. and Widdicombe, J. G.**, The activity of lung irritant receptors during pneumothorax, hyperpnoea and pulmonary vascular congestion, *J. Physiol. (London)*, 203, 359, 1969.

166. **Coleridge, H. M., Coleridge, J. C. G., Baker, D. G., Ginzel, K. H., and Morrison, M. A.**, Comparison of the effects of histamine and prostaglandin on afferent C-fiber endings and irritant receptors in the intrapulmonary airways, *Adv. Exp. Med. Biol.*, 99, 291, 1978.

167. **Sampson, S. R. and Vidruk, E. H.**, Chemical stimulation of rapidly adapting receptors in the airways, *Adv. Exp. Med. Biol.*, 99, 281, 1978.

168. **Vidruk, E. H., Hahn, H. L., Nadel, J., and Sampson, S. R.**, Mechanisms by which histamine stimulates rapidly adapting receptors in dog lungs, *J. Appl. Physiol.*, 43, 397, 1977.

169. **Coleridge, H. M., Coleridge, J. C. G., Ginzel, K. H., Baker, D. G., Banzett, R. B., and Morrison, M. A.**, Stimulation of "irritant" receptors and afferent C-fibers in the lungs by prostaglandins, *Nature*, 264, 451, 1976.

170. **Bergren, D. R. and Sampson, S. R.**, Prostaglandin $F_{2\alpha}$ and bradykinin challenge of intrapulmonary rapidly-adapting receptors in the guinea pig, *Fed. Proc., Fed. Am. Soc. Exp. Biol.*, 40(3), 507, 1981.

171. **Prabhakar, N. R., Runold, M., Yamamoto, Y., Lagercrantz, H., Cherniack, N. S., and von Euler, C.**, Role of the vagal afferents in substance P-induced respiratory responses in anaesthetized rabbits, *Acta Physiol. Scand.*, 131, 63, 1987.

172. **Cherniack, N. S., Runold, M., Prabhakar, N. R., and Mitra, H.**, Effect of adenosine on vagal sensory pulmonary afferents, *Fed. Proc., Fed. Am. Soc. Exp. Biol.*, 43, 825, 1987.

173. **Runold, M., Prabhakar, N. R., Mitra, H., and Cherniack, N. S.**, Adenosine stimulates respiration by acting on vagal receptors, *Fed. Proc., Fed. Am. Soc. Exp. Biol.*, 46(3), 825, 1987.

174. **Matsumoto, S.**, The activities of lung stretch and irritant receptors during cough, *Neurosci. Lett.*, 90, 125, 1988.

175. **Sellick, H. and Widdicombe, J. G.**, Stimulation of lung irritant receptors by cigarette smoke, carbon dust and histamine aerosol, *J. Appl. Physiol.*, 31, 15, 1971.

176. **Coleridge, H. M., Coleridge, J. C. G., Luck, J. C., and Norman, J.**, The effect of four volatile anesthetic agents on the impulse activity of two types of pulmonary receptor, *Br. J. Anaesth.*, 40, 484, 1968.

177. **Dixon, M., Jackson, D. J., Richards, I. M., and Vendy, K.**, The effects of acetylcholine and histamine on total lung resistance, dynamic lung compliance and lung irritant receptor discharge in the anesthetized dog, *J. Physiol. (London)*, 257, 79, 1978.

178. **Shioya, T., Solway, J., Munoz, S. M., Mack, M., and Leff, A. R.,** Distribution of airway contractile responses within the major diameter bronchi during exogenous bronchoconstriction, *Am. Rev. Respir. Dis.,* 135, 1105, 1987.

179. **Hamilton, R. D., Winning, A. J., and Guz, A.,** Blockade of "alveolar" and airway reflexes by local anesthetic aerosol in dogs, *Respir. Physiol.,* 67, 159, 1987.

180. **Kariya, S. T., Shore, S. A., Skornik, W. A., Anderson, K., Ingram, R. H., Jr., and Drazen, J. M.,** Methacoline-induced bronchoconstriction in dogs: effects of lung volume and O_3 exposure, *J. Appl. Physiol.,* 65(6), 2679, 1988.

181. **Hegardt, B., Lowhagen, O., and Svedmyr, N.,** Histamine-induced bronchospasm, *Allergy,* 35, 113, 1980.

182. **Bergren, D. R. and Kincaid, R. J.,** Rapidly-adapting receptor activity and intratracheal pressure in guinea pigs. II. Action of aspirin and salicylic acid in antagonizing mediators of allergic asthma, *Prostaglandins, Leukotriene Med.,* 16, 163, 1984.

183. **Bergren, D. R. and Myers, D. L.,** Leukotriene C_4 rapidly-adapting receptor activity and intratracheal pressure in guinea pigs. I. Action of leukotriene C_4, *Prostaglandins, Leukotriene Med.,* 16, 147, 1984.

184. **Sampson, S. R. and Vidruk, E. H.,** Chemical stimulation of rapidly adapting receptors in the airways, in *The Regulation of Respiration During Sleep and Anesthesia,* Fitzgerald, R. S., Gautier, H., and Lahiri, S., Eds., Plenum Press, New York, 1977, 281.

185. **Peachell, P. T., Columbo, M., Kagey-Sobotka, A., Lichtenstein, L. M., and Marone, G.,** Adenosine potentiates mediator release from human lung mast cells, *Am. Rev. Respir. Dis.,* 138, 1143, 1988.

186. **Bergren, D. R., Vidruk, E. H., and Sampson, S. R.,** Stimulation of rapidly-adapting airway receptors by antigen in allergic dogs, *Fed. Proc., Fed. Am. Soc. Exp. Biol.,* 37, 714, 1978.

187. **Golden, J. A., Nadel, J. A., and Boushey, H. A.,** Bronchial hyperirritability in healthy subjects after exposure to ozone, *Am. Rev. Respir. Dis.,* 118, 287, 1978.

188. **Dumont, C., Lee, L.-Y., and Nadel, J. A.,** Effect of ozone on bronchomotor response to aerosolized prostaglandin $F_{2\alpha}$ in dogs, *Physiologist,* 20, 35, 1977.

189. **Lee, L.-Y., Dumont, C., Djokie, T. D., Monzel, T. E., and Nadel, J. A.,** Mechanism of rapid, shallow breathing after ozone exposure in conscious dogs, *J. Appl. Physiol: Respir. Environ. Exercise Physiol.,* 46(6), 1108, 1979.

190. **Lee, L.-Y., Bleecker, E. R., and Nadel, J. A.,** Effect of ozone on the bronchomotor response to inhaled histamine aerosol in dogs, *J. Appl. Physiol.,* 43, 626, 1977.

191. **Sampson, S. R., Vidruk, E. H., Bergren, D. R., Dumont, C., and Lee, L.-Y.,** Alteration in responsiveness of rapidly-adapting airway receptors to bronchoactive agents by ozone, *Fed. Proc., Fed. Am. Soc. Exp. Biol.,* 37, 712, 1978.

192. **Yu, J., Coleridge, J. C. G., and Coleridge, H. M.,** Influence of lung stiffness on rapidly adapting receptors in rabbits and cats, *Respir. Physiol.,* 68, 161, 1987.

193. **Coleridge, H. M., Coleridge, J. C. G., and Roberts, A. M.,** Rapid shallow breathing evoked by selective stimulation of bronchial C-fibers in dogs, *J. Physiol. (London),* 340, 415, 1983.

194. **Glogowska, M., Richardson, P. S., Widdicombe, J. G., and Winning, A. J.,** The role of the vagus nerves, peripheral chemoreceptors and other afferent pathways in the genesis of augmented breaths in cats and rabbits, *Respir. Physiol.,* 16, 179, 1982.

195. **Knowlton, G. C. and Larrabee, M. G.,** A unitary analysis of pulmonary volume receptors, *Am. J. Physiol.,* 147, 100, 1946.

196. **Nicholas, T. E., Power, J. H. T., and Barr, H. A.,** The pulmonary consequences of a deep breath, *Respir. Physiol.,* 49, 315, 1982.

197. **Pack, A. I., DeLaney, R. G., and Fishman, A. P.,** Augmentation of phrenic neural activity by increased rates of lung inflation, *J. Appl. Physiol.,* 50, 149, 1981.

198. **Widdicombe, J. G.,** Respiratory reflexes excited by inflation of the lungs, *J. Physiol. (London),* 123, 105, 1954.

199. **Patberg, W. R.,** Effect of graded vagal blockade and pulmonary volume on tonic inspiratory activity in rabbits, *Pfluegers Arch.,* 398, 88, 1983.

200. **Davies, A.,** The effect of irritant receptor activity on expiratory time, *J. Physiol. (London),* 275, 39P, 1978.

201. **Sant' Ambrogio, G., Milic-Emili, J., and Camporesi, E.,** Occurrence of a deep breath after a period of airway occlusion, *Arch. Ges. Physiol.,* 327, 95, 1971.

202. **Davies, A. and Roumy, M.,** Changes in the pattern of breathing provoked by irritant receptors, *J. Physiol. (London),* 272, 78P, 1977.

203. **Davies, A. and Roumy, M.,** The inspiratory augmenting effect of lung irritant receptor activity, *J. Physiol. (London),* 275, 14P, 1978.

204. **Paintal, A. S.,** The response of gastric stretch receptors and certain other abdominal and thoracic vagal receptors to some drugs, *J. Physiol. (London),* 271, 1954.

205. **Paintal, A. S.,** The mechanism of excitation of type J receptors, and the J reflex, in *Ciba Found. Symp. Breathing: Hering-Breuer Centenary Symposium,* Porter, R., Ed., Churchill Livingstone, London, 1970, 59.

206. **Hung, K.-S., Hertweck, M. S., Hardy, J. D., and Loosli, C. G.,** Electron microscopic observations of nerve endings in the alveolar walls of mouse lungs, *Am. Rev. Respir. Dis.,* 108, 328, 1973.

207. **Hung, K.-S., Hertweck, M. S., Hardy, J. D., and Loosli, C. G.,** Ultrastructure of nerves and associated cells in bronchiolar epithelium of the mouse lung, *J. Ultrastruct. Mol. Struct. Res.,* 43, 426, 1973.

208. **Trenchard, D., Russell, N. J. W., and Raybould, H. E.,** Non-myelinated vagal lung receptors and their reflex reflects on respiration in rabbits, *Respir. Physiol.,* 55, 63, 1984.

209. **Boushey, H. A., Richardson, P. S., and Widdecombe, J. G.,** The response of laryngeal afferent fibers to mechanical and chemical stimuli, *J. Physiol. (London),* 240, 153, 1974.

210. **Jammes, Y., Barthelemy, P., and Delpierre, S.,** Respiratory effects of cold air breathing in anesthetized cats, *Respir. Physiol.,* 54, 41, 1983.

211. **Lauweryns, J. M. and Van Lommel, A.,** Effect of various vagotomy procedures on the reaction to hypoxia of rabbit neuroepithelial bodies: modulation of intrapulmonary axon reflexes?, *Exp. Lung Res.,* 11, 319, 1986.

212. **Lauweryns, J. M. and Cokelaere, M.,** Hypoxia-sensitive neuro-epithelial bodies. Intrapulmonary secretory neuroreceptors, modulated by the CNS, *Z. Zellforsch. Mikrosk. Anat.,* 145, 521, 1973.

213. **Paintal, A. S.,** Impulses in vagal afferent fibers from specific pulmonary deflation receptors. The response of these receptors to phenyl diguanide, potato starch, 5-hydroxytryptamine and nicotine and their role in respiratory and cardiovascular reflexes, *Q. J. Exp. Physiol.,* 40, 89, 1955.

214. **Paintal, A. S.,** The location and excitation of pulmonary deflation receptors by chemical substances, *Q. J. Exp. Physiol.,* 42, 56, 1957.

215. **Coleridge, H. M., Coleridge, J. C. G., and Luck, J. C.,** Pulmonary afferent fibers of small diameter stimulated by capsaicin and by hyperinflation of the lungs, *J. Physiol. (London),* 179, 248, 1965.

216. **Delpierre, S., Grimaud, C. H., Jammes, Y., and Mei, N.,** Changes in activity of vagal bronchopulmonary C fibers by chemical and physical stimuli in the cat, *J. Physiol. (London),* 316, 61, 1981.

217. **Armstrong, D. J., Luck, J. C., and Martin, V. M.,** The effect of emboli upon intrapulmonary receptors in the cat, *Respir. Physiol.,* 26, 41, 1976.

218. **Coleridge, H. M. and Coleridge, J. C. G.,** Afferent vagal C-fibers in the dog lung: their discharge during spontaneous breathing and their stimulation by alloxan and pulmonary congestion, in *Krogh Centenary Symposium on Respiratory Adaptations, Capillary Exchange and Reflex Mechanisms,* Paintal, A. S., Gill-Kumar, P., Eds., Vallabhbhai Patel Chest Inst., New Delhi, 1977, 396.

219. **Roberts, A. M., Bhattacharya, J., Schultz, H. D., Coleridge, H. M., and Coleridge, J. C. G.,** Stimulation of pulmonary vagal afferent C-fibers by lung edema in dogs, *Circ. Res.,* 58, 512, 1986.

220. **Marshall, R. and Widdicombe, J. S.,** The activity of pulmonary stretch receptors during congestion of the lungs, *Q. J. Exp. Physiol.,* 43, 320, 1958.

221. **Wead, W. B., Cassidy, S. S., and Reynolds, R. C.,** Pulmonary edema in dogs fails to cause reflex responses, *Am. J. Physiol. 252 (Heart Circ. Physiol.),* 21, H89, 1987.

222. **Lloyd, T. C., Jr.,** Cardiopulmonary baroreflexes effects of pulmonary congestion and edema, *J. Appl. Physiol.,* 43, 107, 1977.

223. **Greene, J. F., Schmidt, N. D., Schultz, H. D., Roberts, A. M., Coleridge, H. M., and Coleridge, J. C. G.,** Pulmonary C-fibers evoke both apnea and tachypnea of pulmonary chemoreflex, *J. Appl. Physiol.,* 57, 562, 1984.

224. **Roberts, A. M., Hahn, H. L., Schultz, H. D., Nadel, J. A., Coleridge, H. M., and Coleridge, J. C. G.,** Afferent vagal C-fibers are responsible for the reflex airway constriction and secretion evoked by pulmonary administration of SO_2 in dogs, *Physiologist,* 25(Abstr.), 226, 1982.

225. **Cassidy, S. S., Ashton, J. H., Wead, W. B., Kaufman, M. P., Monsereenusorn, Y., and Whiteside, J. A.,** Reflex cardiovascular responses caused by stimulation of pulmonary C-fibers with capsaicin in dogs, *J. Appl. Physiol.,* 60, 949, 1986.

226. **Jancso, G. and Such, G.,** Effects of capsaicin applied perineurally to the vagus nerve on cardiovascular and respiratory functions in the cat, *J. Physiol. (London),* 341, 359, 1983.

227. **Davis, B., Roberts, A. M., Coleridge, H. M., and Coleridge, J. C. G.,** Reflex tracheal gland secretion evoked by stimulation of bronchial C-fibers in dogs, *J. Appl. Physiol.,* 53, 985, 1982.

228. **Davies, A. M., Koenig, J. S., and Thach, B. T.,** Upper airway chemoreflex responses to saline and water in preterm infants, *J. Appl. Physiol.,* 64, 1412, 1988.

229. **Kaufman, M. P., Coleridge, H. M., Coleridge, J. C. G., and Baker, D. G.,** Differential sensitivity of bronchial and pulmonary C-fibers in dogs to bradykinin, histamine and serotonin, *Fed. Proc., Fed. Am. Soc. Exp. Biol.,* 39(Abstr.), 828, 1980.

230. **Fuller, R. W., Dixon, C. M. S., Cuss, F. M. C., and Barnes, P. J.,** Bradykinin-induced bronchoconstriction in man: mode of action, *Am. Rev. Respir. Dis.,* 135, 176, 1987.

231. **Roberts, A. M., Kaufman, M. P., Baker, D. G., Brown, J. K., Coleridge, H. M., and Coleridge, J. C. G.,** Reflex tracheal contraction induced by stimulation of bronchial C-fibers in dogs, *J. Appl. Physiol,* 51, 485, 1981.

232. **Simonsson, B. G., Skoogh, B. E., Bergh, N. P., Anderson, R., and Svedmyr, N.,** *In vivo* and *in vitro* effect of bradykinin of bronchial motor tone in normal subjects and in patients with airway obstruction, *Respiration,* 30, 378, 1973.

233. **Greene, R., Fowler, J., MacGlasha, D., Jr., and Weinreich, D.,** IgE-challenged lung mast cells excite vagal sensory neurons *in vitro, J. Appl. Physiol.,* 64, 2249, 1988.

234. **Haxhiu, M. A., van Lunteren, E., Deal, E. C., and Cherniack, N. S.,** Effect of stimulation of pulmonary C-fiber receptors on canine respiratory muscles, *J. Appl. Physiol.,* 65(3), 1087, 1988.

235. **Agrawal, S. G. and Evans, R. H.,** The primary afferent depolarizing action of kainate in the rat, *Br. J. Pharmacol.,* 87, 345, 1986.

236. **Lloyd, T. C., Jr.,** Reflex effect of lung inflation and inhalation of halothane, ether, and ammonia, *Am. J. Physiol.: Respir. Environ. Exercise Physiol.,* 45(2), 212, 1978.

237. **Lee, L.-Y., Beck, E. R., Morton, R. F., Kou, Y. R., and Frazier, D. T.,** Role of bronchopulmonary C-fiber afferents in the apneic response to cigarette smoke, *J. Appl. Physiol.,* 63(4), 1366, 1987.

238. **Haas, F., Levin, N., Pasierski, S., Bishop, M., and Axen, K.,** Reduced hyperpnea-induced bronchospasm following repeated cold air challenge, *J. Appl. Physiol.,* 61(1), 210, 1986.

239. **Delpierre, S., Jammes, Y., and Mei, N.,** Effects of hypercapnia, hypoxia and increase in tidal volume on vagal bronchopulmonary C fibers in cat, *J. Physiol. (London),* 298, 48P, 1980.

240. **Anand, A. and Paintal, A. S.,** Reflex effects following selective stimulation of J receptors in the cat, *J. Physiol. (London),* 299, 553, 1980.

241. **Clifford, P. S., Litzow, J. T., and Coon, R. L.,** Pulmonary depressor reflex elicited by capsaicin in conscious intact and lung-denervated dogs, *Am. J. Physiol.,* 252 *(Regulatory Integrative Comp. Physiol.),* 21, R394, 1987.

242. **Coast, J. R., Romeo, R. M., and Cassidy, S. S.,** Diaphragmatic vasodilation elicited by pulmonary C-fiber stimulation, *Respir. Physiol.,* 75, 279, 1989.

243. **Coast, J. R. and Cassidy, S. S.,** Diaphragmatic responses to graded stimulation of pulmonary C-fibers with capsaicin, *J. Appl. Physiol.,* 59(5), 1487, 1985.

244. **Pisarri, T. E., Yu, J., Coleridge, H. M., and Coleridge, J. C. G.,** Background activity in pulmonary vagal C-fibers and its effects on breathing, *Respir. Physiol.,* 64, 29, 1986.

245. **Russell, J. A., and Lai-Fook, S. J.,** Reflex bronchoconstriction induced by capsaicin in the dog, *J. Appl. Physiol.,* 47, 961, 1979.

246. **Bergren, D. R.,** Capsaicin challenge, reflex bronchoconstriction and local action of substance P, *Am. J. Physiol. 254 (Regulatory Integrative Comp. Physiol.),* 23, R845, 1988.

247. **Biggs, D. F. and Goel, V.,** Does capsaicin cause reflex bronchospasm in guinea pigs? *Eur. J. Pharmacol.,* 115, 71, 1985.

248. **Lundberg, J. M., Saria, A., Brodin, E., Rosell, S., and Folkers, K.,** A substance P antagonism inhibits vagally induced increases in vascular permeability and bronchial smooth muscle contraction in the guinea pig, *Proc. Natl. Acad. Sci. U.S.A.,* 80, 1120, 1983.

249. **Mitchell, H. W.,** Analysis by microcomputer of the effect of capsaicin on pulmonary mechanics in the rat and guinea-pig, *Arch. Int. Pharmacodyn. Ther.,* 275, 279, 1985.

250. **Makara, G. B., Gyorgy, L., and Molnar, J.,** Circulatory and respiratory responses to capsaicin, 5-hydroxytryptamine and histamine in rats pretreated with capsaicin, *Arch. Int. Pharmacodyn. Ther.,* 170, 39, 1967.

251. **Collier, J. G. and Fuller, R. W.,** Capsaicin inhalation in man and the effects of sodium cromoglycate, *Br. J. Pharmacol.,* 81, 113, 1984.

252. **Fuller, R. W., Dixon, C. M. S., and Barnes, P. J.,** Bronchoconstrictor response to inhaled capsaicin in humans, *J. Appl. Physiol.,* 58(4), 1080, 1985.

253. **Jancso, N., Kiraly, E., and Jancso-Gabor, A.,** Pharmacologically induced selective degeneration of chemosensitive primary neurons, *Nature,* 270, 741, 1977.

254. **Lundblad, L., Lundberg, J. M., Anggard, A., and Zetterstrom, O.,** Capsaicin pretreatment inhibits the flare component of the cutaneous allergic reaction in man, *Eur. J. Pharmacol.,* 113, 461, 1985.

255. **Winning, A. J., Hamilton, R. D., Shea, S. A., and Guz, A.,** Respiratory and cardiovascular effects of central and peripheral intravenous injections of capsaicin in man: evidence for pulmonary chemosensitivity, *Clin. Sci.,* 71, 519, 1986.

256. **Clozel, J. P., Roberts, A. M., Hoffman, J. I. E., Coleridge, H. M., and Coleridge, J. C. G.,** Vagal chemoreflex coronary vasodilation evoked by stimulating pulmonary C-fibers in dogs, *Circ. Res.,* 57, 450, 1985.

257. **Ordway, G. A. and Pitetti, K. H.,** Stimulation of pulmonary C fibers decreases coronary arterial resistance in dogs, *J. Physiol. (London),* 371, 277, 1986.

258. **Buck, S. H., Walsh, J. H., Yamamura, H. I., and Burks, T. F.,** Neuropeptides in sensory neurons, *Life Sci.,* 30, 1857, 1982.

259. **Cervero, F. and Plenderleith, M. B.,** C-Fiber excitation and tonic descending inhibition of dorsal horn neurons in adult rats treated at birth with capsaicin, *J. Physiol. (London),* 365, 223, 1985.

260. **Cromer, S. P., Young, R. H., and Ivy, A. C.,** On the existence of afferent respiratory impulses mediated by the stellate ganglia, *Am. J. Physiol.,* 104, 468, 1933.

261. **Jammes, Y., Mathiot, M. J., Delpierre, S., and Grimaud, C.,** Role of vagal and spinal sensory pathways on eupneic diaphragmatic activity, *J. Appl. Physiol.,* 60(2), 479, 1986.

262. **Saria, A., Martling, C.-R., Dalsgaard, C.-J., and Lundberg, J. M.,** Evidence for substance P-immunoreactive spinal afferent that mediate bronchoconstriction, *Acta Physiol. Scand,* 125, 407, 1985.

263. **Waldrop, T. G.,** Respiratory response to chemical activation of left ventricular receptors, *Respir. Physiol.,* 63, 383, 1986.

264. **Anard, P., Bloom, S. R., and McGregor, G. P.,** Topical capsaicin pretreatment inhibits axon reflex vasodilation caused by somatostatin and vasoactive intestinal polypeptide in human skin, *Br. J. Pharmacol.,* 78, 665, 1983.

265. **Barnes, P. J.,** Asthma as an axon reflex, *Lancet,* 1, 242, 1986.

266. **Foreman, J. C.,** Peptides and neurogenic inflammation, *Br. Med. Bull.,* 43(2), 386, 1987.

267. **Lundberg, J. M. and Saria, A.,** Bronchial smooth muscle contraction induced by stimulation of capsaicin-sensitive sensory neurons, *Acta Physiol. Scand.,* 116, 473, 1982.

268. **Lundberg, J. M. and Saria, A.,** Capsaicin-induced desensitization of airway mucosa to cigarette smoke, mechanical and chemical irritants, *Nature,* 302, 251, 1983.

269. **Lundberg, J. M., Martling, C.-R., and Saria, A.,** Substance P and capsaicin-induced contraction of human bronchi, *Acta Physiol. Scand.,* 119, 49, 1983.

270. **Lundberg, J. M., Franco-Cereceda, A., Hua, X., Hokfelt, T., and Fischer, J. A.,** Co-existence of substance P and calcitonin gene-related peptide-like immunoreactivities in sensory nerve in relation to cardiovascular and bronchoconstrictor effects of capsaicin, *Eur. J. Pharmacol.,* 108, 315, 1985.

271. **Lundberg, J. M., Hokfelt, T., Martling, C.-R., Saria, A., and Cuello, C.,** Sensory substance P-immunoreactive nerves in the lower respiratory tract of various mammals including man, *Cell Tissue Res.,* 235, 251, 1984.

272. **Palmer, J. B. D. and Barnes, P. J.,** Neuropeptides and airway smooth muscle function, *Am. Rev. Respir. Dis.,* 136, S5, 1987.

273. **Palmer, J. B. D., Cuss, F. M. C., Mulderry, P. K., Ghatei, M. A., Springall, D. R., Cadieux, A., Blood, S. R., Polak, J. M., and Barnes, P. J.,** Calcitonin gene-related peptide localized to human airway nerves and potently constricts human airway smooth muscle, *Br. J. Pharmacol.,* 91, 95, 1987.

274. **Jancso, G., Kiraly, E., and Jancso-Gabor, A.,** Pharmacologically induced selective degeneration of chemosensitive primary sensory neurones, *Nature,* 270, 741, 1977.

275. **Gamse, R., Holzer, P., and Lembeck, F.,** Decrease of substance P in primary afferent neurons and impairment of neurogenic plasma extravasation by capsaicin, *Br. J. Pharamacol.,* 68, 207, 1980.

276. **Helke, C. J., Jacobwitz, D. M., and Thoa, N. B.,** Capsaicin and potassium blocked substance P release from the nucleus tractus solitarius and spinal trigeminal nucleus *in vitro, Life Sci.,* 29, 1779, 1981.

277. **Towle, A. C., Mueller, R. A., Breese, G. R., and Lauder, J.,** Altered respiratory response to substance P in capsaicin-treated rats, *J. Neurosci. Res.,* 14, 239, 1985.

278. **Sheppard, D., Rizk, N. W., Boushey, H. A., and Bethel, R. A.,** Mechanism of cough and bronchoconstriction induced by distilled water aerosol, *Am. Rev. Respir. Dis.,* 127, 691, 1983.

279. **Harries, M. G., Parkes, P. E. G., Lessof, M. H., and Orr, T. S. C.,** Role of bronchial irritant receptors in asthma, *Lancet,* January 3, 5, 1981.

280. **Karlsson, J.-A., Zackrisson, C., and Forsberg, K.,** Hyperresponsiveness to irritant induced cough but not bronchoconstriction in guinea pigs exposed to cigarette smoke for 2 weeks, *Br. J. Pharmacol.,* 93, 550, 1988.

281. **Forsberg, S. and Karlsson, J. A.,** Cough induced by stimulation of capsaicin-sensitive sensory neurons in conscious guinea pigs, *Acta Physiol. Scand.,* 128, 319, 1986.

282. **Dixon, M., Jackson, D. M., and Richards, I. M.,** The action of sodium cromoglycate on "C" fibre endings in the dog lung, *Br. J. Pharmacol.,* 70, 11, 1980.

283. **Coleridge, J. C. G., Poore, E. R., Roberts, A. M., and Coleridge, H. M.,** Effect of sodium cromoglycate on afferent vagal C-fibers and cardiopulmonary chemoreflexes in dogs, *Fed. Proc., Fed. Am. Soc. Exp. Biol.,* 41, 986, 1982.

284. **Dixon, M., Jackson, D. M., and Richards, I. M.,** The effects of sodium cromoglycate on lung irritant receptors and left ventricular cardiac receptors in the anesthetized dog, *Br. J. Pharmacol.,* 67, 569, 1979.

285. **Jackson, D. M. and Richards, I. M.,** The effects of sodium cromoglycate on histamine aerosol-induced reflex bronchoconstriction in the anesthetized dog, *Br. J. Pharmacol.,* 61, 257, 1977.

286. **Mathe, A. A., Hedqvist, P., Holmgren, A., and Svanborg, N.,** Bronchial hyperreactivity to prostaglandin $F_{2\alpha}$ and histamine in patients with asthma, *Br. Med. J.,* 1, 193, 1973.

287. **Head, H.,** On the regulation of respiration. Part I. Experimental, *J. Physiol. (London),* 10, 1, 1889.
288. **Koller, E. A. and Kohl, J.,** The Hering-Breuer reflexes in the bronchial asthma attach, *Pfluegers Arch.,* 357, 165, 1975.
289. **Averill, D. G., Cameron, W. E., and Berger, A. J.,** Monosynaptic excitation of dorsal medullary respiratory neurons by slowly adapting pulmonary stretch receptors, *J. Neurophysiol.,* 52, 771, 1984.
290. **Averill, D. B., Cameron, W. E., and Berger, A. J.,** Neural elements subserving pulmonary stretch receptor-mediated facilitation of phrenic motorneurons, *Brain Res.,* 346, 378, 1985.
291. **Backman, S. B., Anders, C., Ballantyne, D., Rohrig, N., Camerer, H., Mifflin, S., Jordan, D., Dickhaus, H., Spyer, K. M., and Richter, D. W.,** Evidence for a monosynaptic connection between slowly adapting pulmonary stretch receptor afferents and inspiratory beta neurones, *Pfluegers Arch.,* 402, 129, 1984.
292. **Davies, R. O., Metzler, J., Siluge, D. A., and Pack, A. I.,** Effects of lung inflation on the excitability of dorsal respiratory group neurons, *Brain Res.,* 366, 2236, 1986.
293. **Donoghue, S., Garcia, M., Jordan, D., and Spyer, K. M.,** The brain-stem projections of pulmonary stretch afferent neurones in cats and rabbits, *J. Physiol. (London),* 322, 353, 1982.
294. **Kubin, L. and Davies, R. O.,** Bilateral convergence of pulmonary stretch receptor inputs in I_B-neurons in the cat, *J. Appl. Physiol.,* 62(4), 1488, 1987.
295. **Kalia, M. and Richter, D.,** Morphology of physiologically identified slowly adapting lung stretch receptor afferents stained with intra-axonal horseradish peroxidase in the nucleus of the tractus solitarius of the cat. I. A light microscopic analysis, *J. Comp. Neurol.,* 241, 503, 1985.
296. **Kalia, M. and Richter, D.,** Morphology of physiologically identified slowly adapting lung stretch receptor afferents stained with intra-axonal horseradish peroxidase in the nucleus of the tractus solitarius of the cat. II. An ultrastructural analysis, *J. Comp. Neurol.,* 241, 521, 1985.
297. **Kalia, M. and Richter, D.,** Rapidly adapting pulmonary receptor afferents. I. Aborization in the nucleus of the tractus solitarius, *J. Comp. Neurol.,* 274, 560, 1988.
298. **Kalia, M. and Richter, D.,** Rapidly adapting pulmonary receptor afferents. II. Fine structure and synaptic organization of central terminal processes in the nucleus of the tractus solitarius, *J. Comp. Neurol.,* 274, 574, 1988.
299. **Davies, R. O. and Kubin, L.,** Projection of pulmonary rapidly adapting receptors to the medulla of the cat: an antidromic mapping study, *J. Physiol. (London),* 373, 63, 1986.
300. **Kubin, L. and Davies, R. O.,** Sites of termination and relay of pulmonary rapidly adapting receptors as studied by spike-triggered averaging, *Brain Res.,* 443, 215, 1988.
301. **McCrimmion, D. R., Speck, D. F., and Feldman, J. L.,** Role of the ventro-lateral region of the nucleus of the tractus solitarius in processing respiratory afferent input from vagus and superior laryngeal nerves, *Exp. Brain Res.,* 67, 449, 1987.
302. **Millhorn, D. E. and Kiley, J. P.,** Effect of graded cooling of intermediate areas on respiratory response to vagal input, *Respir. Physiol.,* 58, 51, 1984.
303. **Agonstoni, E., Chinnock, J. E., Daly, M. De Burgh, and Murray, J. G.,** Functional and histological studies on the vagus and its branches to the heart, lungs and abdominal viscera in the cat, *J. Physiol. (London),* 135, 182, 1957.
304. **Camporesi, E. M., Mortola, M. P., Sant' Ambrogio, F., and Sant' Ambrogio, G.,** Topical anesthesia of trachea receptors, *J. Appl. Physiol.: Respir. Environ. Exercise Physiol.,* 47(5), 1123, 1979.
305. **Fuller, R. W. and Collier, J. G.,** Sodium cromoglycate and atropine block the fall in FEV, but not the cough induced by hypotonic mist, *Thorax,* 39, 766, 1984.
306. **Thomson, N. C.,** The effect of different pharmacological agents on respiratory reflexes in normal and asthmatic subjects, *Clin. Sci.,* 56, 235, 1979.
306a. **Bergren, D. R.,** unpublished observations.

Chapter 10

ADRENERGIC AND CHOLINERGIC RECEPTORS AND AIRWAY RESPONSIVENESS

Robert G. Townley and Devendra K. Agrawal

TABLE OF CONTENTS

I. Bronchial Hyperresponsiveness 230

II. Adrenergic Innervation of the Airways 230

III. Classification of Adrenergic Receptors..232

IV. Cholinergic Innervation and Function...233

V. Cholinergic Receptors in the Airways...234

VI. Cholinergic Receptors and Bronchial Asthma.................................235

VII. β-Adrenoreceptors in the Airways and Lungs.................................236
    A.   β-Adrenoreceptors in Trachea and Lungs 236
    B.   β-Adrenoreceptors in Airway Epithelium.............................237
    C.   β-Adrenoreceptors in Glands 237
    D.   β-Adrenoreceptors on Mast Cells....................................238
    E.   β-Adrenoreceptors on Alveolar Macrophages 238

VIII. Pulmonary β-Adrenoreceptors in Bronchial Asthma 239

IX. Effect of Glucocorticoids on Pulmonary β-Adrenergic
     Receptors and Responses 243

X. α-Adrenoreceptors in the Airways 245

XI. α-Adrenoreceptors and Bronchial Asthma 245

XII. Conclusions...246

References...247

I. BRONCHIAL HYPERRESPONSIVENESS

A characteristic feature of bronchial asthma is the hypersensitivity of the airways to a number of specific and nonspecific stimuli. Bronchospasm can be precipitated by antigens infection, exercise, fumes, sulfur dioxide, and chemical mediators such as methacholine, histamine, serotonin, leukotrienes C_4 and D_4, and prostaglandins D_2 and $F_{2\alpha}$. Asthmatics are from 100- to 1000-fold more sensitive to these chemical mediators.

Although inflammation is present in the airways of asthmatics and can increase airway responsiveness by about threefold, it is unlikely to be the primary mechanism for airway hyperresponsiveness. Prolonged treatment with inhaled steroids significantly reduced the number of inflammatory cells in the airways and was not significantly different from control biopsies.[1] Despite the absence of inflammation and reduced epithelial damage during treatment, all patients still had bronchial hyperresponsiveness.

This "hypersensitivity" of the airways is used to define asthma and as a possible genetic marker. Methacholine and histamine are the mediators most commonly used at the present time to test for airway hypersensitivity. Exercise-induced asthma results from loss of water and the cooling effect of hyperventilation in the airways. The loss of water results in a hypertonicity of the fluid in the airway mucosa. Bronchial hypersensitivity can be tested by exercise or inhalation challenge with hypertonic saline or by hyperventilation of cold dry air.[2] Whereas histamine and methacholine cause bronchoconstriction by a direct effect on airway smooth muscle, exercise, inhalation of hypertonic saline, or hyperventilation of cold dry air cause bronchoconstriction indirectly through release of mediators.[2] The former tests are virtually 100% sensitive for asthma, but are not as specific as the latter tests. The latter tests, however, are positive in only about 75% of subjects with asthma, but are very specific (see Chapter 8 for clinical methods to evaluate airway reactivity).

Most asthmatics who cease to have attacks remain methacholine positive for many years after their last attack, though the degree of their sensitivity is only one tenth of current asthmatics.[1-4]

Although 25% of allergic rhinitis subjects show a 20% fall in forced expiration volume (FEV_1) to 200 breath units and have a medium positive response, less than 5% of allergic rhinitis or nonatopic normal subjects (normals) show a response to 50 breath units or less and have a high positive methacholine response.[2,3] These subjects may well be potential candidates for developing asthma.

Of the more than 2900 symptomatic asthmatics tested, bronchial sensitivity to methacholine has been observed in all of them.[2] A number of studies have shown a very good correlation between methacholine and histamine sensitivities.[5,6] Bronchial sensitivity may be due to a functional imbalance in the autonomic nervous system of the bronchial tree. Constriction of bronchial smooth muscle by allergens or exercise and subsequent mediator release is essentially unopposed in a situation where there is loss of the normal counterregulatory bronchodilating effect such as loss of nonadrenergic inhibitory activity or as occurs with blockade of the β-adrenergic receptors (Figure 1).

In this chapter, we will discuss the autonomic enervation and the characteristics of α- and β-adrenoreceptors and the cholinergic receptors in the airways and their involvement in the pathophysiology of the airways. These concepts are relevant to the rational therapeutic application of potent pharmacologic agents such as bronchodilator catecholamines (β-adrenoreceptor agonists) and cholinergic antagonists in various pulmonary diseases, and in particular in bronchial asthma.

II. ADRENERGIC INNERVATION OF THE AIRWAYS

The autonomic systems supplying the airways include the sympathetic, parasympathetic, and nonadrenergic inhibitory nervous systems. β-adrenergic agonists and activation of non-

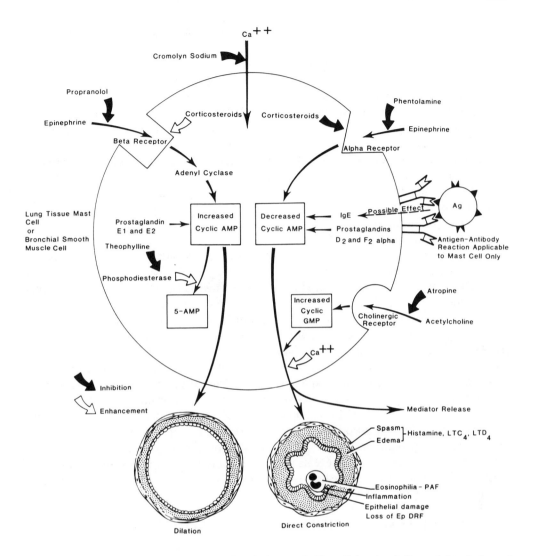

FIGURE 1. Schematic presentation of the pharmacologic control of bronchial tone and allergen-induced release of chemical mediators. Cholinergic or α-adrenergic stimulation in the presence of α-adrenergic blockade results in bronchial constriction directly, as well as enhanced release of mediators from lung tissue. This may result in an amplification phenomenon since there is both enhanced release of mediators as a result of allergens reacting with IgE and an enhanced bronchoconstricting effect of such mediators on the bronchi.

Such an autonomic imbalance could explain the exquisite sensitivity to mediators seen in patients with bronchial asthma. Normally, the intact β-adrenergic system can readily maintain the bronchi in a dilated state even in the presence of cholinergic or α-adrenergic stimulation; this explains the failure of methacholine and histamine to induce bronchoconstriction in the normal individual. The synthesis and release of PAF and leukotrienes from eosinophils may also increase sensitivity to other mediators since PAF has been shown to block β-receptors and decrease the β-adrenergic bronchodilating response in human lung. Finally, the release of toxic proteins such as major basic protein and eosinophil peroxidase may result in epithelial damage and loss of EpiDRF and loss of β-receptors in the epithelium. (From Townley, R. G., *Adv. Asthma Allergy,* 2, 9, 1975. With permission.)

adrenergic inhibitory nerves relax airway smooth muscle, whereas α-adrenergic and muscarinic agonists contract airway smooth muscle. Thus, airway hyperreactivity could be due to decreased β-adrenergic or nonadrenergic inhibitory activity or to increased α-adrenergic or parasympathetic activity.

The lungs receive their sympathetic nerve supply from upper thoracic preganglionic fibers that end in the extrapulmonary stellate ganglia. The postganglionic nerve fibers extend to the hila of the lung, where they intermingle with the cholinergic nerves to form a dense plexus around the airways and blood vessels.[7-9] Evidence of functional sympathetic innervation of intrinsic ganglia in lung is minimal. Adrenergic innervation differs markedly among species. The airways of cats and guinea pigs have a more pronounced sympathetic innervation than other species.[10] Sympathetic innervation to the airway smooth muscle in human trachea is sparse.[10] In comparison to trachea, human bronchi are more densely and closely innervated by nerves with varicosities containing mostly small agranular vesicles, and are considered to be cholinergic in nature.[11] In human lung samples obtained at surgery, axon profiles containing small granular vesicles (30 to 50 nm diameter), characteristics of adrenergic nerves, both in the smooth-muscle layer and in bronchial glands, have also been demonstrated.[8,9] These studies indicate the presence of adrenergic nerves in human peripheral airways. The adrenergic nature of some nerves of human bronchi has been shown by Pack and Richardson[7] using both fluorescence of catecholamines with light microscopy and 5-hydroxydopamine loading with electron microscopy.

These morphological studies suggest that muscles of smaller bronchi and peripheral airways may be organized for more neural and less myogenic control of activity and that large central airways may be organized for a major myogenic control of activity with neural modulation.

There is some evidence for adrenergic control of airway smooth-muscle responses in humans. Pretreatment with propranolol in asthmatic subjects may potentiate the bronchoconstriction caused by histamine,[12] methacholine,[13] acetylcholine,[14] and cigarette smoke.[15] However, the bronchomotor response to methacholine[16] or to histamine[17] was not increased in normal subjects by pretreatment with propranolol given either intravenously or by aerosol. In contrast, allergic rhinitis subjects who were insensitive to methacholine developed transient sensitivity to methacholine and symptoms of asthma after propranolol inhalation.[16] Asthmatics do develop bronchoconstriction after administration of beta-blockers alone. It is believed that unopposed parasympathetic tone may be involved in propranolol-induced bronchoconstriction, since atropine prevents and reverses this effect in most asthmatics.[18] However, vasoactive intestinal peptide has been reported to be at least as effective as ipratropium, an atropinelike agent, in this regard.[19]

III. CLASSIFICATION OF ADRENERGIC RECEPTORS

Epinephrine is a major adrenomedullary hormone. Norepinephrine is the major neurotransmitter substance released from sympathetic nerve terminals. Both catecholamines are known to elicit excitatory and inhibitory responses in various smooth-muscle cells. The sites at which catecholamines act are known as "adrenoreceptors". Adrenoreceptors have been divided historically into two major subtypes that are termed α- and β-adrenoreceptors. α-Adrenoreceptors (at which norepinephrine and epinephrine are roughly equipotent and both are very much more potent than isopropylnorepinephrine) were considered to mediate excitatory effects. β-Adrenoreceptors (at which the rank order potency of the agonists is isopropylnorepinephrine > epinephrine > norepinephrine) were considered to mediate inhibitory effects. The further subdivision of β-adrenoreceptors into β_1 and β_2 receptor subtypes is based on their pharmacological characteristics.[20,21]

Similarly α-adrenoreceptors were subdivided into α_1 and α_2 receptor subtypes.[22-25] Initially, prejunctional α-adrenoreceptors were termed as α_2, and postjunctional α-adrenoreceptors were termed as α_1 receptor subtypes. This classification of α-adrenoreceptors was based partly on the anatomical location and partly on the differences in the order of potency of α-adrenoreceptor agonists and antagonists. Later α-adrenoreceptors were classified on the basis of their pharmacological profile, as demonstrated using selective α-adrenoreceptor agonists and antagonists, independent of their anatomical location or function.[26,27] Postjunctional α-adrenoreceptors may be regulated by circulating catecholamines, whereas post-junctional α_1-adrenoreceptors are more responsive to neuronally released norepinephrine.[28]

α-Adrenoreceptors were subdivided into prejunctional α-adrenoreceptors and postjunctional α_1- and α_2-adrenoreceptors on the basis of their interaction with selective agonists and antagonists. Recently, α-adrenoreceptors have been further divided by the demonstration of subtypes of α_1-adrenoreceptors[29] and subtypes of α_2-adrenoreceptors.[30] This latter classification of α_1- and α_2-adrenoreceptors is not yet convincing and requires further clarification.

IV. CHOLINERGIC INNERVATION AND FUNCTION

The parasympathetic or cholinergic nerve supply to the lungs arises from cells in the brain stem and sacral regions of the spinal cord. Efferent cholinergic fibers may be found in cranial nerves III, VII, IX, and X.

Ganglia of the parasympathetic system are located within the walls of the organs innervated. Most tissue with autonomic innervation receive both sympathetic and parasympathetic nerves. In general, the effects of the two systems are antagonistic.

Cholinergic fibers include all preganglionic neurons of the autonomic nervous system, all postganglionic neurons of the craniosacral division, some postganglionic fibers of the thoracolumbar division, and all somatic motor neurons.

Four classes of cholinergic fibers and at least three types of receptors have been described. The receptors of autonomic effector cells are classified as muscarinic, and those of autonomic ganglion cells and striated muscle are classified as nicotinic. The cholinoceptive neurons of the central nervous system have either nicotinic or muscarinic receptors.[31]

Cholinergic postganglionic fibers are in the vagus nerve and are found in the smooth muscles and glands of the upper tracheobronchial tree down to the level of the small airways.[32] These vagal efferent fibers maintain resting bronchial smooth-muscle tone. If the vagus nerve in animals is stimulated, diffuse bronchoconstriction results and removal of vagal innervation results in mild bronchodilation.[32]

The cholinergic receptors on airway smooth muscle mediates bronchoconstriction, and acetylcholine is the neurotransmitter. Cutting the sympathetic nerves in animals causes only a slight increase in airflow resistance[33] and even maximal stimulation of the nerves only partially reverses the bronchoconstriction caused by simultaneous vagal stimulation.[34]

An increase in cholinergic activity could possibly be responsible for the increased smooth-muscle contraction in asthmatic patients. In this regard, virtually every asthmatic patient demonstrates airway hyperresponsiveness to muscarinic agonists,[1-4,35] and airflow obstruction in asthmatic patients is partially reversed by treatment with muscarinic antagonists.[36-37]

Reflex bronchodilation results from stimulation of sensory endings in the nose or epipharynx and is caused by decreasing parasympathetic motor activity. Bronchoconstriction by increasing parasympathetic motor activity results from stimulating sensory endings in the larynx and lower airways or in central and peripheral chemoreceptors. Parasympathetic reflex bronchoconstriction also occurs by stimulation of C-fiber endings in the airways.[38]

The sensory pathways have been analyzed by studying the cough provoked in asthmatic subjects by inhalation of distilled water aerosol. This cough can be blocked by pretreatment with lidocaine aerosol. However, the bronchoconstriction provoked by distilled water aerosol is not provoked by an aerosolized isotonic solution of sodium gluconate and is not blocked by pretreatment with lidocaine aerosol.[39,40]

In vivo methods for identifying tracheal ganglion cells[41] and for direct recordings of their membrane potentials[42] have been developed. Catechol-containing varicosities have been identified in parasympathetic ganglia of the airway in some species,[43-45] and small dense-core vesicles are found in axons within ganglia in human airways.[46] There is evidence that norepinephrine has a hyperpolarizing inhibitory effect on neurons in airway ganglia.[42] Thus, sympathetic neurotransmitters could modulate parasympathetic ganglionic transmission.

A specific inhibitory role of the sympathetic nerves on vagal nervous output has been shown in canine bronchi *in vitro*. It has been shown that electric field stimulation caused the release of norepinephrine, which inhibits bronchoconstriction produced by stimulation of the parasympathetic nerves.[47] This inhibitory action appears to be reciprocal and could play a role in regulating airways. This is suggested by the fact that acetylcholine inhibits the release of norepinephrine from nerve endings in canine airway smooth muscle.[49,50]

V. CHOLINERGIC RECEPTORS IN THE AIRWAYS

The development of radioligands possessing both high affinity and high specific radioactivity has enabled investigators to identify and characterize muscarinic receptors located in the airways. The relative intensity of physiologic responsiveness to muscarinic agonists and antagonists is related to the concentration of muscarinic receptors among various organs. A greater density of muscarinic receptors in large central airways than in small peripheral airways has been shown by the use of autoradiography.[51] The relative physiologic responses to muscarinic agonists may correlate with these differences in receptor density.

Inhibitory muscarinic receptors, also known as autoreceptors, on cholinergic nerves of human airways have been described.[52] These receptors limit vagal bronchoconstriction by inhibiting acetylcholine release. These muscarinic autoreceptors are of the M_2 subtype, whereas those on airway smooth muscle are classified as M_3 receptors. M_1 receptors are present in human airway ganglia. Pirenzipine blocks these M_1 receptors and inhibits reflex bronchoconstriction.[53]

Activation of muscarinic cholinergic and α-adrenergic receptors is associated with an increase in the turnover of phosphatidylinositol, which causes a rise in cytosolic calcium. The rise in cytosolic Ca^{++}, possibly through the phosphorylation of specific proteins by a Ca^{++}-calmodulin-dependent protein kinase, is responsible for the physiologic responses.[54]

The sequence of physiologic events following stimulation of muscarinic receptors includes activation of guanylate cyclase with a concomitant rise in the cyclic guanosine monophosphate (cGMP).[55] This is followed by an increased permeability of monovalent cations[56] and an increased turnover of phosphatidylinositol.[57] (For a more detailed description of the signal-transduction mechanism following stimulation of receptors see Chapter 2.)

The immunologic release of mast-cell mediators is directly related to intracellular cGMP levels and inversely related to cAMP levels.[58,59] This is supported by data showing that cholinergic stimulation of muscarinic receptors with carbachol increases total lung cGMP levels[58] and increases the immunologic release of mediators[58,59] (Figure 1). Cholinergic stimulation also increases mucus release, and this effect is blocked by pretreatment with atropine.[60]

To determine if receptor density correlates with the physiologic response, we compared the activity of muscarinic and β-adrenergic receptors in bovine peripheral lung to the corresponding receptor activity in tracheal smooth muscle.[61] We found that the concentration of muscarinic receptor binding sites was 37-fold greater in the tracheal muscle preparation (2805 ± 309 fmol/mg protein) than in the peripheral lung preparation (76 ± 28 fmol/mg protein). However, the peripheral lung contained an eightfold higher concentration of the $beta_2$ adrenergic receptors than did the tracheal muscle (1588 ± 17 vs. 199 ± 42 fmol/mg protein). The affinity for either receptor binding site, however, was not significantly different between the two tissues. *In vitro* studies showed that the muscle, but not the peripheral lung strip, exhibited a relaxing response to epinephrine. Furthermore, *in vitro* contraction studies showed that the response of tracheal muscle strips to methacholine was markedly greater than the response of peripheral lung strips, a finding consistent with the muscarinic receptor-binding result. Our data indicate a striking quantitative difference in muscarinic and β-adrenergic receptors between lung tissue and tracheal muscle.

The modulatory role of sympathomimetics on muscarinic receptors or muscarinic agents on β-receptors[62] can be investigated because of the existence of relatively high concentrations of both muscarinic and β-adrenergic receptors in the bovine tracheal muscle.[61] *In vitro* studies suggest a modulatory role for cholinergic agonists on adrenergic receptor activity in many systems.[63-67]

Catecholamines also appear to influence cholinergic receptor activity.[68] Lee et al.[63] found that norepinephrine partly reduced the bethanechol-induced increase in cGMP in the ileum. All of these findings may be of significance in relation of the *in vivo* interaction of the muscarinic and β-adrenergic receptors in airway smooth muscle.

It appears that exogenous and endogenous catecholamines could directly down-regulate the activity of adrenergic receptors.[69] A decrease in β-adrenergic receptors is generally related to an increase in α_2-adrenergic receptors.[70] It is unclear whether or not decreasing β-adrenergic receptors could also be associated with an increase in the muscarinic receptors.

VI. CHOLINERGIC RECEPTORS AND BRONCHIAL ASTHMA

Currently, there are three schools of thought as to the pharmacological cause of hypersensitivity in asthma. First is a "beta receptor blockade theory",[71,72] and the second is the neurogenic theory which states that the predominant factor in bronchial constrictor response to mediators such as histamine is a vagally mediated reflex arising from epithelial irritant receptors within the airways.[73,74] Third is an absence or deficiency of the nonadrenergic, noncholinergic bronchodilator system in the airways with a loss of the neuropeptide vasoactive intestinal peptide or its receptors.[75]

Holtzman et al.[76] have attempted to determine which site in the parasympathetic pathway is responsible for bronchial hypersensitivity. They treated five atopic subjects with aerosols of hexamethonium, a ganglionic blocker. After hexamethonium, patients' baseline specific airway resistance (SRaw) was decreased and the increase in their SRaw produced by histamine aerosols was blocked. However, the increase in the SRaw by methacholine aerosols was not significantly affected, suggesting that the hypersensitivity to methacholine may have been due to a change in the efferent cholinergic pathway distal to the ganglion, possibly at airway smooth muscle. The three following studies tend to support this possibility. Studies in animals have revealed little effect of acetylcholine on electrophysiological properties of vagal sensory nerve endings[77] and no effect of vagal blockade with cooling on acetylcholine induced bronchoconstriction.[78] Studies in patients with mild allergic asthma indicate an increase in the methacholine response of their pupillary muscle, a muscarinic organ.[79]

Thus, abnormal end-organ hyperresponsiveness to methacholine in asthmatics might indicate that some lesion is present in the muscarinic cholinergic system at the level of the receptor. However, it is difficult to evaluate the role of airway smooth-muscle muscarinic receptors in asthmatics by conventional *in vivo* or *in vitro* pharmacological techniques since the response may be modified by factors such as reflex activity, muscle function, and endogenous humoral substance.

Measurements of the muscarinic receptor concentration may be correlated with physiological responses and clinical phenomena (such as Huntington's disease).[80] Moreover, binding studies performed on circulating cells[81-84] from normal subjects vs. patients with pulmonary disease may serve as tools to help elucidate the mechanism of airway hypersensitivity.

The relative importance of neural mechanisms in the bronchial hyperresponsiveness of asthma have involved comparing the responses to an inhaled material before and after pharmacologic blockade of neural pathways. Most studies have used postganglionic (muscarinic) antagonists, such as atropine sulfate or ipratropium bromide, rather than ganglionic blocking agents. The results of these studies are inconsistent; some show that muscarinic antagonists effectively inhibit the bronchomotor response to histamine,[85-87] to sulfur dioxide,[88] to antigen,[89,90] and to exercise,[91] whereas other studies show muscarinic antagonists to have little inhibitory effect.[92-94]

To further investigate if histamine sensitivity is mediated by vagal effects, we compared the ability of two drugs, metaproterenol and ipratropium bromide, to antagonize the effects of both histamine and methacholine.[95]

Ipratropium bromide is an anticholinergic drug with bronchospasmolytic activity, especially by the aerosol route. In the methacholine challenges, both ipratropium bromide and metaproterenol had significant protection as compared to placebo ($p < 0.001$). There was no statistical difference in the degree of protection against methacholine between ipratropium bromide and metaproterenol. In histamine challenges, metaproterenol had significant protection as compared to the placebo, while ipratropium bromide did not protect against histamine.

If the mechanisms of bronchoconstriction after histamine are mediated solely by enhanced vagal tone, then ipratropium bromide, which is anticholinergic, should have blocked this action. Indeed, this was not the case in our study.[95] In contrast to this, after metaproterenol premedication, a beta agonist, all patients had comparable protection to both methacholine and histamine challenges. While we cannot as yet precisely define the mechanisms of asthma, we can say that the bronchoconstriction effect of histamine in an asthmatic is not solely vagally mediated.

In asthmatic patients exercise has long been known to precipitate bronchospasm.[96] Early studies of parasympathetic neural reflexes in exercise-induced asthma were hampered by ignorance of the role of heat or water loss as a stimulus to bronchospasm.

Tinkleman et al.[97] reported that aerosolized atropine sulfate prevented the fall in forced expiration volume (FEV_1) caused by exercise in 17 of 18 asthmatic children. Other have since shown that when postexercise values are expressed as a percentage of the postatropine values, the apparent protective effects are seen to be an artifact of the bronchodilation caused by atropine.[98] Because the doses of atropine that inhibited the response to a parasympathomimetic drug did not inhibit exercise-induced asthma, these studies were interpreted as showing that parasympathetic pathways were not involved.

VII. β-ADRENORECEPTORS IN THE AIRWAYS AND LUNGS

A. β-ADRENORECEPTORS IN TRACHEA AND LUNGS

β-Adrenoreceptors in the airways have been studied extensively because they influence many aspects of lung function. β-adrenoreceptor agonists are potent bronchodilators. In addition, they act on secretion of inflammatory mediators from mast cells, secretion of surfactant, secretion of mucus from airway glands, increase ciliary beat frequency and thus mucociliary flow, tone and permeability of pulmonary blood vessels, neurotransmission, and fluid movement across airway epithelium.

The characteristics of β-adrenoreceptors in the airways as revealed by the radioligand-receptor binding studies have been reported.[99-111] Radioligand binding studies have demonstrated the presence of a high density of β-adrenoreceptors in the lungs of experimental animals and humans as determined by direct receptor-binding studies. A majority of β-adrenoreceptors in airway smooth muscle are of the β_2-subtype. Functional studies of canine tracheal smooth-muscle tissue showed that the relaxation to exogenous β-adrenoreceptor agonists is mediated almost entirely by β_2-adrenoreceptors, whereas the relaxation by sympathetic nerve stimulation is mediated predominantly by β_1-adrenoreceptors.[112] In guinea pig trachea, 15% of β-adrenoreceptors are of the β_1 subtype, whereas in parenchymal lung strips mechanical responses are mediated entirely by β_2-adrenoreceptors.[106] The pattern of adrenergic innervation to airway smooth muscle in guinea pig is consistent with these findings.[113]

Relaxation of human central and peripheral airways is mediated only by β_2-adenoreceptors.[114,115] A β_1-selective agonist (prenalterol) *in vivo* has no bronchodilator action in asthmatic subjects, despite significant cardiovascular effects.[116] Secondly, the β-adrenoreceptor agonist isoproterenol, which is nonselective, has no greater bronchodilator effect than the selective β-adrenoreceptor agonist salbutamol.[117] Autoradiography of human airways has shown that the density of these β_2-adrenoreceptors progressively increases from trachea to terminal bronchioles.[118]

The hypothesis that β_2-adrenoreceptors are regulated by circulated epinephrine and β_1-adrenoreceptors are regulated by sympathetic nerves is consistent with these findings on the correlation between the degree of adrenergic innervation and the distribution of subtypes of β-adrenoreceptors in the airways.

B. β-ADRENORECEPTORS IN AIRWAY EPITHELIUM

Airway epithelial cells have a high density of β-adrenoreceptors, and β-adrenoreceptor agonists may influence ion and fluid transport across these cells. Autoradiographic visualization in human lung showed that β-adrenoreceptors were densely located in airway epithelium, alveolar walls, and submucosal glands, while in lower density over airway and vascular smooth muscle.[119,120] The density of β-adrenoreceptors was determined to be significantly greater (about twofold higher) in bovine epithelial membranes than in bovine tracheal smooth muscles.[105] Furthermore, we have also demonstrated that the affinity of β-adrenoreceptors was about sixfold greater in the epithelial membranes as compared to those in the smooth-muscle membranes of bovine trachea. In addition, the small airways and parenchyma contained an eightfold higher density of β-receptors than the trachea.[61]

The function of β-adrenoreceptors in airway epithelium is not well established yet. The integrity of airway epithelium is very important for pulmonary function. Isoproterenol is a more potent relaxant in the presence of intact airway epithelium, which suggests that β-agonist may release a relaxant factor (yet to be identified) from epithelial cells.[121] Increased responsiveness of airway smooth-muscle cells to various mediators occurs as a result of damage to or dysfunction of airway epithelial cells in isolated canine bronchi,[121] rabbit trachea and bronchi,[122,123] and guinea pig trachea.[107] This increased bronchial reactivity[87] has also been shown *in vivo* following experimentally induced epithelial damage. A high percentage of eosinophils, which are capable of damaging epithelial cells, are present in the sputum of the asthmatics.[124] Laitinen and colleagues[129] observed epithelial damage at various sites in fresh biopsy specimens from airway mucosa in asthmatic patients. Asthmatics with mild to severe airway hyperresponsiveness showed this epithelial damage in the respiratory tract which was prominent enough to expose the epithelial nerves.

The airway epithelium elaborates an unidentified relaxant or inhibitory factor, called epithelium-derived relaxing factor or EpiDRF.[125] The regulation of the release of such a relaxing factor and/or movement of inflammatory mediators across the epithelial membrane may be regulated by β-adrenoreceptors on airway epithelium. cAMP has been shown to regulate the permeabilty of epithelial tight junctions. Increased cAMP levels, by altering the structure of the tight junctions,[126] reduces the ion or mediator permeability in the epithelium. Airway epithelium is densely populated with β-adrenoreceptors, and the activation of β-adrenoreceptors increases cAMP levels in the cell. It is therefore possible that, under normal conditions, when airway epithelium is intact, β-adrenoreceptors on the epithelium maintain the integrity of tight junction and thus regulate the ion and fluid transport across epithelial cells. The physiological role of β-adrenoreceptors in airway epithelium requires further studies.

C. β-ADRENORECEPTORS IN GLANDS

β-adrenoreceptor agonists, including epinephrine, isoproterenol, salbutamol, terbutaline, and metaproterenol, stimulate secretion of airway mucus in animals and humans.[127,128]

However, submucosal glands are sparsely innervated by sympathetic nerves.[18,129] Autoradiographic studies have shown a high density of β-adrenoreceptors in airway glands; the β-adrenoreceptors of submucosal glands were predominantly of the β_2 subtype. A larger density of β-adrenoreceptors was found on mucous than on serous cells.[118,119,130] Some studies reported that β-adrenoreceptor agonists increased mucociliary clearance in normal and asthmatic subjects, while other studies observed little effect.[131,132] The beat frequency of respiratory tract ciliated cells was increased in a dose-dependent manner by isoproterenol.[133] An increase in intracellular free calcium as determined by changes in the fluorescence of cells loaded with fura-2 accompanied the communication of the frequency response between cells.[133] These results suggest that ciliated cells have at least two independent mechanisms for the control of respiratory tract ciliary beat frequency; one probably utilizing calcium, the other probably cAMP.

A possible mechanism of β-agonists-induced therapeutic effects in asthma is the increased mucociliary clearance. β-adrenoreceptor agonists can also stimulate Clara cells, which are nonciliated cells present in small airways.[134] Stimulation of Clara cells secretes a lipid into the lumen which acts as a surfactant to prevent small-airway collapse.[135]

D. β-ADRENORECEPTORS ON MAST CELLS

β-Adrenoreceptor agonists inhibit the release of antigen-induced mast-cell mediator release from passively sensitized human lung fragments and isolated lung mast cells[136] (Figure 1). These β-adrenoreceptors are of the β_2 subtype.[137] Functional β-adrenoreceptors have also been demonstrated in mast cells isolated from human lung by enzymatic digestion or mechanical dispersion.[138,139] β-Adrenoreceptor agonists inhibit release of histamine from rat peritoneal mast cell[140] and from canine trachea.[141] Antigen-mediated respiratory mast-cell degranulation in canine bronchus *in situ* was inhibited by sympathetic stimulation elicited by infused dimethylpiperazinium.[142] This effect of sympathetic stimulation was completely abolished by the blockade of β-adrenoreceptors; however, β-adrenoreceptor stimulation in this system did not cause significant augmentation of mast-cell secretion.[143]

In subjects with nocturnal asthma the plasma histamine concentration is lowered by the infusion of low doses of epinephrine.[144] The early bronchoconstriction occurring after antigen challenge and the accompanying increase in circulating mast cell-associated mediators, histamine and neutrophil chemotactic factor, are both inhibited by the inhaled β_2-agonist salbutamol.[145] These studies suggest that β-adrenoreceptor agonists are capable of preventing mediator release from mast cells. This is consistent with the theory that increased cAMP levels in mast cells decrease mast-cell degranulation, possibly through cAMP-induced inhibition of phospholipid methylation and Ca^{++} influx[146,147] (Figure 1).

E. β-ADRENORECEPTORS ON ALVEOLAR MACROPHAGES

Radioligand binding studies and the functional response in various experimental animals have shown the existence of β-adrenoreceptors in alveolar macrophages. Similar studies have also been used to characterize β-adrenoreceptors on human alveolar macrophages, obtained by bronchoalveolar lavage.[148] The density of β-adrenoreceptors was 42 ± 9 fmol/mg protein with an apparent equilibrium dissociation constant (k_D) of 44 ± 9 pM using alveolar macrophage membranes. With intact macrophages, each cell contained about 5600 β_2-adrenoreceptors with a K_D of about 29 pM.[148] When the cells were incubated with isoproterenol the functional activity of the β-adrenoreceptors on alveolar macrophages was shown by a sixfold increase in cAMP production. We can conclude from these studies that human alveolar macrophages possess high-affinity functional β_2-adrenoreceptors.

Macrophages are capable of releasing various mediators including interleukin-1, tumor necrosis factor, leukotrienes, etc., and play an important role in the immunological and pathological processes in the lung.[149] An increase in intracellular cAMP via the activation of β-adrenoreceptors may inhibit migration and the release of lysosomal enzymes and mediators from alveolar macrophages.[150,151] A decrease in macrophage phagocytosis of immune complexes[152] and fibronectin-mediated phagocytosis[153] is also caused by β-adrenoreceptor agonists or cAMP analogs. Macrophage expression of Fc-mediated phagocytosis in immunocompetent mice[154] has also been shown to be modulated by cAMP. The stimulation of β-adrenoreceptor inhibits calcium-dependent potassium channels in mouse macrophages.[155] These studies demonstrate that β-adrenoreceptors may regulate the function of alveolar macrophages. The effect of β₂-adrenoreceptor agonists in asthma may also be due to their effect on alveolar macrophages, since macrophages have also been implicated to play a significant role in the pathogenesis of bronchial asthma.[266]

VIII. PULMONARY β-ADRENORECEPTORS IN BRONCHIAL ASTHMA

The effect of bronchial challenge on airway obstruction in bronchial asthma may be characterized in two phases occurring in sequence, an immediate and the late asthmatic response. Acute bronchoconstriction with the immediate asthmatic reaction begins 15 to 30 min after exposure; the late-phase inflammatory response begins hours later.[156] This late-phase response can last for many hours or sometimes for days and matches the prolonged symptoms seen in chronic asthma. Corticosteroids consistently block the late-phase response, but have little or no effect on the immediate reaction. In contrast, β-adrenoreceptor agonists are very effective in treating an immediate asthmatic reaction, but have less effect on a late-phase response.

Although the beneficial effect of β₂-adrenoreceptor agonists has been attributed mainly to their property to relax airway smooth muscle, there is evidence to suggest that this is not the only reason for the therapeutic benefit of β₂-adrenoreceptor agonists taken prophylactically.[157] In previous sections we have discussed that β-adrenoreceptor agonists may also inhibit the release of histamine and other mediators from mast cells and basophils, and possibly the mediators from eosinophils, macrophages, and lymphocytes. Other studies have shown that β₂-adrenoreceptor agonists are also able to improve mucociliary transport in asthmatics.[158,159] The increases in microvascular permeability caused by histamine and bradykinin (see above) are also inhibited by these drugs. The microvascular permeability induced by platelet-activating factor (PAF) could not be attenuated by β-adrenoreceptor agonists in one species (guinea pig), yet they could be attenuated in another (mice). Nevertheless, many of the factors which have been implicated in the pathogenesis of bronchial asthma can be affected by the activation of β₂-adrenoreceptors in the airways.

As discussed in the previous sections, functional β-adrenoreceptors are present in various cells in the airways. Furthermore, the bronchodilating β-adrenoreceptor activity is determined by β-adrenoreceptor function and circulating catecholamines. It is therefore possible that an abnormality in β-adrenoreceptor function and/or circulating catecholamines may underlie or contribute to airway hyperresponsiveness in bronchial asthma. Szentivanyi[71] postulated that bronchial asthma might in part be due to impaired β-adrenoreceptor function. However, the question of whether or not a defect in airway β-adrenoreceptor function is present in bronchial asthma has not been answered conclusively. Nevertheless, there are several reports detailing altered adrenergic responsiveness and decreased number of leukocyte β-adrenoreceptors in asthmatics.[160-163] In lung membranes of a guinea pig model of asthma, we observed a down-regulation of β-adrenoreceptors and an up-regulation of α-adrenoreceptors.[164] Other laboratories have also reported similar results.[165,166] Meurs and colleagues[167,168] have reported that the lymphocyte β-adrenoreceptor density was reduced after an allergen-induced asthmatic reaction.[267] Yukawa and co-workers[169] have recently reported that anaphylactic challenge of the sensitized guinea pig tracheal muscle diminishes relaxing effects of isoproterenol, prostaglandin E$_1$ (PGE$_1$), and forskolin, but not of aminophylline. These results suggest an impairment in adenylate cyclase system in the airways after anaphylactic reaction.[267] These studies support the theory of an altered β-adrenoreceptor function in asthmatics. However, the mechanism of this phenomenon is not known.

Cheng and Townley[61] and Mita and colleagues[170] demonstrated significant decreases in β-adrenoreceptors in lung membrane fractions from animals exposed to chronic histamine or antigen aerosols. On the basis of these data, the investigators speculated that recurrent bronchoconstriction could result in the loss of pulmonary β-adrenoreceptors, perhaps as a result of down-regulation secondary to catecholamine release. However, the role of other chemical mediators which are generated as a consequence of immunological responses in the airways is also possible. We have examined the effect of PAF (PAF-acether) on β-adrenoreceptor function in the airways. PAF can cause marked bronchoconstriction, acute inflammation and edema, and chemotaxis to neutrophils and eosinophils.[171-173] Interestingly, PAF is the only mediator known so far which produces airway hyperresponsiveness in man and experimental animals.[174,175] Recently, we have observed that the *in vitro* incubation of the human lung tissue with PAF decreased the density of β-adrenoreceptors in human lung membranes without any change in the receptor sensitivity.[176,177] Braquet and colleagues[178] have also reported a PAF-induced decrease in the number of β-adrenoreceptors in the homogenate of rat cerebellum. However, in guinea pig lung tissue, *in vitro* exposure of the lung tissue to PAF did not affect the β-adrenoreceptor density or the affinity.[179] In the functional studies in the isolated trachea and lung parenchyma of guinea pig or human, PAF significantly reduced the potency of isoproterenol to reverse methacholine- or histamine-induced contraction. BN 52021, a PAF receptor antagonist, protected against these PAF-induced changes.

On the basis of these results, we first proposed a hypothesis that PAF by itself and/or through the release of other mediators down-regulates the β-adrenoreceptor responses in the airways, which in turn produces nonspecific airway hyperresponsiveness. However, in our *in vivo* studies in conscious guinea pigs, we observed that PAF aerosol potentiated the specific airway resistance produced by methacholine, and this airway obstruction was not reversed by isoproterenol or PGE$_2$.[179] Since PAF also desensitized the responses to PGE$_2$ in the same way as it did to isoproterenol, it is possible that PAF desensitizes the responses to bronchodilators nonspecifically, possibly through a postreceptor site which is involved in the responses to bronchodilators. This may lead to a nonspecific airway hyperresponsiveness.

PAF had also been reported to induce activation of phospholipase A$_2$ in rabbit platelets. Therefore, our results on the PAF-induced desensitization of β-adrenoreceptor responses may also be due to an increase in phospholipase A$_2$ activity.

Sensitivity to methacholine, histamine, and antigen can be markedly increased, as reported in a variety of animal and human studies, when the β-adrenergic receptors are blocked.[24,27,72] Therefore, when histamine, leukotrienes, and other mediators are released due to an allergic reaction, they are able to cause bronchoconstriction which is unopposed by the usually present intact β-receptors which normally serve to maintain bronchodilation. In the normal individuals, the presence of catecholamines provides a constant tone of the β-adrenergic receptors, maintaining the bronchi in a dilated state. The adrenergic imbalance resulting from β-adrenergic blockade deprives the bronchial tissue of its normal counter-regulatory adjustment (Figure 1).

In asthma subjects this adrenergic imbalance induced by the noncardioselective drugs propranolol and oxprenolol, 100 mg each, caused a 26 to 35% decrease in FEV$_1$ at 2 h, which was not reversed by the usual doses of isoproterenol. In contrast, the cardioselective β$_1$-adrenergic blocking agent atenolol (100 mg) caused only a slight fall in FEV$_1$ and was reversed by isoproterenol.[180]

Patients with bronchial asthma have markedly increased reactivity to immunologically released pharmacologic mediators as well as an abnormal immunologic mechanism for the release of mediators.[2-6] Patients with allergic rhinitis may have the same immunologic mechanisms for reaginic antibody production and for release of these mediators. However, the effect of these mediators on the bronchial tree in these patients is markedly diminished in comparison with the effect in asthmatic subjects.[3-6]

In order to determine if β-adrenergic blockade alters the sensitivity to mediators in nonasthmatic atopic individuals, we studied the effect of propranolol by inhalation on the sensitivity to methacholine inhalation in normal and allergic rhinitis subjects.[27] In terms of their initial unresponsiveness to methacholine, the two groups were equally matched. A second group of allergic rhinitis subjects who showed a positive response to methacholine was also included in the study. Neither of these groups of allergic rhinitis subjects had ever experienced any asthma symptoms.

We obtained mean decreases in FEV_1 of 11 and 20.6% in the normal subjects and the allergic rhinitis patients, respectively ($p < 0.05$), following aerosol administration of both propranolol and methacholine. In six allergic rhinitis patients, this decrease in FEV_1 following propranolol was associated with clinical symptoms of asthma, i.e., wheezing, coughing, and tightness in the chest for the first time in their lives. The hayfever subjects who were sensitive to methacholine even before propranolol developed an even more marked sensitivity to methacholine. Following propranolol these subjects experienced a mean decrease in FEV_1 of 43%, and all of them developed transient symptoms of asthma for the first time in their lives. The fact that the airway reactivity to methacholine was increased and that these symptoms were produced by propranolol could suggest a partial β-adrenergic blockade as being instrumental in asthma.

Apold and Aksenes[181] studied 21 children with moderate bronchial asthma in whom the use of bronchodilators had been discontinued for at least 8 d. They reported a statistically significant correlation between a high respiratory sensitivity to histamine and a low plasma cAMP response to epinephrine. Likewise, Makino et al.[182] reported that cAMP production in lymphocytes from asthmatic subjects was significantly less than in normal subjects after exposure to salbutamol, a β_2-receptor stimulant. These findings suggest that the more defective the β-adrenergic cAMP activity, the more hyperresponsive is the airway and the more severe is the asthma.

As illustrated in Figure 1, the bronchospasm and the release of chemical mediators[183-185] seen in asthma culd be explained by β-adrenergic hyporesponsiveness with normal or elevated cholinergic or α-adrenergic responsiveness. There are many reports about β-adrenergic hyporesponsiveness in asthma.[186-189] The correlation of decreased β-adrenergic receptor function and disease severity might also be caused by repeated and prolonged β-agonist treatment rather than by the disease itself, and several investigators[160,161,190] have reported this observation.

Measurement of beta-adrenergic receptor density and affinity has been made in various tissues including the mononuclear leukocyte cell pool (MNC),[191,192] and the polymorphonuclear leukocytes (PMNC).[193,194] Some investigators have reported that asthmatic patients have a lower density of beta-adrenergic receptors in lymphocyte membranes;[195,196] others report no difference in beta-adrenergic receptor density in granulocyte membranes between controls and subjects with asthma or atopic eczema.[194,197] These conflicting observations are used to argue for and against the beta adrenergic defect hypothesis in asthma. The difference, however, may be due solely to the different tissues used by the different investigators. To our knowledge there are no prior reports of simultaneous determination of beta-adrenergic receptor densities and affinities in MNC and PMNC.[198]

We compared the densities and affinities of beta adrenergic receptors among 12 nonatopic controls (Group I), 13 mild asthmatics off drugs (Group II), and 8 asthmatics on chronic beta-agonist therapy (Group III).

Scatchard analysis of the data resulted in a single line indicating the presence of a single population of binding sites. We found that: (1) Asthmatics off drugs (Group II) have significantly lower mean mononuclear leukocyte beta-adrenergic receptor density ($p < 0.001$), but no significant difference in mean polymorphonuclear leukocyte beta adrenergic receptor density than the control group. (2) Asthmatics on chronic beta agonist treatment (Group

III) had significantly lower mean beta adrenergic receptor density in all three cell fractions compared to Group I and Group II ($p < 0.001$). (3) Group I and II females had a higher mean beta adrenergic receptor density in mixed leukocyte and polymorphonuclear cell fractions than males ($p < 0.05$). Mean dissociation constants (Kd) were not significantly different among the groups for all three cell types. (4) Terbutaline sulfate clearly caused desensitization of beta-adrenergic receptors in human leukocyte membranes *in vivo* and a decrease in the MNC intracellular cAMP response to ($-$) isoproterenol.[163]

These results show that bronchial asthma itself is associated with lower lymphocyte β-receptor density. They also show that β-adrenergic receptor density is influenced by cell type, β-adrenergic agonist administration, and sex. Kariman and Lefkowitz[195] also reported lower density on β-receptors on lymphocytes in subjects with asthma. Szentivanyi et al.[196] measured α- and β-adrenergic receptors in human lymphocytes and lung tissue. They reported lower β-receptor density and higher α-receptor density in subjects with asthma. However, Wolfe et al.[199] reported no difference between a group of aspirin-sensitive asthmatics and a control group in the number or infinity of lymphocyte β-adrenergic receptors.

Lymphocytes are a heterogenous group of cells and have important roles in immunological aspects of many diseases. Thus it is possible that the different observations in MNC and PMNC β-adrenergic receptors may be due to differences in tissue. A characteristic of extrinsic asthma is increased serum IgE, which is associated with the interactions of T and B lymphocytes. The β-adrenergic receptor density has been studied and compared on T and B lymphocytes in human peripheral blood.[192,200,201] However, there is no clear consensus in the literature, suggesting that further study in this area is needed.

Szentivanyi[71] hypothesized that an autonomic nerve imbalance in association with decreased β-adrenergic responsiveness caused bronchial hyperresponsiveness. Several investigators supported this hypothesis by showing β-adrenergic hyporesponsiveness in different tissues of asthmatics.[202,203]

Szentivanyi[196] also reported increased α-adrenergic receptors and decreased β-receptors in the lung of asthmatic patients. This phenomenon was also confirmed in experimental animal studies.[165,186,187]

Human platelets have α_2-receptors.[204,205] Several investigators[206,207] have found an abnormal platelet response to α-agonists in asthma patients, whereas another investigator found normal responses.[208] It is unclear whether or not these blood cells reflect the characteristics of adrenergic receptors of human lung.

Therefore, we studied the adrenergic receptor system by measuring α- and β-receptor-binding characteristics and cAMP response to different stimuli including PAF in mononuclear cells and platelets.[209]

We studied normals, asthma patients who had not received beta agonist or steroid hormone for more than two weeks and a group of non-asthmatic subjects who show positive responses to methacholine inhalation challenge (NAMS). Studies of adrenergic receptors in these groups might explain the role of these receptors in non-specific bronchial hyperreactivity.

Our findings were as follows: (1) asthmatics had a significantly lower density of beta receptors as compared to normal subjects, (2) asthmatics had a significantly lower cAMP response to isoproterenol stimulation as compared to the two other groups, (3) in non-asthmatic subjects, PAF decreased the basal cAMP level and significantly inhibited the response to isoproterenol stimulation, (4) there was no difference in density and affinity of platelet alpha receptors or in platelet cAMP responses to stimulation by alpha agonists among these three groups, (5) neither density nor cAMP response of beta receptors on mononuclear cells were significantly correlated with pulmonary function tests ($FEV_1/FVC \times 100$), sensitivity to methacholine or cold-air inhalation.

These results suggest that asthma patients may have a decreased density of beta adrenergic receptors on mononuclear cells in the absence of beta agonist therapy. It is speculated that release of PAF and other mediators secondary to allergen exposure, even in the absence of overt attacks of asthma, may inhibit the response to endogenous or exogenous beta adrenergic agonists.[209]

Many factors have been reported to alter the density and affinity of adrenergic receptors on various tissues. For this reason, the asthma subjects and normal subjects were carefully matched. Therefore, young subjects were studied to avoid the aging influence.[210] To avoid the influence of female hormones, only males were studied.[211] Adrenergic receptors are reported to be affected by endogenous catecholamines.[212,213] Thus, special attention was paid to avoid patients under excessive physical and psychological stress.

The asthmatic patients studied had not taken oral β-agonist or steroid hormone for more than 2 weeks. Although four asthmatics did use a few inhalations of β-agonists, the results were no different from the rest of the asthmatics. A 2-week period is sufficient to recover from acquired down-regulation of receptors due to previous β-agonist therapy.[162,163,167,214]

Hoffman et al.[215] reported three types of desensitization of β-receptors: (1) loss of β-receptors,[216] (2) loss of high-affinity receptors,[217] and (3) loss of physiological response without loss of β-receptors. Recently, Davies and Lefkowitz[218] demonstrated uncoupling (reduction in density) of β-receptors after catecholamine exposure in human neutrophils. Feldman et al.[213] reported an uncoupling of β-receptor in lymphocytes without down-regulation due to the change of posture from supine to ambulation.

Heterologous desensitization of the cAMP system in lymphocytes of patients with atopic dermatitis and in vitro heterologous desensitization induced by isoproterenol, PGE_1, and histamine were reported by Safko et al.[219] Heterologous desensitization in granulocytes of patients with bronchial asthma has also been reported.[220] In atopic diseases as described above, elevated leukocyte phosphodiesterase was reported.[221,222] This is important because of its influence on cAMP levels. High spontaneous histamine release from basophils isolated in MNC fraction of asthmatic patients in vitro has been reported by Akagi and Townley.[223] This spontaneous histamine release was inhibited in vitro by β-agonists and other agents which increased the intracellular cAMP levels.[224] These reports indicate that asthmatic patients may have an impaired cAMP system. Whether or not the abnormal β-receptor cAMP system in asthmatics is a primary or secondary phenomenon is still not clear.

Recently, Meurs et al.[167,168] have reported that reduced β-adrenergic responsiveness in lymphocytes of asthmatic patients was accompanied by an increased bronchial reactivity to propranolol after an allergen challenge. These reports suggest that reduced β-adrenergic function in lymphocytes of asthmatic patients may reflect a reduced adrenergic function of airways. Bryan et al.[225] proposed that $β_2$-receptors of both lymphocytes and bronchial smooth muscle may be regulated by circulating catecholamines. Conversely, a discrepancy in sub-sensitization of β-receptors between airways and lymphocytes[214,226] or between lung and spleen[227] (which consists largely of lymphocytes) after administration of β-agonist has been demonstrated.

IX. EFFECT OF GLUCOCORTICOIDS ON PULMONARY β-ADRENERGIC RECEPTORS AND RESPONSES

In the treatment of allergic disease, corticosteroids, in addition to their anti-inflammatory effects, increase the density of β-adrenergic receptors in animal lung tissue.[229] We examined the time-course changes in lymphocyte and granulocyte β-adrenergic receptors to evaluate mechanisms of action of corticosteroid hormone. We used ^{125}I-Iodohydroxybenzylpindolol (IHYP)-binding assay during and after oral prednisone 15 mg t.i.d. for 5 d to six subjects.[230] Beginning on day 2 of prednisone administration we observed a significant increase ($p < 0.001$) in β-adrenergic receptor density (by Scatchard analysis). The dissociation constant of IHYP did not show a significant change. Pulmonary function improved, granulocyte cAMP doubled, and white blood cell counts changed as expected. Our results suggest that the therapeutic effect of corticosteroids in asthma may be due to their enhancement of β-adrenergic receptors.

A difference in the response of lymphocytes and granulocytes to corticosteroids was also observed. The time-course changes in the density of β-adrenergic receptors of lymphocytes and polymorphonuclear cells may be simultaneously regulated differently from each other following the administration of corticosteroids.[231] Specific reactions to hormones such as the granulocytosis and lymphopenia associated with corticosteroid administration is another example of such cell- or tissue-specific responses.

Glucocorticoid hormones have been shown to lower the threshold of relaxation response of β-adrenergic receptors and to inhibit the α-adrenergic contractile response to catecholamines in isolated tracheas from humans and guinea pigs.[288,232,233] The decreased responsiveness to β-adrenergic agonists induced by chronic treatment with β-agonist drugs in normal[234] and asthmatic airways can also be reversed by glucocorticoid hormones.[235] They can also potentiate the stimulation of adenylate cyclase by β-adrenergic agonists in human leukocytes and canine tracheal smooth muscle.[236,237]

This potentiating action of glucocorticoids was investigated by examining the effect of glucocorticoids on the number and affinity of β-adrenergic receptors in animal lung tissues.[229] The density of β-adrenergic receptors after chronic administration of hydrocortisone increased by 70% from 386 fmol to 657 fmol/mg protein with no significant change in the affinity of ^{125}I-IHYP for β-adrenergic receptors. Adrenalectomy produced an opposite effect with a 29% fall in the number of β-adrenergic receptors without altering the affinity of ^{125}I-IHYP for β-receptors. Furthermore, this change induced by adrenalectomy was reversed by exogenous administration of hydrocortisone. This suggests that glucocorticoids potentiate β-adrenergic receptors stimulation, at least in part by increasing β-receptor density in tissue membranes.

Surfactant production is increased in type 2 pneumocytes by pulmonary β-adrenergic responses. Epinephrine and other β-adrenergic agonists stimulate the release of surfactant in rabbit and sheep fetal lungs.[238,239] Epinephrine also decreases secretion of the lung fluid in fetal sheep.[240] That increased sensitivity of β-adrenergic responses accompanies lung maturation is suggested by the fact that these responses are most evident toward the end of gestation.[239,240]

The development of pulmonary β-adrenergic receptors in fetal rabbit has been examined to quantitate the effect of betamethasone (0.17 mg/kg) treatment on the β-adrenergic receptor concentration.[241] After glucocorticoid treatment the concentration of pulmonary β-receptors increased in fetal rabbit at term and this increase occurs precociously. However, the β-receptor binding sites in the fetal rabbit heart or the affinity in either tissue was not affected by this treatment. Glucocorticoid treatment increased adrenergic responsiveness[242] and β-receptor concentration[243] in transformed human lung cells.

Cortisone can alter the affinity for a β-agonist even though cortisone did not alter the affinity of the β-receptor for the DHA ligand or other antagonists. In this regard the affinity for isoproterenol increased after hydrocortisone injection, that is, the isoproterenol competition curve shifted to the left and the curve became shallow with a slope factor of 0.54 compared with a factor of 0.89 in control lymphocytes.[231]

In contrast to corticosteroids, which increase β-adrenergic receptors in certain tissues, β-agonists cause a decrease in several tissues, as mentioned previously. In this regard in *in vitro* studies, we observed reduced β-receptor density in spleen cells, but not in lung parenchyma after incubation of these tissues with terbutaline.[227] The isoproterenol competition curve for [^{3}H]dihydroalprenolol binding shifted to the right and steepened, suggesting reduced affinity of the receptors for isoproterenol. This suggests that there was agonist-specific alterations in lung β-receptors. We used whole lung and we did not examine bronchial smooth muscle per se, nor were functional studies performed.

The above studies show a difference in the susceptibility of β-receptors to desensitization by an adrenergic agonist between lung parenchyma and spleen tissue. They also show that chronic administration of β-agonist decreases its affinity for the β-receptor, whereas corticosteroids increase this affinity. Thus, endogenous release or exogenous administration of corticosteroids may exert their therapeutic effect by increasing the density of β-receptors and the affinity of β-agonist for these receptors. In addition, hydrocortisone has an inhibitory effect on the α-adrenergic contraction responses of human and guinea pig respiratory smooth muscle.[228]

X. α-ADRENORECEPTORS IN THE AIRWAYS

Although studies on α-adrenoreceptors in the airways to date are limited, great progress has been made with the cloning and sequence analysis of genes encoding adrenergic receptors. This should provide important structural and functional information of these receptors. Both α_1- and α_2-receptors have a wide distribution. α_1-Receptors predominate on postsynaptic effector cells, whereas α_2-receptors are found both pre- and postsynaptically. Stimulation of these presynaptic α_2-receptors attenuates the release of norepinephrine from neurons. Characteristics of α-adrenoreceptors as revealed by the radioligand-receptor binding studies in the airways have been described.[112,130,164,165,244-250] Most of the studies have been done in lung tissue for α_1-adrenoreceptors and few on α_2-receptors. Two distinct bindings sites of α-adrenoreceptors have been observed in canine tracheal smooth muscle.[112,251] Activation of α-adrenoreceptors in tracheal smooth muscle elicits contraction which is mediated predominantly by α_2-adrenoreceptors. This has been demonstrated by the contractile studies using α-adrenoreceptor agonists and antagonists (yohimbine). This is consistent with the finding that the density of α_2-adrenoreceptors predominates over α_1-adrenoreceptors in canine trachealis.[112,118,130]

It is possible that the density of α_1- and α_2-adrenoreceptors could be different in smaller airways, since most of the functional and radioligand-binding studies have been done in large airways. In this regard it has been shown that the density of α_1-adrenoreceptors in canine peripheral lung was very much greater than that of α_2-adrenoreceptors.[112,118,248] The majority of α-adrenoreceptors in human lung membranes were also of α_1 in nature.[118,252] Neonatal rat lung contained a high density of α_2-adrenoreceptors.[249,250] However, in 5-week-old rat lung there was no detectable level of α_2-adrenoreceptors, suggesting that α_2-adrenoreceptors decreased rapidly with age. In rat lung membranes at birth the density of α_1-adrenoreceptors was higher than the adult rat lung.[250]

The presence of a high density of α_1-adrenoreceptors in the lung is shown by the above studies. However, the precise localization of these receptors within the lung using autoradiographic localization of α_1-adrenoreceptors in frozen sections of ferret lung has been shown by Barnes and colleagues.[130] Autoradiographs showed that α_1-adrenoreceptors were present in highest density in vascular tissues (small vessels > large vessels). These α_1-receptors were also present in airway epithelium and submucosal glands. Stimulation of these receptors produced a watery secretion from these glands. In marked contrast to the very low density of α-adrenoreceptors in large-airway smooth muscle (bronchi), smooth muscles of small airways (bronchioles) were very rich in α_1-adrenoreceptors. This suggests that the high density of α_1-adrenoreceptors in small airways may be relevant in pulmonary diseases such as asthma. The presence of α-receptors on human lung mast cells is suggested by the fact that α-agonists facilitate histamine release.[59]

XI. α-ADRENORECEPTORS AND BRONCHIAL ASTHMA

Hyperresponsiveness to α-adrenergic stimulation contributes to the pathogenesis of asthma.[59] Inhalation of α-adrenoreceptor agonists (methoxamine or phenylephrine) has no effect on normal subjects, but causes airway narrowing in asthmatic subjects.[253,254] The involvement of α_1-adrenoreceptors is suggested because the effect of methoxamine on asthmatic airways is prazosin-sensitive.[254] A selective α_2-adrenoreceptor agonist, clonidine, has been reported to protect against allergen-induced bronchoconstriction in man.[255] These studies suggest a role of α-adrenoreceptors in asthma. Furthermore, the sensitivity of airway α-adrenergic receptors may increase following exercise or exposure to cold. We would anticipate a beneficial effect of α-adrenoreceptor antagonists if α-adrenoreceptor stimulation contributed to bronchoconstriction in asthma.

In patients with airway obstruction, studies of the airway effects of α-adrenoreceptor antagonists have revealed conflicting results. Increased airway-specific conductance (SGaw) after administration of aerosolized α-adrenoreceptor antagonists has been demonstrated by Gould and Dilieto[256] and Patel and Kerr.[257] An improvement in the pulmonary functions (as determined by an increased FEV_1 and SGaw) after giving indoramin, an α-adrenergic blocking agent, to subjects with exercise-induced asthma has been observed by Bianco and co-workers.[258] Beil and de Kock[259] have also reported similar results on the protective effect of phentolamine on exercise-induced bronchoconstriction in seven out of nine patients. These effects of α-adrenoreceptor antagonists in exercise-induced asthma could be explained by their effect on bronchial blood flow which may counteract airway cooling. The combination of isoproterenol with alpha-blocking drugs such as thymoxamine or phentolamine produced significantly greater improvement than isoproterenol alone.[257] They also reported that thymoxamine restored the bronchodilating response to albuterol in patients who did not respond to albuterol alone. However, Barnes and co-workers[260] found no significant change in lung function or effect on histamine responsiveness in other asthmatic subjects 1 h after inhaled prazosin, a selective α_1-adrenoreceptor antagonist. Similarly, Utting[261] reported that 39 asthmatics showed no response to indoramine during a double-blind trial.

The controversial results on the effect of α-adrenoreceptor antagonists in the airways prevent us from reaching any conclusion on the role of α-adrenoreceptors in the pathogenesis of asthma. The additional antiserotonergic and antimuscarinic effects of α-adrenoreceptor antagonists as therapeutic agents make the interpretation difficult. Nevertheless, the observations that bronchoconstriction in response to α-adrenoreceptor agonists in the presence, and even in the absence, of prior beta-blockade occurs in asthmatics, but not in normal subjects,[253,262] could be relevant to human bronchial asthma. Consistent with these observations is the finding of decreased β- and increased α-receptors in the lung of asthmatics.[197] These asthmatics also showed a reduced capacity of lung tissue to synthesize cAMP in response to β-adrenergic stimulation.[263] The idea of an imbalance between α- and β-receptor function in asthmatic tissue is supported by the observations that phentolamine[264] and thymoxamine restore the capacity of asthmatic leukocytes to synthesize cAMP in response to β-agonists. It is also possible that various mediators from inflammatory cells may prime α-adrenoreceptors on airway smooth muscle in asthmatics, resulting in increased α-adrenergic responses.

Autonomic dysfunction has been shown to be a concomitant of asthma in many studies. Increased α-adrenergic sensitivity of pupillary dilator and skin vasoconstrictor muscles has been shown in asthma patients. These systems are thought to be largely α-adrenergic in character because they are responsive to phenylephrine, unresponsive to clonidine, and inhibited by prazosin. Furthermore, the threshold-response dose of exogenous phenylephrine is lower for asthmatic subjects than for controls.[265]

XII. CONCLUSIONS

The characteristics of α- and β-adrenoreceptors in the airways have been summarized. Furthermore, the role of these receptors in the pathogenesis of bronchial asthma has been discussed. Bronchial smooth muscle is relaxed by β-adrenergic stimulation at mostly non-neural β_2-adrenergic receptors. β-adrenoreceptor agonists regulate many aspects of the lung function in addition to their potent relaxatory effect on airway smooth muscle. These include inhibition of mast-cell degranulation, regulation of ion and fluid transport across epithelial cells, stimulation of secretion from submucosal glands and Clara cells, relaxation of vascular smooth muscle, and inhibition of microvascular permeability. In the presence of preexisting bronchoconstriction and/or blockage of the homeostatic β-adrenergic relaxant mechanisms, α-adrenergic stimulation may cause further bronchoconstriction.[233] However, the pharmacologic class and physiologic importance of α-adrenergic receptors have not been established in human.

Electrogenic flux of chloride into the trachea and bronchi is stimulated by β-adrenergic and other systems mediated by cAMP.[264] α-Adrenergic agents do not have an effect on chloride flux, but their effect on other ions awaits further studies.

In the late-phase reaction of bronchial asthma, inflammation in the airways depends on recruitment of inflammatory cells to the airways. Margination and adherence of neutrophils can be attenuated by β-adrenergic agents *in vitro*. The inflammatory process is associated with the release of oxygen radicals and lytic enzymes from neutrophils. This process is enhanced by α-adrenergic and cholinergic agents and reduced by α-adrenergic agonists.[264] These changes are consistent with the therapeutic and anti-inflammatory effect of corticosteroids in the lung[230] and in the airways where corticosteroids increase β-adrenergic responses[232] and decrease α-adrenergic responses (Figure 1).[228,233]

An imbalance of autonomic function could contribute to asthma. In this regard a decrease of β-adrenergic responses could result in diminished bronchial smooth-muscle relaxation, impaired mucociliary clearance, and a blockade of the mechanisms that attenuate mast-cell degranulation and neutrophil lysosomal enzyme release.[264] An increase in α-adrenergic responses could result in bronchoconstriction, enhanced release of inflammatory mediators from mast cells, and increased glandular secretion. An increased response to cholinergic stimuli could result in increased bronchial constriction, enhanced mast-cell mediator release, and increased secretion by tracheobronchial glands.

PAF appears to cause a further derangement of autonomic function by decreasing the β-adrenergic and increasing the cholinergic response in the airways.[265] This is in addition to its inflammatory effect of edema, mucus secretion, and airway eosinophilia.

REFERENCES

1. **Lundgren, R., Soderberg, M., Horsledt, P., and Stenling, R.,** Morphological studies of bronchial mucosal biopsies from asthmatics before and after ten years of treatment with inhaled steroids, *Eur. Respir. J.,* 1, 883, 1989.
2. **Townley, R. G. and Hopp, R. J.,** Inhalation methods for the study of airway responsiveness, *J. Allergy Clin. Immunol.,* 80, 111, 1987.
3. **Townley, R. G., Ryo, U. Y., Kolotkin, B. M., and Kang, B.,** Bronchial sensitivity to methacholine in current and former asthmatics and allergic rhinitis patients and control subjects, *J. Allergy Clin. Immunol.,* 56, 429, 1975.
4. **Reed, C. E. and Townley, R. G.,** Asthma: classification and pathogenesis, in *Allergy — Principles and Practice,* Middleton, R., Reed, C. E., and Ellis, E. F., Eds., C. V. Mosby, St. Louis, 1978, 659.
5. **Townley, R. G., Dennis, M., and Itkin, I. H.,** Comparative action of acetyl-beta-methacholine, histamine, and pollen antigens in subjects with hay fever and patients with bronchial asthma, *J. Allergy,* 36, 121, 1965.
6. **Itkin, I. H.,** Bronchial hypersensitivity to mecholyl and histamine in asthma subjects, *J. Allergy,* 40, 245, 1967.
7. **Pack, R. J. and Richardson, P. S.,** The adrenergic innervation of the human bronchus: a light and electron microscopic study, *J. Anat.,* 138, 493, 1984.
8. **Laitinen, L. A. and Laitinen, A.,** Innervation of airway smooth muscle, *Am. Rev. Respir. Dis.,* 136, S38, 1987.
9. **Laitinen, L. A., Heino, M., Laitinen, A., Kava, T., and Haahtela, T.,** Damage of the airway epithelium and bronchial reactivity in patients with asthma, *Am. Rev. Respir. Dis.,* 131, 599, 1985.

10. **Daniel, E. E., Davis, C., Jones, T. R., and Kannan, M. S.,** Control of airway smooth muscle, in *Airway Reactivity,* Hargreave, F. E., Ed., Astra Pharmaceuticals, Mississauga, Ontario, 1980, 80.

11. **Daniels, E. E., Kannan, M., Davis, C., and Posey-Daniels, V.,** Ultrastructural studies on the neuromuscular control of human tracheal and bronchial muscle, *Respir. Physiol.,* 63, 109, 1986.

12. **Ploy-Song-Sang, U., Corbin, R. P., and Engel, L. A.,** Effects of intravenous histamine on lung mechanics in man after beta-blockade, *J. Appl. Physiol.,* 44, 690, 1978.

13. **Ryo, U. and Townley, R. G.,** Comparison of respiratory and cardiovascular effects of isoproterenol, propranolol, and practolol in asthmatic and normal subjects, *Clin. Res.,* 19, 519, 1976.

14. **Orehek, J., Gayrard, P., Grimaud, C., and Charpin, J.,** Effect of maximal respiratory maneuvers on bronchial sensitivity of asthmatic patients as compared to normal people, *Br. Med. J.,* 1, 123, 1975.

15. **Zuskin, E., Mitchell, C. A., and Bouhuys, A.,** Interaction between effects of beta blockade and cigarette smoke on airways, *J. Appl. Physiol.,* 36, 449, 1974.

16. **Townley, R. G., McGeady, S., and Bewtra, A.,** The effect of beta-adrenergic blockade on bronchial sensitivity to methacholine in normal and allergic rhinitis subjects, *J. Allergy Clin. Immunol.,* 57, 358, 1976.

17. **Zaid, G. and Beall, G. N.,** Bronchial response to beta-adrenergic blockade, *N. Engl. J. Med.,* 275, 580, 1966.

18. **Grieco, M. H. and Pierson, R. N., Jr.,** Mechanism of bronchoconstriction due to beta-adrenergic blockade, *J. Allergy Clin. Immunol.,* 48, 143, 1971.

19. **Crimi, N., Palermo, F., Oliveri, R., Palerrmo, B., Bancheri, C., Polosa, R., and Mistretta, A.,** Effect of vasoactive intestinal peptide (VIP) on propranolol-induced bronchoconstriction, *J. Allergy Clin. Immunol.,* 82, 617, 1988.

20. **Furchgott, R. F.,** The pharmacological differentiation of adrenergic receptors, *Ann. N.Y. Acad. Sci.,* 139, 553, 1969.

21. **Lands, A. M., Arnold, A., McAuliff, J. P., Luduena, F. P., and Brown, T. G.,** Differentiation of receptor systems activated by sympathomimetic amines, *Nature,* 214, 597, 1967.

22. **Langer, S. Z.,** Presynaptic regulation of catecholamine release, *Biochem. Pharmacol.,* 23, 1793, 1974.

23. **Langer, S. Z.,** Presynaptic receptors and their role in the regulation of transmitter release, *Br. J. Pharmacol.,* 60, 481, 1977.

24. **Starke, K.,** Regulation of noradrenaline release by presynaptic receptor systems, *Rev. Physiol. Biochem. Pharmacol.,* 77, 1, 1977.

25. **Agrawal, D. K., Crankshaw, D. J., and Daniel, E. E.,** Postsynaptic alpha adrenoceptors in vascular smooth muscle, in *Sarcolemmal Biochemistry,* Vol. II, Kidwai, A. M., Ed., CRC Press, Boca Raton, FL, 1987, 89.

26. **Langer, S. Z.,** Presynaptic regulation of the release of catecholamines, *Pharmacol. Rev.,* 32, 337, 1981.

27. **Starke, K.,** Presynaptic receptors, *Annu. Rev. Pharmacol. Toxicol.,* 21, 7, 1981.

28. **Langer, S. Z., Massinghan, R., and Shepperson, N. B.,** Presence of postsynaptic alpha$_2$-adrenoceptors of predominantly extrasynaptic location in the vascular smooth muscle of the dog hind limb, *Clin. Sci.,* 59, 2255, 1980.

29. **Han, C., Abel, P. W., and Minneman, K. P.,** Alpha$_1$ adrenoreceptor subtype linked to different mechanisms for increasing intracellular calcium in smooth muscle, *Nature,* 329, 333, 1987.

30. **Bylund, D. B., Ray-Prenger, C., and Murphy, T. J.,** Alpha-2A and alpha-2B adrenergic receptor subtype: antagonist binding in tissues and cell lines containing only one subtype, *J. Pharmacol. Exp. Ther.,* 245, 600, 1988.

31. **Lemanske, R. G., Casale, T. B., and Kaliner, M.,** The autonomic nervous system in allergic disease, in *Allergy,* Kaplan, A. P., Ed., Churchill Livingstone, New York, 1985, 199.

32. **Richardson, J. B.,** Nerve supply to the lungs, *Am. Rev. Respir. Dis.,* 119, 785, 1979.

33. **Woolcock, A. J., Macklem, P. T., Hogg, J. C., and Wilson, N. J.,** Influence of autonomic nervous system on airway resistance and elastic recoil, *J. Appl. Physiol.* 26, 814, 1969.

34. **Cabezas, G. A., Graf, P. D., and Nadel, J. A.,** Sympathetic versus parasympathetic nervous regulation of airways in dogs, *J. Appl. Physiol.* 31, 651, 1971.

35. **Laitinen, L. A.,** Histamine and methacholine challenge in the testing of bronchial reactivity, *Scand. J. Respir. Dis.,* 86, 1, 1974.

36. **Cavanaugh, M. J. and Cooper, D. M.,** Inhaled atropine sufate: dose response characteristics, *Am. Rev. Respir. Dis.,* 114, 517, 1976.

37. **Chamberlain, D. A., Muir, D. C. F., and Kennedy, K. P.,** Atropine methonitrate and isoprenaline in bronchial asthma, *Lancet,* 2, 1019, 1962.

38. **Roberts, A. M., Kaufman, M. P., Baker, D. G., Brown, J. K., Coleridge, H. M., and Coleridge, J. C.,** Reflex tracheal contraction induced by stimulation of bronchial C-fibers in dogs, *J. Appl. Physiol.,* 51, 485, 1981.

39. **Eschenbacher, W. L., Boushey, H. A., and Sheppard, D.,** The effect of osmolarity and ion content of nebulized solution on cough and bronchoconstriction in human subjects, *Am. Rev. Respir. Dis.,* 127, 240, 1983.

40. **Sheppard, D., Rizk, N. W., Boushey, H. A., and Bethel, R. A.,** Mechanism of cough and broncho-constriction induced by distilled water aerosol, *Am. Rev. Respir. Dis.,* 127, 691, 1983.

41. **Grillo, M. A. and Nadel, J. A.,** Vital staining of tracheal ganglia, *Physiologist,* 178, 77, 1980.

42. **Baker, D. G., Herbert, D. A., and Mitchell, R. A.,** Cholinergic neurotransmission in airway ganglia: inhibition by norepinephrine, *Physiologist,* 25, 225, 1982.

43. **Blumcke, S.,** Experimental and morphological studies on the efferent bronchial innervation. I. The peri-bronchial plexus, *Beitr. Pathol. Anat. Allg. Pathol.,* 137, 239, 1968.

44. **Jacobwitz, D., Kent, K. M., Fleisch, J. H., and Cooper, T.,** Histofluorescent study of catecholamine containing elements in cholinergic ganglia from the calf and dog lung, *Proc. Soc. Exp. Biol. Med.,* 144, 464, 1973.

45. **Mann, S. P.,** The innervation of mammalian bronchial smooth muscle: the localization of catecholamines and cholinesterases, *Histochem. J.,* 3, 319, 1971.

46. **Richardson, J. and Beland, J.,** Nonadrenergic inhibitory nervous system in human airways, *J. Appl. Physiol.,* 41, 764, 1976.

47. **Vermiere, P. A. and Vanhoutte, P. M.,** Inhibitory effects of catecholamines in isolated canine bronchial smooth muscle, *J. Appl. Physiol.,* 46, 787, 1979.

48. **Russell, J. A. and Bartlett, S.,** Inhibition of adrenergic neurotransmission in airway smooth muscle by acetylcholine, *Fed. Proc., Fed. Am. Soc. Exp. Biol.,* 38, 1111, 1979.

49. **Murlas, C., Nadel, J. A., and Basbaum, C. B. A.,** A morphometric analysis of the autonomic innervation of cat tracheal glands, *J. Auton. Nerv. Syst.,* 2, 23, 1980.

50. **Silva, D. G. and Ross, G.,** Ultrastructure and fluorescence histochemical studies on the innervation of the tracheobronchial muscle of normal cats and cats treated with 6-hydroxydopamine, *J. Ultrastruct. Res.,* 47, 310, 1980.

51. **Barnes, P. J., Nadel, J. A., Roberts, J., M., and Basbaum, C. B.,** Muscarinic receptors in lung and trachea: autoradiographic localization using ^{3}H quinuclidinyl benzilate, *Eur. J. Pharmacol.,* 86, 103, 1983.

52. **Minette, P., Lammers, J-W., and Barnes, P. J.,** Is there a defect in inhibitory muscarinic receptors in asthma?, *Am. Rev. Respir. Dis.,* 137, 239, 1988.

53. **Lammers, J. W., Minette, P., McCusker, M., and Barnes, P. J.,** The role of pirenzepine in vagally mediated bronchoconstriction in humans, *Am. Rev. Respir. Dis.,* 139, 446, 1989.

54. **Exton, J. H.,** Molecular mechanisms involved in alpha-adrenergic responses, *Trends Pharmacol. Sci.,* 3, 111, 1982.

55. **George, W. J., Polson, J. B., O'Toole, A. G., and Goldberg, N. D.,** Elevation of guanosine 3', 5' cyclic phosphate in rat heart after perfusion with acetylcholine, *Proc. Natl. Acad. Sci. U.S.A.,* 66, 398, 1970.

56. **Burgen, A. S. V. and Spero, L.,** The action of acetylcholine and other drugs on the efflux of potassium and rubidium from smooth muscle of guinea pig intestine, *Br. J. Pharmacol.,* 34, 99, 1968.

57. **Jafferji, S. S. and Michell, R. H.,** Muscarinic cholinergic stimulation of phosphoinositol turnover in longitudinal smooth muscle of guinea pig illeum, *Biochem. J.,* 154, 63, 1976.

58. **Kaliner, M.,** Human lung tissue and anaphylaxis. I. The role of cyclic GMP as a modulator of the immunologically induced secretory process, *J. Allergy Clin. Immunol.,* 60, 204, 1977.

59. **Kaliner, M., Orange, R. P., and Austen, K. F.,** Immunological release of histamine and slow-reacting substance from human lung. IV. Enhancement by cholinergic and alpha adrenergic stimulation, *J. Exp. Med.,* 136, 556, 1972.

60. **Shelhamer, J. H., Marom, Z., and Kaliner, M.,** Immunologic and neuropharmacologic stimulation of mucous glycoprotein release from human airways in vitro, *J. Clin. Invest.,* 66, 1400, 1980.

61. **Cheng, J. B. and Townley, R. G.,** Comparison of muscarinic and beta adrenergic receptors between bovine peripheral lung and tracheal smooth muscles: a striking difference in the receptor concentration, *Life Sci.,* 30, 2079, 1982.

62. **Ehlert, F. J., Roeske, W. R., and Yamamura, H. I.,** Muscarinic receptor: regulation by guanine nucleotides, ions, and N-ethylmaleimide, *Fed. Proc., Fed. Am. Soc. Exp. Biol.,* 40, 153, 1981.

63. **Lee, T. P., Kuo, J. F., and Greegard, P.,** Role of muscarinic cholinergic receptors in regulation of guanosine 3', 5' cyclic monophosphate content in mammalian brain, heart muscle, and intestinal smooth muscle, *Proc. Natl. Acad. Sci.,* 69, 3287, 1981.

64. **Murad, F., Chi, Y. M., Rall, T. W., and Sutherland, E. W.,** Adenylate cyclase. IV. The effect of catecholamines and choline esters on the formation of adenosine 3', 5' phosphate by preparations from cardiac muscle and liver, *J. Biol. Chem.,* 237, 1233, 1962.

65. **Gardner, R. M. and Allen, D. O.,** Regulation of cyclic nucleotide levels and glycogen phosphorylase activity by acetylcholine and epinephrine in perfused rat heart, *J. Pharmacol. Exp Ther.,* 198, 412, 1976.

66. **Gross, R. A. and Clark, R. B.,** Regulation of adenosine 3', 5' monophosphate content in human astro-cytoma cells by isoproterenol and carbachol, *Mol. Pharmacol.,* 13, 242, 1977.

67. **Watanabe, A. M., McConnaughey, M. M., Strawbridge, R. A., Fleming, J. W., Jones, L. R., and Besch, H. R., Jr.,** Muscarinic cholinergic receptor modulation of beta-adrenergic receptor affinity for catecholamines, *J. Biol. Chem.,* 253, 4833, 1978.

68. **Roeske, W. R. and Yamamura, H. I.**, Muscarinic cholinergic receptor regulation, in *Psychopharmacology and Biochemistry of Neurotransmitter Receptors*, Yamamura, H. I., Olson, H. I., and Usdin, E., Eds., Elsevier/North-Holland, New York, 1980, 101.

69. **Lefkowitz, R. J.**, Direct binding studies of adrenergic receptors: biochemical, physiological and clinical implications, *Ann. Int. Med.*, 91, 450, 1979.

70. **Maggi, A., U'Prichard, D. C., and Enna, S. J.**, Beta adrenergic regulation of alpha$_2$-adrenergic receptors in the central nervous system, *Science*, 207, 645, 1980.

71. **Szentivanyi, A.**, The beta adrenergic theory of the atopic abnormality in bronchial asthma, *J. Allergy*, 42, 203, 1968.

72. **Townley, R. G., Trapani, I. L., and Szentivanyi, A.**, Sensitization to anaphylaxis and to some of its pharmacological mediators by blockage of the beta adrenergic receptors, *J. Allergy*, 39, 117, 1967.

73. **Boushey, H. A., Holtzman, M. J., Sheller, J. R., and Nadel, J. A.**, Bronchial hyperreactivity, *Am. Rev. Respir. Dis.*, 121, 389, 1980.

74. **Middleton, E., Jr.**, Antiasthmatic drug therapy and calcium ions: review of pathogenesis and role of calcium, *J. Pharmaceut. Sci.*, 69, 243, 1980.

75. **Said, S. I.**, Vasoactive intestinal peptide and asthma, *N. Engl. J. Med.*, 320, 1271, 1989.

76. **Holtzman, M. J., Scheller, J. R., Dimeo, M., Nadel, J. A., and Boushey, H. A.**, Effect of ganglionic blockade on bronchial reactivity in atopic subject, *Am. Rev. Respir. Dis.*, 123, 17, 1980.

77. **Vidruk, E. H., Hahn, H. L., Nadel, J. A., and Sampson, S. R.**, Mechanism by which histamine stimulates rapidly adapting receptors in dog lungs, *J. Appl. Physiol.*, 43, 397, 1977.

78. **Hahn, H. L., Wilson, A. G., Graf, P. D., Fischer, S. P., and Nadel, J. A.**, Intreaction between serotonin and efferent vagus nerves in dog lungs, *J. Appl. Physiol.*, 44, 144, 1978.

79. **Smith, L. J., Shelhamer, J. R., Metcalfe, D. D., Evans, R. E., III, and Kaliner, M.**, The array of autonomic abnormalities in allergic asthmatic patients, *J. Allergy Clin. Immunol.*, 63, 141, 1979.

80. **Wastek, G. J. and Yamamura, H. I.**, Biochemical characterization of the muscarinic receptor in human brain: alterations is Huntington's disease, *Mol. Pharmacol.*, 14, 768, 1980.

81. **Lopker, A., Abood, L. G., Hoss, W., and Lioneth, F.**, Stereoselective muscarinic acetylcholine and opiate receptors in human phagocytic leukocytes, *Biochem. Pharmacol.*, 29, 1361, 1980.

82. **Zalcman, S. J., Neckers, L. M., Kaayalp, O., and Wyatt, R. J.**, Muscarinic cholinergic binding sites on intact human lymphocytes, *Life Sci.*, 29, 69, 1981.

83. **Richman, D. P. and Arnason, B. G. W.**, Nicotinic acetylcholine receptor: evidence for a functionally distinct receptor on human lymphocytes, *Proc. Natl. Acad. Sci.*, 76, 4632, 1979.

84. **Dulis, B. H., Gordon, M. A., and Wilson, I. B.**, Identification of muscarinic binding sites in human neutrophils by directed binding, *Mol. Pharmacol.*, 15, 28, 1979.

85. **Empey, D. W., Laitinen, L. A., Jacobs, L., Gold, W. M., and Nadel, J. A.**, Mechanisms of bronchial hyperreactivity in normal subjects after upper respiratory tract infection, *Am. Rev. Respir. Dis.*, 113, 131, 1976.

86. **Golden, J. A., Nadel, J. A., and Boushey, H. A.**, Bronchial hyperirritability in healthy subjects after exposure to ozone, *Am. Rev. Respir. Dis.*, 118, 287, 1978.

87. **Holtzman, M. J., Sheller, J. R., Dimeo, M., Nadel, J. A., and Boushey, H. A.**, Effect of ganglionic blockade on bronchial reactivity in atopic subjects, *Am. Rev. Respir. Dis.*, 122, 17, 1980.

88. **Nadel, J. A., Salem, H., Tamplin, B., and Tokeiva**, Mechanism of bronchoconstriction during inhalation of sulfur dioxide, *J. Appl. Physiol.*, 20, 164, 1965.

89. **Kersten, W.**, Protektive wirkung von ipratropium-bromid (Sch 1000) bei akuten bronchokonstriktionen durch allergeninhalation, *Respiration*, 31, 412, 1974.

90. **Woolcock, A. J., Macklem, P. T., Hogg, J. C., Wilson, N. J., Nadel, J. A., Frank, N. R., and Brain J.**, Effect of vagal stimulation on central and peripheral airway in dogs, *J. Appl. Physiol.*, 26, 806, 1969.

91. **Chen, W. Y., Brenner, A. M., Weiser, P. C., and Chai, H.**, Atropine and exercise-induced bronchoconstriction, *Chest*, 79, 651, 1981.

92. **Altounyan, R. E. C.**, Variation of drug action on airway obstruction in man, *Thorax*, 19, 406, 1964.

93. **Bandouvakis, J., Cartier, A., Roberts, R., Ryan, G., and Hargreave, F. E.**, The effect of ipratropium and fenoterol on methacholine- and histamine-induced bronchoconstriction, *Br. J. Dis. Chest*, 75, 295, 1981.

94. **Casterline, C. L., Evans, R., III, and Ward, G. W., Jr.**, The effect of atropine and albuterol aerosols on the human bronchial response to histamine, *J. Allergy Clin. Immunol.*, 58, 607, 1976.

95. **Townley, R. G., Bewtra, A. K., Nair, N. M., Brodkey, F. D., Watt, G., and Burke, K.**, Methacholine inhalation challenge studies, *J. Allergy Clin. Immunol.*, 64, 569, 1979.

96. **Godfrey, S.**, Exercise-induced asthma — clinical, physiological, and therapeutic implications, *J. Allergy Clin. Immunol.*, 56, 1, 1975.

97. **Tinkelman, D. G., Cavanaugh, M. J., and Cooper, D. M.**, Inhibition of exercise-induced bronchospasm by atropine, *Am. Rev. Respir. Dis.*, 114, 87, 1976.

98. **Deal, E. C., Jr., McFadden, E. R., Jr., Ingram, R. H., Jr., and Jaeger, J. J.,** Effects of atropine on potentiation of exercise-induced bronshospasm by cold air, *J. Appl. Physiol.,* 45, 238, 1978.

99. **van Koppen, C. J., Hermanussen, M. W., Verrijp, K. N., Rodrigues de Miranda, J. F., Beld, A. J., Lammers, J-W. J., and Ginneken, C. A. M.,** Beta-adrenoceptors in human tracheal smooth muscle: characteristics of binding and relaxation, *Life Sci.,* 40, 2561, 1987.

100. **Casale, T. B. and Hart, J. E.,** (−) [^{125}I]Pindolol binding to human peripheral lung beta-receptors, *Biochem. Pharmacol.,* 36, 2557, 1987.

101. **Engel, G.,** Subclasses of beta-adrenoreceptors — a quantitative estimation of beta$_1$- and beta$_2$-adrenoceptors in guinea pig and human lung, *Postgrad. Med.,* 57(Suppl. 1), 77, 1981.

102. **Davis, D. J., Dattel, B. J., Ballard, P. L., and Roberts, J. M.,** Beta-adrenergic and cyclic adenosine monophosphate generation in human fetal lung, *Pediatr. Res.,* 21, 142, 1986.

103. **Falkay, G., Nemeth, G., and Kovaca, L.,** Binding properties of beta-adrenergic receptors in early human fetal lung, *Biochem. Biophys. Res. Commun.,* 135, 816, 1986.

104. **Minneman, K. P., Puckett, A. M., Jensen, A. D., and Rinard, G. A.,** Regional variation in beta adrenergic receptors in dog trachea: correlation of receptor density and *in vitro* relaxation, *J. Pharmacol. Exp. Ther.,* 226, 140, 1983.

105. **Agrawal, D. K., Schugel, J. W., and Townley, R. G.,** Comparison of beta adrenoceptors in bovine airway epithelium and smooth muscle cells, *Biochem. Biophys. Res. Commun.,* 148, 178, 1987.

106. **Carswell, H. and Nahorski, S. R.,** Beta-adrenoreceptor heterogeneity in guinea-pig airways: comparison of functional and receptor labeling studies, *Br. J. Pharmacol.,* 79, 965, 1983.

107. **Goldie, R. G., Papadimitriou, J. M., Paterson, J. W., Rigby, P. J., Self, H. M., and Spina, D.,** Influence of the epithelium on responsiveness of guinea pig isolated trachea to contractile and relaxant agonists, *Br. J. Pharmacol.,* 87, 5, 1986.

108. **Taki, F., Takagi, K., Satake, T., Sugiyama, S., and Ozawa, T.,** The role of phospholipase in reduced beta-adrenergic responsiveness in experimental asthma, *Am. Rev. Respir. Dis.,* 133, 362, 1986.

109. **Suzuki, K., Sugiyama, S., Takagi, K., Satake, T., and Ozawa, T.,** The role of phospholipase in beta-agonist-induced down regulation in guinea pig lungs, *Biochem. Med.. Metab. Biol.,* 37, 157, 1987.

110. **Koshino, T., Agrawal, D. K., Townley, T. A., and Townley, R. G.,** Ketotifen prevents terbutaline-induced down-regulation of beta-adrenoreceptors in guinea pig lung, *Biochem. Biophys. Res. Commun.,* 152, 1221, 1988.

111. **van Heuven-Nolsen, D., Folkerts, G., de Wildt, D. J., and Nijkamp, F. P.,** The influence of bordetella purtussis and its constituents on the beta-adrenergic receptor in the guinea pig respiratory system, *Life Sci.,* 38, 677, 1986.

112. **Barnes, P. J., Skoogh, B. E., Nadel, J. A., and Roberts, J. M.,** Postsynaptic alpha$_2$-adrenoceptors predominate over alpha$_1$-adrenoceptors in canine tracheal smooth muscle and mediate neuronal and humoral alpha-adrenergic contraction, *Mol. Pharmacol.,* 23, 570, 1983.

113. **O'Donnel, S. R., Saar, N., and Wood, L. J.,** The density of adrenergic nerves at various levels in the guinea-pig lung, *Clin. Exp. Pharmacol. Physiol.,* 5, 325, 1978.

114. **Zaagsma, J., van der Heijden, P. M. C. M., van der Schaar, M. W. G., and Bank, C. M. C.,** Comparison of functional beta-adrenoceptor heterogeneity in central and peripheral airway smooth muscle of guinea pig and man, *J. Recep. Res.,* 3, 89, 1983.

115. **Goldie, R. G., Paterson, J. W., Spira, D., and Wale, J. L.,** Classification of beta-adrenoceptors in human and porcine bronchus, *Br. J. Pharmacol.,* 81, 611, 1984.

116. **Lofdahl, C. G. and Suedmyr, N.,** Effects of prenalterol in asthmatic patients, *Eur. J. Clin. Pharmacol.,* 23, 297, 1982.

117. **Barnes, P. J. and Pride, N. B.,** Dose-response curves to inhaled beta-adrenoceptor agonist in normal and asthmatic subjects, *Br. J. Clin. Pharmacol.,* 15, 677, 1983.

118. **Barnes, P. J., Basbaum, B. J., and Nadel, J. A.,** Autoradiography localization of autonomic receptors in airway smooth muscle. Marked differences between large and small airways, *Am. Rev. Respir. Dis.,* 127, 758, 1983.

119. **Carstairs, J. R., Nimmo, A. J., and Barnes, P. J.,** Autoradiographic visualization of beta-adrenoceptor subtypes in human lung, *Am. Rev. Respir. Dis.,* 132, 541, 1985.

120. **Knowles, M., Murray, G., and Shallal, J.,** Bioelectric properties and ion flow across excised human bronchi, *J. Appl. Physiol.,* 56, 868, 1984.

121. **Flavahan, N. A., Aarhus, L. L., Rimele, T. J., and Vanhoutte, P. M.,** Respiratory epithelium inhibits bronchial smooth muscle tone, *J. Appl. Physiol.,* 58, 834, 1985.

122. **Raeburn, D., Hay, D. W. P., Farmer, S. G., and Fedan, J. S.,** Epithelium removal increases the reactivity of human isolated tracheal muscle to methacholine and reduces the effect of verapamil, *Eur. J. Pharmacol.,* 123, 451, 1986.

123. **Szarek, J. L., Gillespie, M. N., Altiere, R. J., and Diamond, L.,** Reflex activation of the nonadrenergic noncholinergic inhbitory nervous system in airways, *Am. Rev. Respir. Dis.,* 133, 1159, 1986.

124. **Townley, R. G., Hopp, R., Weiss, S., Lang, D., and McCall, M. B.,** Mechanisms and management of bronchial asthma, in *Clinical Medicine,* Spittel, J. A., Jr., Ed., Harper & Row, Philadelphia, 1986, 1.

125. **Vanhoutte, P. M.,** Epithelium-derived relaxing factor(s) and bronchial reactivity, *Am. Rev. Respir. Dis.,* 138, S24, 1988.

126. **Smith, P. L., Welsh, M. J., Stoff, J. S., and Frizzell, R. A.,** Chloride secretion by canine tracheal epithelium: role of intracellular cAMP levels, *J. Membr. Biol.,* 70, 217, 1982.

127. **Phipps, R. J., Williams, I. P., Richardson, P. S., Pell, L., Pack, R. J., and Wright, N.,** Sympathetic drugs stimulate the output of secretory glycoprotein from human bronchi in vitro, *Clin. Sci.,* 63, 23, 1982.

128. **Leikhauf, G. D., Ueki, I. F., and Nadel, J. A.,** Selective autonomic regulation of the viscoelastic properties of submucosal gland secretions from cat trachea, *J. Appl. Physiol.,* 56, 426, 1984.

129. **Partanen, M., Laitinen, A., Hervonen, A., Toivanen, M., and Laitinen, L. A.,** Catecholamine and acetylcholinesterase containing nerves in human lower respiratory tract, *Histochemistry,* 76, 175, 1982.

130. **Barnes, P. J., Basbaum, C. B., Nadel, J. A., and Roberts, J. M.,** Pulmonary alpha-adrenoceptors: autoradiographic localization using [^{3}H]prazosin, *Eur. J. Pharmacol.,* 88, 57, 1983.

131. **Camner, P., Strandberg, K., and Philipson, K.,** Increased mucociliary transport by cholinergic stimulation, *Arch. Environ. Health,* 29, 220, 1974.

132. **Foster, W. M., Bergofsky, E. H., Bohning, D. E., Lippmann, M., and Albert, R. E.,** Effect of adrenergic agents and their mode of action on mucociliary clearance in man, *J. Appl. Physiol.,* 41, 146, 1976.

133. **Sanderson, M. J. and Dirksen, E. R.,** Mechano-sensitive and beta-adrenergic control of the ciliary beta frequency of mammalian respiratory tract cells in culture, *Am. Rev. Respir. Dis.,* 139, 432, 1989.

134. **Massaro, G. D., Fischman, C. M., Chiang, M. J., Amado, C., and Massaro, D.,** Regulation of secretion in Clara cells, Studies using isolated perfused lung, *J. Clin. Invet.,* 67, 345, 1981.

135. **Widdicombe, J. G. and Pack, R. J.,** The Clara cell, *Eur. J. Respir. Dis.,* 63, 202, 1982.

136. **Orange, R. P., Austen, W. G., and Austen, K. F.,** Immunological release of histamine and slow reacting substance of anaphylaxis from human lung. I. Modulation by agents influencing cellular levels of cyclic-3',5'-adenosine monophosphate, *J. Exp. Med.,* 134, 136, 1971.

137. **Butchers, P. R., Skidmore, I. F., Vardey, C. J., and Wheeldon, A. M.,** Characterization of the receptor mediating the anti-anaphylactic effects of beta-adrenoceptor agonists in human lung tissue in vitro, *Br. J. Pharmacol.,* 71, 663, 1980.

138. **Peters, S. P., Schulman, E. S., Schleimer, R. P., MacGlashan, D. W., Jr., Newball, H. H., and Litchtenstein, L. N.,** Dispersed human lung mast cells: pharmacologic aspects amd comparison with human lung tissue fragments, *Am Rev. Respir. Dis.,* 126, 1034, 1982.

139. **Church, M. K., Holgate, S. T., and Pao, G. J. K.,** Histamine release from mechanically and enzymatically dispersed human lung mast cells: inhibition by salbutamol and cromoglycate, *Br. J. Pharmacol.,* 79 (Suppl.), 374, 1983.

140. **Donlon, M., Hunt, W. A., Catravas, G. N., and Kaliner, M. A.,** Characterization of beta-adrenergic receptors on cellular and perigranular membranes of rat peritoneal mast cells, *Life Sci.,* 31, 411, 1982.

141. **Brown, M. J., Ind, P. W., Causon, R., and Lee, T. H.,** A novel double-isotope technique for the enzymatic assay of plasma histamine: application to stimulation of mast cell activation assessed by antigen challenge in asthmatics, *J. Allergy Clin. Immunol.,* 69, 20, 1982.

142. **Garrity, E. R., Stimler, N. P., Munoz, N. M., Tallet, J., David, A. C., and Leff, A. R.,** Sympathetic modulation of biochemical and physiological response to immune degranulation in canine bronchial airways in vivo, *J. Clin. Invest.,* 75, 2038, 1985.

143. **White, S. R., Stimler-Gerard, N. P., Munoz, N. M., Popovich, K. J., Murphy, T. M., Blake, J. S., Mack, M. M., and Leff, A. R.,** Effect of beta-adrenergic blockade and sympathetic stimulation on canine bronchial mast cell response to immune degranulation in vivo, *Am. Rev. Respir. Dis.,* 139, 73, 1989.

144. **Barnes, P. J., Fitzgerald, G., Brown, M., and Dollery, C.,** Nocturnal asthma and changes in circulating epinephrine, histamine and cortisol, *N. Engl. J. Med.,* 303, 263, 1980.

145. **Howarth, P. H., Durham, S. R., Lee, T. H., Kay, A. B., Church, M. K., and Holgate, S. T.,** Influence of albuterol, cromolyn sodium and ipratropium bromide on the airway and circulating mediator response to allergen bronchial provocation in asthma, *Am. Rev. Respir. Dis.,* 132, 986, 1985.

146. **Ishizaka, T.,** Analysis of triggering events in mast cells for immunoglobulin E-mediated histamine release, *J. Allergy Clin. Immunol.,* 67, 90, 1981.

147. **Siraganian, R. P.,** Histamine secretion from mast cells and basophils, *Trends Pharmacol. Sci.,* 4, 432, 1983.

148. **Liggett, S. B.,** Identification and characterization of a homogenous population of beta$_2$-adrenergic receptors on human alveolar macrophages, *Am. Rev. Respir. Dis.,* 139, 552, 1989.

149. **Fels, A. O.. and Cohn, Z. A.,** The alveolar macrophage, *J. Appl. Physiol.,* 60, 353, 1986.

150. **Pick, E.,** Cyclic AMP affects macrophage migration, *Nature,* 238, 176, 1972.

151. **Lowrie, D B., Jackett, P. S., and Ratcliff, N. A.,** Mycobacterium microti may protect itself from intracellular destruction by releasing cyclic AMP into phagosomes, *Nature,* 254, 600, 1975.

152. **Abrass, C. K., O'Conner, S. W., Scarpace, P. J., and Abrass, I. B.,** Characterization of the beta-adrenergic receptor of the rat peritoneal macrophage, *J. Immunol.,* 135, 1338, 1985.

153. **Gudewicz, P. W., Cabelman, L. B., Lai, M. Z., and Molnar, J.,** A role for anti-inflammatory agents and cyclic AMP in regulating fibronectin-mediated phagocytosis, *J. Immunopharmacol.,* 3, 193, 1981.

154. **Vogel, S. N., Weedon, L. L., Oppenheim, J. J., and Rosenstreich, D. L.,** Defective Fc-mediated phagocytosis in C3H/HeJ macrophage. II. Correction by cAMP agonists, *J. Immunol.,* 126, 441, 1981.

155. **Rosati, C., Hanneart, P., Daussse, J., Braquet, P., and Garay, R.,** Stimulation of beta-adrenoceptor inhibits calcium-dependent potassium-channels in mouse macrophage, *J. Cell. Physiol.,* 129, 310, 1986.

156. **Cockcroft, D. W., Killian, D. N., Mellon, J. J. A., and Hargreave, F. E.,** Bronchial reactivity to inhaled histamine: a method and clinical survey, *Clin. Allergy,* 7, 235, 1977.

157. **Skidmore, I. F.,** Allergic asthma and rhinitis: the relationship between pathophysiology and treatment, *Trends Pharmacol. Sci.,* 3, 66, 1982.

158. **Paterson, J. W., Woolcock, A. J., and Shenfield, G. M.,** Bronchodilator drugs, *Am. Rev. Respir. Dis.,* 120, 1149, 1979.

159. **Sackner, M. A.,** Effect of respiratory drugs on mucociliary clearance, *Chest,* 73, 958, 1978.

160. **Conolly, M. E. and Greenacre, J. K.,** The lymphocyte beta-adrenoceptor in normal subjects and with patients with bronchial asthma, *J. Clin. Invest.,* 58, 1307, 1976.

161. **Morris, H. G., Rusnake, S. A., Selner, J. C., Barzens, K., and Barnes, P. J.,** Adrenergic desensitization in leukocytes of normal and asthmatic subjects, *J. Cyclic Nucleotide Res.,* 3, 439, 1977.

162. **Tashkin, D. P., Conolly, M. E., Deutsch, R. I., Hui, K. K., Littner, M., Scarpace, P., and Abrass, I.,** Subsensitization of beta-adrenoceptors in airways and lymphocytes of healthy and asthmatic subjects, *Am. Rev. Respir. Dis.,* 125, 185, 1982.

163. **Sano, Y., Watt, G., and Townley, R. G.,** Decreased mononuclear cell beta-adrenergic receptors in bronchial asthma: parallel studies of lymphocyte and granulocyte desensitization, *J. Allergy Clin. Immunol.,* 72, 495, 1983.

164. **Takeyama, H. F., Agrawal, D. K., and Townley, R. G.,** Both allergen and histamine-induced bronchoconstriction cause increased $alpha_1$ and decreased beta-adrenergic receptors in guinea pig lung, submitted.

165. **Barnes, P. J., Dollery, C. T., and Macdermot, J.,** Increased pulmonary alpha-adrenergic and reduced beta-adrenergic receptors in experimental asthma, *Nature,* 285, 569, 1980.

166. **Gatto, C., Green, T. P., Johnson, M. G., Marchessault, R. P., Seybold, V., and Johnson, D. E.,** Localization of quantitative changes in pulmonary beta-receptors in ovalbumin-sensitized guinea pigs, *Am. Rev. Respir. Dis.,* 136, 150, 1987.

167. **Meurs, H., Koeter, G. H., de Vries, K., and Kauffman, H. F.,** The beta-adrenergic system and allergic bronchial asthma: changes in lymphocyte beta adrenergic receptor number and adenylate cyclase activity after an allergen-induced asthmatic attack, *J. Allergy Clin. Immunol.,* 70, 272, 1982.

168. **Meurs, H., Kauffman, H. F., Timmermans, A., de Monchy, J. D. R., Koeter, G. H., and de Vries, K.,** Specific immunological modulation of lymphocyte adenylate cyclase in asthmatic patients after allergenic bronchial provocation, *Int. Arch. Allergy Appl. Immunol.,* 81, 224, 1986.

169. **Yukawa, T., Makino, S., Fukuda, T., and Kamikawa, Y.,** Experimental model of anaphylaxis-induced beta-adrenergic blockade in the airways, *Ann. Allergy,* 57, 219, 1986.

170. **Mita, H., Yui, Y., Yasueda, H., and Shida, T.,** Changes in $alpha_1$- and beta-adrenergic and cholinergic muscarinic reeptors in guinea pig lung sensitized with ovalbumin, *Int. Arch. Allergy Appl. Immunol.,* 70, 225, 1983.

171. **Tamura, N., Agrawal, D. K., Suliaman, F. A., and Townley, R. G.,** Effects of platelet-activating factor on the chemotaxis of normodense eosinophils from normal subjects, *Biochem. Biophys. Res. Commun.,* 142, 638, 1987.

172. **Tamura, N., Agrawal, D. K., Townley, R. G., and Braquet, P. G.,** Platelet-activating factor, human eosinophils, and ginkgolide B (BN 52021), in *Ginkgolides — Chemistry, Biology, Pharmacology, and Clinical Perspectives,* Vol. 1, Braquet, P., Ed., J.R. Prous Publishers, Barcelona, Spain, 1988, 217.

173. **Braquet, P., Touqui, L., Shen, T. Y., and Vargaftig, B. B.,** Perspectives in platelet-activating factor research, *Pharmacol. Rev.,* 39, 97, 1987.

174. **Barnes, P. J. and Chung, K. F.,** PAF closely mimics pathology of asthma, *Trend Pharmacol. Sci.,* 8, 285, 1987.

175. **Townley, R. G., Hopp, R., Agrawal, D. K., and Bewtra, A. K.,** Human airway responses to platelet-activating factor, *Am. Rev. Respir. Dis.,* 137, 429, 1988.

176. **Agrawal, D. K. and Townley, R. G.,** Effect of platelet-activating on beta-adrenoceptors in human lung, *Biochem. Biophys. Res. Commun.,* 143, 1, 1987.

177. **Agrawal, D. K. and Townley, R. G.,** PAF, human lung beta-adrenoceptors and ginkgolide B (BN 52021), in *Ginkgolides — Chemistry, Biology, Pharmacology, and Clinical Perspectives,* Vol. 1, Braquet, P., Ed., J.R. Prous Publishers, Barcelona, Spain, 1988, 217.

178. **Braquet, P., Etienne, A., and Clostre, F.,** Down-regulation of $beta_2$ adrenergic receptors by Paf-acether and its inhibition by the Paf-acether antagonist BN 52021, *Prostaglandins,* 30, 721, 1985.

179. **Agrawal, D. K., Bergren, D. R., Byorth, P. J., and Townley, R. G.,** Platelet-activating factor induces non-specific desensitization to bronchodilators in guinea pigs, *Am. Rev. Respir. Dis.,* in press.
180. **Benson, M. K., Berrill, W. T., Sterling, G. M., Decalmer, P. B., Chatterjee, S. S., Croson, R. S., and Cruickshank, J. M.,** Cardioselective and non-cardioselective beta-blockers in reversible obstructive airways disease, *Postgrad. Med. J.,* 53 (Suppl. 3), 146, 1977.
181. **Apold, J. and Aksenes, L.,** Correlation between increased bronchial responsiveness to histamine and diminished plasma cyclic adenosine monophosphate response after epinephrine in asthmatic children, *J. Allergy Clin. Immunol.,* 59, 343, 1977.
182. **Makino, S., Ikemori, K., Kashima, T., and Fuxuda, T.,** Comparison of cyclic adenosine monophosphate response of lymphocytes in normal and asthmatic subjects to norepinephrine and salbutamol, *J. Allergy Clin. Immunol.,* 59, 348, 1977.
183. **Kaliner, M. and Austen, K. J.,** A sequence of biochemical events in the antigen-induced release of chemical mediators from sensitized human lung tissue, *J. Exp. Med.,* 138, 1077, 1973.
184. **Coffey, R. G. and Middleton, E., Jr.,** Mechanisms of action of antiallergic drugs and relationship of cyclic nucleotide to allergy. Comprehensive immunology, in *Immunopharmacology,* Harden, J. W., Coffey, R. G., and Spreatico, J., Eds., Plenum Press, New York, 1977, 203.
185. **Henderson, R. W., Shelhamer, H. J., Reingold, B. D., Smith, J. L., Evans, R., III, and Kaliner, M.,** Alpha-adrenergic hyper-responsiveness in asthma, *N. Engl. J. Med.,* 300, 642, 1979.
186. **Parker, C. and Smith, J.,** Alterations in cyclic adenosine monophosphate metabolism in human bronchial asthma. 1. Leukocyte reponsiveness to beta-adrenergic agents, *J. Clin. Invest.,* 52, 48, 1973.
187. **Gillespie, Z., Valentine, M. D., and Lichtenstein, L. M.,** Cyclic AMP metabolism in asthma: studies with leukocytes and lymphocytes, *J. Allergy Clin. Immunol.,* 53, 27, 1974.
188. **Logsdon, P. J., Carnright, D. B., Middleton, E., Jr., and Coffey, R. G.,** The effect of phentolamine on adenylate cyclase and on isoproterenol stimulation on asthmatic subjects, *J. Allergy Clin. Immunol.,* 53, 148, 1974.
189. **Alston, W. C., Patel, K. R., and Kerr, J. W.,** Response of leukocyte adenyl cyclase to isoprenaline and effect of alpha blocking drugs in extrinsic bronchial asthma, *Br. Med. J.,* 1, 90, 1974.
190. **Morris, H. G., Rusnak, S. A., and Barzens, K.,** Leukocyte cylic adenosine monophosphate in asthmatic children: effect of adrenergic therapy, *Clin. Pharmacol. Ther.,* 22, 352, 1977.
191. **Williams, L. T., Snyderman, R., and Lefkowitz, R. J.,** Identification of beta adrenergic receptors in human leukocytes with (−) ³H-dihydroalprenolol, *J. Clin. Invest.,* 57, 149, 1976.
192. **Pochet, R., Delespesse, G., Gausset, P. W., and Collet, J.,** Distribution of beta adrenergic receptors on human lymphocyte subpopulations, *Clin. Exp. Immunol.,* 38, 578, 1978.
193. **Galant, S. P., Underwood, S., Duriseti, L., and Insel, P. A.,** Characterization of high affinity beta₂-adrenergic receptor binding of (−) ³H-dihydroalprenolol to human polymorphonuclear cell particulates, *J. Lab. Clin. Med.,* 92, 613, 1978.
194. **Ruoho, A. E., DeClerque, J. L., and Busse, W. W.,** Characterizations of granulocyte beta-adrenergic receptors in atopic eczema, *J. Allergy Clin. Immunol.,* 66, 46, 1980.
195. **Kariman, K. and Lefkowitz, R. J.,** Beta-adrenergic receptor binding in lymphocytes from patients with bronchial asthma, *Lung,* 158, 41, 1980.
196. **Szentivanyi, A., Heim, O., and Schultze, P.,** Changes in adrenergic receptor density in membranes of lung tissue and lymphocyte from patients with atopic disease, *Ann. N.Y. Acad. Sci.,* 332, 295, 1979.
197. **Galant, S., Underwood, S., Allred, S., and Hanifin, J. M.,** Beta-adrenergic receptor of polymorpho-nuclear particulates in bronchial asthma, *J. Clin. Invest.,* 65, 577, 1980.
198. **Townley, R. G.,** Receptors and non-specific bronchial reactivity, in *Proc. Invited Symposia, XI Int. Congress of Allergology and Clinical Immunology,* Kerr, J. W. and Ganderton, M. A., Eds., Macmillan, London, 1983, 197.
199. **Wolfe, R. N., Hui, K. K., Conolly, M. E., Tashkin, D. P., and Fisher, H. K.,** A study of beta-adrenergic and prostaglandin receptors in patients with aspirin induced bronchospasm, *J. Allergy Clin. Immunol.,* 69, 46, 1982.
200. **Sheppard, J. R., Gormus, Q., and Moldow, C. F.,** Catecholamine hormone receptors are reduced on chronic lymphocytic leukemic lymphocytes, *Nature,* 269, 693, 1977.
201. **Bishopric, H. N., Cohen, H. J., and Lefkowitz, R. J.,** Beta adrenergic receptors in lymphocyte sub-populations, *J. Allergy Clin. Immunol.,* 65, 29, 1980.
202. **Shelhamer, J. H., Maron, A., and Kaliner, M.,** Abnormal beta-adrenergic responsiveness in allergic subjects. II. The role of selective beta₂-adrenergic hyporeactivity, *J. Allergy Clin. Immunol.,* 57, 12, 1976.
203. **Lockey, S. D., Glennon, J. A., and Reed, C. E.,** Comparison of some metabolic responses in normal and asthmatic subjects to epinephrine and glucagon, *J. Allergy,* 40, 349, 1967.
204. **Hoffman, B. B., Lean, A., Wood, C. L., Schocken, D. D., and Lefkowitz, R. J.,** Alpha-adrenergic receptor subtypes: quantitative assessment by ligand binding, *Life Sci.,* 24, 1739, 1979.
205. **Motulsky, H. J. and Insel, P. A.,** [³H]Dihydroergocryptine binding to alpha-adrenergic receptor of human platelets: a reassessment using the selective radioligands [³H]Prazosin, [³H]Yohimbine and [³H]Rauwolscine, *Biochem. Pharmacol.,* 31, 2591, 1982.

206. **Solinger, A., Bernstein, L., and Glueck, H. I.,** The effect of epinephrine on platelet aggregation in normal and atopic subjects, *J. Allergy Clin. Immunol.,* 59, 29, 1973.

207. **Maccia, C. A., Gallagher, J. S., Ataman, G., Glueck, H. I., Brooks, S. M., and Berstein, I. L.,** Platelet thrombopathy in asthmatic patients with elevated immunoglobin E, *J. Allergy Clin. Immunol.,* 59, 101, 1977.

208. **McDonald, J. R., Tan, E. M., Stevenson, D. D., and Vaughan, J. H.,** Platelet aggregation in asthmatic and normal subjects, *J. Allergy Clin. Immunol.,* 54, 200, 1973.

209. **Sato, T., Bewtra, A. K., Hopp, R. J., and Townley, R. G.,** Alpha and beta adrenergic receptor systems in bronchial asthma and non-asthmatic subjects: reduced mononuclear cell beta receptors in bronchial asthma, *J. Allergy Clin. Immunol.,* in press.

210. **Schocken, D. D. and Roth, G. S.,** Reduced beta-adrenergic receptor concentration in aging man, *Nature,* 267, 856, 1979.

211. **Jones, S. B., Bylund, D. B., Rieser, C. A., Shekim, W. O., Byer, J. A., and Carr, G. W.,** Alpha$_2$-adrenergic receptor binding in human platelets: alterations during the menstrual cycle, *Clin. Pharmacol. Ther.,* 34, 90, 1983.

212. **Frazer, J., Nadeau, J., Robertson, D., and Wood, A. J. J.,** Regulation of human leukocyte beta receptors by endogenous catecholamines, *J. Clin. Invet.,* 67, 1777, 1981.

213. **Feldman, R. D., Limbird, L. E., Nadeau, J., Fiztzgerald, G. A., Robertson, D., and Wood, A. J.,** Dynamic regulation of leukocyte beta adrenergic receptor-agonist interactions by physiological changes in circulating catecholamines, *J. Clin. Invest.,* 72, 164, 1983.

214. **Kariman, K.,** Beta adrenergic receptor binding in lymphocytes from patients with asthma, *Lung,* 158, 41, 1980.

215. **Hoffman, B. B., Mullikin-Kilpatrick, D., and Lefkowitz, R. J.,** Desensitization of beta adrenergic stimulated adenylate cyclase in turkey erythrocytes, *J. Cyclic Nucleotide Res.,* 5, 355, 1979.

216. **Johnson, G. L., Wolfe, B. B., Harden, T. K., Molinoff, P. B., and Perkins, J. P.,** Role of beta adrenergic receptors in catecholamine-induced desensitization of adenylate cyclase in human astrocytoma cells, *J. Biol. Chem.,* 253, 1472, 1978.

217. **Wessels, M. R., Mullikin, D., and Lefkowitz, R. J.,** Selective alteration in high affinity agonist bindings: a mechanism of beta adrenergic receptor desensitization, *Mol. Pharmacol.,* 16, 10, 1979.

218. **Davies, A. O. and Lefkowitz, R. J.,** In vitro desensitization of beta adrenergic receptors in human neutrophils, *J. Clin. Invest.,* 71, 565, 1983.

219. **Safko, M. J., Chan, S. C., Cooper, K. D., and Hanifin, J. M.,** Heterologous desensitization of leukocytes: a possible mechanism of beta-adrenergic blockade in atopic dermatitis, *J. Allergy Clin. Immunol.,* 68, 218, 1981.

220. **Busse, W. W. and Sosmanm, J.,** Decreased H$_2$ histamine response of granulocytes of asthmatic patients, *J. Clin. Invest.,* 59, 1080, 1977.

221. **Grewe, S. R., Chan, S. C., and Hanifin, J. M.,** Elevated leukocyte cyclic AMP-phosphodiesterase in atopic disease: a possible mechanism for cyclic AMP-agonist hyporesponsiveness, *J. Allergy Clin. Immunol.,* 70, 452, 1982.

222. **Butler, J. M., Chan, S. C., Stevens, S., and Hanifin, J. M.,** Increased leukocyte histamine release with elevated cyclic AMP-phosphodiesterase activity in atopic dermatitis, *J. Allergy Clin. Immunol.,* 74, 490, 1983.

223. **Akagi, K. and Townley, R. G.,** Spontaneous histamine release and histamine content in normal and asthmatic subjects, *J. Allergy Clin. Immunol.,* 83, 742, 1989.

224. **Akagi, K., Kohi, F., Trivedi, R., and Townley, R. G.,** Pharmacologic modulation of spontaneous histamine release, *Ann. Allergy,* 63, 39, 1989.

225. **Bryan, L. J., Cole, J. J., O'Donnel, S. R., and Wanstoll, J. C.,** A study designed to explore the hypothesis that beta$_1$-adrenoceptors are ''innervated'' receptors and beta$_2$-adrenoceptors are ''hormonal'' receptors, *J. Pharmacol. Exp. Ther.,* 216, 395, 1981.

226. **Van den Berg, W., Leferink, J. G., Fokkens, J. K., Kreukneit, J., Maes, R. A., and Bruynzeel, P. L.,** Clinical implication of drug-induced desensitization of beta receptor after continuous oral use of terbutaline, *J. Allergy Clin. Immunol.,* 69, 410, 1982.

227. **Hasegawa, M. and Townley, R. G.,** Difference between lung and spleen susceptibility of beta-adrenergic receptors to desensitization by terbutaline, *J. Allergy Clin. Immunol.,* 71, 230, 1983.

228. **Townley, R. G., Honrath, I., and Guirgis, H. M.,** The inhibitory effect of hydrocortisone on the alpha-adrenergic responses of human and guinea pig isolated respiratory smooth muscle, *J. Allergy Clin. Immunol.,* 49, 88, 1972.

229. **Mano, K., Akbarzadeh, A., and Townley, R. G.,** Effect of hydrocortisone on beta-adrenergic receptors in lung membranes, *Life Sci.,* 25, 195, 1979.

230. **Sano, Y., Ford, L., Begley, M., Watt, G., Townley, R. G., Tsai, H., and Bewtra, A. K.,** Effect of in vivo asthma drugs on human leukocyte beta-adrenergic receptors, *Clin. Res.,* 28 (Abstr.), 431A, 1980.

231. **Davis, A. W. and Lefkowitz, R. J.,** Steroid-induced regulation of human leukocyte beta-adrenergic receptors, *J. Clin. Endocrinol. Metab.,* 51, 599, 1980.

232. **Townley, R. G., Reeb, R., Fitzgibbons, T., and Adolphson, R. L.,** The effect of corticosteroids on the beta-adrenergic receptors in bronchial smooth muscle, *J. Allergy,* 40, 118, 1970.

233. **Townley, R. G., Honrath, I., and Guirgis, H. M.,** The inhibitory effect of hydrocortisone on the alpha-adrenergic responses of human and guinea pig isolated respiratory smooth muscle, *J. Allergy Clin. Immunol.,* 49, 88, 1972.

234. **Holgate, S. T., Baldwin, C. J., and Tattersfield, A. E.,** Beta-adrenergic agonist resistance in normal human airways, *Lancet,* 11, 375, 1977.

235. **Ellul-Micallef, R. and Fenech, F F.,** Effect of intravenous prednisone in asthmatics with diminished adrenergic responsiveness, *Lancet,* 27, 1269, 1975.

236. **Coffey, R. G., Logsdon, P. J., and Middleton, E., Jr.,** Effects of glucocorticoids on leukocyte adenylate cyclase and ATPase of asthmatic and normal children, *J. Allergy Clin. Immunol.,* 49, 87, 1972.

237. **Rinand, G. A.,** Effects of hydrocortisone and isoproterenol on cyclic AMP formation and relaxation in canine trachea smooth muscle, *Fed. Proc., Fed. Am Soc. Exp. Biol.,* 38, 1082, 1979.

238. **Hayden, W., Olson, E. B., Jr., and Zachman, R. D.,** Effect of maternal isoxsuprine on fetal rabbit lung biochemical maturation, *Am. J. Obstet. Gynecol.,* 129, 691, 1977.

239. **Lawson, E. E., Brown, E. R., Torday, J. S., Madansky, D. L., and Taeusch, H. W., Jr.,** The effect of epinephrine on tracheal fluid flow and surfactant flux in fetal sheep, *Am. Rev. Respir. Dis.,* 118, 1023, 1978.

240. **Walters, D. V. and Oliver, R. E.,** The role of catecholamines in lung liquid absorption at birth, *Pediatr. Res.,* 12, 239, 1978.

241. **Cheng, J. B., Goldfien, A., Ballard, P. L., and Roberts, J. M.,** Glucocorticoid increase pulmonary beta-adrenergic receptors in fetal rabbit, *Endocrinology,* 107, 1646, 1980.

242. **Smith, B. T.,** Cell line A 549: a model system for the study of alveolar type II cell function, *Am. Rev. Respir. Dis.,* 115, 285, 1977.

243. **Fraser, C. M. and Venter, J. C.,** The synthesis of β-adrenergic receptors in cultured human lung cells: induction by glucocorticoids, *Biochem. Biphys. Res. Commun.,* 94, 390, 1980.

244. **Raaijmakers, J. A. M., Wassink, G. A., Kreukniet, J., and Terpstra, G. K.,** Adrenoreceptors in lung tissue: characterization, modulation and relations with pulmonary function, in *Receptors and Cold,* Kerrebijn, K. F., Sluiter, H. J., and Wams, H. W. A., Eds., *Excerpta Med.,* Amsterdam, 1984, 215.

245. **Barnes, P. J., Karliner, J. S., and Dollery, C. T.,** Human lung adrenoceptors studied by radioligand binding, *Clin. Sci.,* 58, 457, 1980.

246. **Barnes, P. J.,** Adrenoceptors in bronchial asthma, in *Pharmacology of Adrenoceptors,* Szbadi, E., Bradshaw, C. M., and Nahorski, S. R., Eds., Macmillan, London, 1985, 205.

247. **Hayashi, K., Taki, F., Sugiyama, S., Takagi, K., Satake, T., and Ozawa, T.,** Mechanism responsible for alterations in numbers of autonomic nerve receptors in experimental asthma, *Int. Arch. Allergy Appl. Immunol.,* 86, 170, 1988.

248. **Hasegawa, M. and Townley, R. G.,** Alpha and beta adrenergic receptors of canine lung tissue: identification and characterization of alpha adrenergic receptors by two different ligands, *Life Sci.,* 30, 1035, 1982.

249. **Latifpour, J., Jones, S. B., and Bylund, D. B.,** Characterization of [³H] yohimbine binding to putative alpha-2 adrenergic receptors in neonatal rat lung, *J. Pharmacol. Exp. Ther.,* 223, 606, 1982.

250. **Latifpour, J. and Bylund, D. B.,** Characterization of adrenergic receptor binding in rat lung: physiological regulation, *J. Pharmacol. Exp. Ther.,* 224, 186, 1983.

251. **Leff, A. R. and Munoz, N. M.,** Selective autonomic stimulation of canine trachealis with dimethylphenylpiperazinium, *J. Appl. Physiol.,* 51, 428, 1981.

252. **Liggett, S. B., Marker, J. C., Shah, S. D., Roper, C. L., and Cryer, P. E.,** Direct relationship between mononuclear leukocyte and lung beta-adrenergic receptors and apparent reciprocal regulation of extravascular, but not intravascular alpha- and beta-adrenergic receptors by the sympathochromaffin system in humans, *J. Clin. Invest.,* 82, 48, 1988.

253. **Snashall, R., Boother, F. A., and Sterling, G. M.,** The effect of alpha-adrenergic stimulation on the airways of normal and asthmatic man, *Clin. Sci.,* 54, 283, 1978.

254. **Black, J. L., Salome, C., Yan, K., and Shaw, J.,** The action of prazosin and propylene glycol on methoxamine-induced bronchoconstriction in asthmatic subjects, *Br. J. Clin. Pharmacol.,* 18, 349, 1984.

255. **Lindgren, B. R., Ekstrom, T., and Andersson, R. G. G.,** The effect of inhaled clonidine in patients with asthma, *Am. Rev. Respir. Dis.,* 134, 266, 1986.

256. **Gould, L. and Dilieto, M.,** Phentolamine, new bronchodilator, *N.Y. J. Med.,* 70, 2332, 1970.

257. **Patel, K. R. and Kerr, J. W.,** Alpha-receptor-blocking drugs in bronchial asthma, *Lancet,* 1, 348, 1975.

258. **Bianco, S., Griffin, J. P., Kamburoff, P. L., and Prime, F. J.,** Prevention of exercise-induced asthma by indoramin, *Br. Med. J.,* 4, 18, 1974.

259. **Beil, M. and de Kock, A.,** Role of alpha-adrenergic receptors in exercise-induced bronchoconstriction, *Respiration,* 35, 78, 1978.

260. **Barnes, P. J., Ind, P. W., and Dollery, C. T.,** Inhaled prazosin in asthma, *Thorax,* 36, 378, 1981.
261. **Utting, J. A.,** Alpha-adrenegic blockade in severe asthma, *Br. J. Dis. Chest.,* 73, 317, 1979.
262. **Black, J. L., Salome, C. M., Yan, K., and Shaw, J.,** Comparison between airways response to an alpha adrenoceptor agonist and histamine in asthmatic and non-asthmatic subjects, *Br. J. Clin. Pharmacol.,* 14, 464, 1982.
263. **Kaliner, M., Shelhamer, J. H., Davis, P. B., Smith, L. J., and Venter, J. C.,** NIH conference: autonomic nervous system abnormalities and allergy, *Ann. Intern. Med.,* 96, 349, 1982.
264. **Davis, P.,** Autonomic function in patients with airway obstruction, in *The Airways: Neural Control in Health and Disease,* Kaliner, M. A. and Barnes, P. J., Eds., Marcel Dekker, New York, 1988.
265. **Townley, R. G., Hopp, R. J., Agrawal, D. K., and Bewtra, A. K.,** Platelet-activating factor and airway reactivity, *J. Allergy Clin. Immunol.,* 83, 997, 1989.
266. **Meurs, H. and Zaagsma, J.,** Pharmacological and biochemical changes in airway smooth muscle in relation to bronchial hyperresponsiveness, in *Inflammatory Cells and Mediators in Bronchial Asthma,* Agrawal, D. K. and Townley, R. G., Eds., CRC Press, Boca Raton, FL, Chap. 1, in press.
267. **Rankin, J. A.,** Macrophages and their potential role in hyperreactive airways disease, in *Inflammatory Cells and Mediators in Bronchial Asthma,* Agrawal, D. K. and Townley, R. G., Eds., CRC Press, Boca Raton, FL, Chap. 5, in press.

Chapter 11

AIRWAY HISTAMINE RECEPTORS AND THEIR SIGNIFICANCE IN ALLERGIC LUNG DISEASES

N. Chand, W. Diamantis, and R. D. Sofia

TABLE OF CONTENTS

I.   Summary 260

II.   Introduction 260
        A.   Distribution and Classification of Histamine Receptor in
                Airway Smooth Muscle 261
        B.   Possible Mechanisms of Action of Histamine in the Airways
                and Lungs 264
        C.   Significance of Histamine and Histamine Receptors in Allergic
                Airway Diseases 264

III.   Antihistamines in Asthma 267

Acknowledgments 267

References 267

I. SUMMARY

Histamine is a biogenic amine which is found in large quantities in lung mast cells. It is one of the most important mediators of allergic bronchoconstriction and airway inflammation. Allergic histamine secretion in the immediate vicinity of respiratory smooth muscles, mucous glands, and epithelial and endothelial cells produces airway constriction, bronchial secretion, edema, and inflammatory reactions, mostly via H_1-histamine receptor activation. It is well established that there is an abundance of histamine H_1-receptors which mediate constrictions in the airway smooth muscles of man, swine, langur monkey, dog, horse, cattle, goat, ferret, and guinea pig. The biochemical effects of histamine, such as increased phosphatidylinositol breakdown, influx of Ca^{2+} (elevation of the cytoplasmic Ca^{2+}), formation of thromboxane A_2 (TXA_2), prostaglandin $F_{2\alpha}$ ($PGF_{2\alpha}$), or the products of lipoxygenase pathway are also mediated via H_1-receptor activation in airway smooth muscles.

The tracheobronchial smooth muscle of rhesus monkey, trachea of rabbit and cat, and sheep bronchus possess a preponderance of histamine H_2-receptors which mediate bronchodilatation. A small population of H_2-histamine receptors also exists in the bronchial smooth muscle of man, horse, and guinea pig.

The H_2-histamine receptor activation could play a modulatory role in allergic reactions in the lung of sheep, cat, horse, guinea pig, and man. Tachyphylaxis to histamine which involves PGE_2 release is also mediated via histamine H_2-receptor activation in certain respiratory smooth muscles. This could be an important protective mechanism in asthma. The physiological significance of histamine H_2-receptors in asthmatics is controversial.

Epithelium-derived contractile factor(s) (epithelin?) seem to produce a functional defect in Ca^{2+} homeostasis in airway smooth muscles which induces remarkable airway hyperreactivity to histamine in guinea pig tracheal rings. The importance of the synthesis/secretion of epithelin and its role in the induction of nonspecific airway hyperreactivity and interactions with histamine and other mediators in airways of different species remain to be established. Furthermore, the release of histamine-releasing factors (lymphokines, cytokines, interleukins, O_2^-, major basic proteins [MBP], anaphylatoxins, etc.) from inflammatory cells (lymphocytes, macrophages, monocytes, eosinophils, and PMN) could play an important role in the pathogenesis of late-phase asthmatic responses.

The development and introduction of newer, potent, orally effective, long-acting, and nonsedating H_1-receptor antagonists seem to provide an impetus to reevaluate the important role of histamine in the pathogenesis of airway inflammation (rhinitis and asthma).

II. INTRODUCTION

The lung mast cells, which contain large amounts of histamine, play a central role in the pathogenesis of asthma since this mediator is released during allergic reactions. Asthmatics exhibit remarkable airway hyperreactivity to histamine.[1-3] In addition, histamine produces diverse responses such as bronchoconstriction, lung edema, and bronchial hypersecretion (Table 1). In this chapter we will briefly summarize the recent literature on the distribution, classification, and significance of airway histamine receptors and introduce some of the newer and safer histamine H_1-receptor antagonists which offer a basis to reevaluate the role of histamine in allergic inflammatory diseases of the total airway (rhinitis and asthma). A vast amount of data on mast cells, histamine, histamine receptor agonists and antagonists, and pulmonary histamine receptors have been reviewed by several investigators.[1-3,5-7]

TABLE 1
Diverse Pharmacologic Effects of Histamine in the Lungs

Airway effects	Receptor subtype
Nose	
Tickling	H_1
Sneezing	H_1
Mucus secretion	H_1
Increased postcapillary venule permeability	H_1
Lung	
Bronchoconstriction	H_1
Increased lung epithelial permeability	H_1, H_2
Increased capillary permeability (edema)	H_1, H_2
Bronchial vasodilatation	
Bronchodilatation (small)[a]	H_2
Mucus (tracheobronchial) secretion	H_1, H_2

[a] Evident after H_1-receptor blockade in certain tissues in some species.

TABLE 2
Relatively Specific H_1- and H_2-Agonists and Antagonists

Histamine receptor subtype	Agonist	Antagonist
H_1	2-Methylhistamine	Pyrilamine
		Diphenhydramine
	Betahistine	Chlorpheniramine
	2-Pyridylethylamine	Azelastine
		Terfenadine
	Histamine	Astemizole
		Ketotifen
		Cetirizine
		Clemastine
		Azatidine
		Mequitazine
		Oxatomide
		SKF-93944
		Tazifylline
H_2	4-Methylhistamine	Burimamide
	Dimaprit	Metiamide
	Impromidine	Cimetidine
	Histamine	Ranitidine
		Oxmetidine
		YM-11170

A. DISTRIBUTION AND CLASSIFICATION OF HISTAMINE RECEPTOR IN AIRWAY SMOOTH MUSCLE

Soon after the introduction of selective H_1- and H_2-receptor agonists and antagonists[8-12] (Table 2), it was established that the overall effect of histamine on respiratory smooth muscle is very complex. It depends on the algebraic sum of a mixed population of histamine H_1- and H_2-receptors, which generally exert opposite effects. Remarkable qualitative and quantitative species and regional differences in the airway responses to histamine have been reported[5] (Table 3). There is a preponderance of H_1-receptors in the airways of swine,[13] dog,[14] guinea pig,[15,16] horse,[17] cattle,[18] langur monkey,[19] goat,[20] and man.[6,7] H_1-receptor stimulation produces constriction of tracheobronchial smooth muscle and peripheral airways of most of the species studied thus far. The H_2-receptors, which exist in preponderance in

TABLE 3
**Species and Regional Differences in the Responsiveness of the Airway
Smooth Muscle to Histamine**

	Region of the airways		
Species	Trachea	Bronchus	Lung strip (bronchioalveolar tissue)
Rat	Unresponsive Contraction	Unresponsive Contraction	Unresponsive
Ferret	Contraction	Contraction	Contraction
Rabbit	Unresponsive Relaxation[a]	Contraction	Contraction
Cat	Unresponsive Contraction Relaxation[a]	Unresponsive Contraction Relaxation[a]	Contraction
Rhesus monkey	Unresponsive Contraction	Contraction Relaxation[a]	Contraction
Swine	Unresponsive Contraction	Contraction	Contraction
Sheep	Contraction	Primary: contraction Intermediate: relaxation[a] Terminal: relaxation[a]	Contraction

[a]   Relaxation in precontracted tissues.

From Chand, N., *Adv. Pharmacol. Chemother.*, 17, 103, 1980. With permission.

the tracheobronchial smooth muscle of rhesus monkey,[21] cat[18] and rabbit[22] trachea, sheep bronchus,[18] and, to some extent, in human[5,23] and horse[5,17] bronchi as well as in guinea pig airways,[24,25] mediate relaxation (Table 4).

A dual histamine receptor mechanism exists in the lung and airways of guinea pigs.[24,25] The addition of H_2-agonists (dimaprit, impromidine) to guinea pig tracheobronchial and lung strips which were contracted with H_1-agonist (2-methylhistamine or 2-pyridylethylamine) produces concentration-dependent relaxations which were antagonized by H_2-receptor antagonists.

The lung parenchyma strips of man, cat, rabbit, horse, sheep, goat, dog, swine, cattle, and rhesus and langur monkey possess only H_1-receptors, producing peripheral airway contractions.[5] The nonrespiratory elements in lung strips, such as vascular and other contractile tissue, may also contribute to histamine effects. Thus, caution must be exercised when interpreting the data obtained in studies utilizing lung strips as a model of peripheral airway pharmacology.

The isolated tracheobronchial smooth muscle of rats, neonatal dog, calf, and swine is relatively insensitive to histamine.[5] This does not appear to be related to the existence of H_2-receptors in these tissues. These findings may suggest that the functional maturation of H_1-receptors takes place during postnatal life.[5,15]

A novel class of H_3-histamine receptors has been shown to exist at the prejunctional (presynaptic) sites of the autonomic and central nervous systems.[26] However, thus far there is no concrete evidence supporting the existence of H_3-histamine receptors in the lung. The possibility of the existence of H_2- or H_3-receptors in prejunctional (presynaptic) sites of the autonomic nervous system in the lung and their pathophysiological significance in the modulation of irritant lung receptors and cholinergic-adrenergic control of pulmonary function remain unknown.

Acidic solutions of histamine could produce airway relaxation which is not blocked by H_1- and H_2-antagonists.[5] Therefore, it is recommended that histamine and antagonists should

TABLE 4
Classification and Distribution of the Histamine Receptors in the Respiratory Smooth Muscle

Species	Respiratory smooth muscle		
	Tracheal	Bronchial	Peripheral airways (lung strip)
Guinea pig	H_1	H_1 H_2	H_1 H_2
Horse	H_1	H_1 H_2	H_1
Man	—	H_1 H_2	H_1
Rhesus monkey	H_1 H_2	H_1, H_2	H_1
Langur monkey	H_1	H_1	H_1
Swine	H_1	H_1	H_1
Neonatal piglet	H_1	H_1	H_1
Rabbit	H_1 H_2	H_1	H_1
Dog	H_1	H_1	H_1
Cat	H_1 H_2	H_1	H_1
Ferret	H_1	H_1	H_1
Chicken	—	H_1	H_1
Sheep	H_1	H_1 H_2	H_1
Goat	H_1	H_1	H_1
Cattle	H_1	H_1	H_1

Note: H_1 = contraction; H_2 = relaxation.

Updated and modified after Chand, N., *Adv. Pharmacol. Chemother.*, 17, 103, 1980. With permission.

be solubilized in phosphate buffer and/or neutralized by the addition of NaOH solution. Histamine solutions (37°C) should be used in small doses/concentrations at sufficient time intervals to prevent the development of tachyphylaxis.[27,28] The use of small doses/concentrations of indomethacin, propranolol, and atropine will eliminate the possible involvement of prostaglandins,[5,27,28] catecholamines,[5,29] and cholinergic mechanisms,[30] especially in experiments demonstrating the direct activation of histamine receptors in a biological system. The H_2-agonists (dimaprit, impromidine, and 4-methylhistamine), when used as airway relaxants, should be tested in the presence of H_1-receptor blockade in tissues which are partially precontracted with a spasmogen(s).[5,25]

Besides the species,[5] age,[15] sex,[31] and the region of the airways,[5] other factors may contribute to the differences in airway responsiveness to histamine. These include factors such as season, state of health (sensitization, asthma),[5] hormonal status, method of procurement of tissue (autopsy, postmortem, abattoir), and method of euthanasia (anesthetics,[32] ketamine, shooting, electricity, stunning, cervical dislocation, thoracotomy). Additional factors may include the duration of storage of tissue at room or cold temperatures, type of preparation (rings, chains, helical strips), absence or presence of epithelium,[36,37] resting loading tensions, recording systems (isotonic/isometric responses), composition and pH of physiological solution(s) and air or mixture of CO_2 and O_2, spontaneous tone or induced tone, the magnitude of tone, and the nature and concentration of spasmogen used to induce tone. Furthermore, dose (concentration), route of administration (aerosol, i.v.), frequency of administration of histamine, the degree of blockade of one receptor type or the presence of inhibitor of catecholamine or prostaglandin/leukotriene synthesis/release, and experimental design (*in vitro/in vivo*) may also contribute to the differences in airway histamine responses.[5]

B. POSSIBLE MECHANISMS OF ACTION OF HISTAMINE IN THE AIRWAYS AND LUNGS

The direct activation of H_1-histamine receptors on respiratory smooth muscle leads to bronchoconstriction. The blockage of H_1-receptors could unmask H_2-receptors,[5] which may be associated with adenylate cyclase activation, leading to an increase in cAMP in smooth muscles.[7,16] In addition, histamine causes bronchoconstriction by a vagal reflex mechanism in intact animals and man which is susceptible to atropine blockade.[5,30] Some airway effects of histamine are also mediated/modulated by TXA_2,[33] prostaglandin release,[27,28] and synthesis/secretion of the products of the 5-lipoxygenase pathway of arachidonic acid metabolism.[5,13,35] The increased phosphatidylinositol breakdown and increased Ca^{2+} influx/mobilization (elevation of cytoplasmic Ca^{2+}), and elevation of cGMP in response to histamine is mediated via H_1-receptor activation.[7] These biochemical changes could play an important role in the pathogenesis of allergic lung diseases (Figure 1).

C. SIGNIFICANCE OF HISTAMINE AND HISTAMINE RECEPTORS IN ALLERGIC AIRWAY DISEASES

The mechanism for the development of exclusive airway hyperreactivity to histamine and other nonspecific stimuli is not known. Epithelium removal produces a fourfold shift in the concentration-effect curve of histamine in isolated guinea pig tracheal rings (ED_{50} of histamine, intact epithelium = $2 \times 10^{-5} M$ and rubbed rings = $5 \times 10^{-6} M$). However, the exposure of guinea pig tracheal rings to subthreshold concentration of epithelial-conditioned buffer produced remarkable airway hyperreactivity to histamine (EC_{50} in intact rings = $10^{-11} M$ and in epithelial-denuded rings = $10^{-12} M$).[36] These recent experiments seem to suggest the synthesis/secretion of a contractile factor(s) (polypeptides or epithelin?) by the epithelial cells, which, perhaps, causes depolarization,[32] a defect in Ca^{2+} homeostasis, and increased phosphatidyl inositol turnover, leading to the development of exclusive airway hyperreactivity to histamine. It remains to be established whether epithelial-derived factors (epithelin?) in different animal species and man cause nonspecific airway hyperresponsiveness to other mediators (leukotrienes, acetylcholine, platelet activating factor [PAF]), or other stimuli such as cold, exercise, ozone, SO_2, viral/bacterial infections, antigens, etc.

Histamine released from perivascular and submucosal mast cells during early (immediate) allergic reactions in the lungs produces increased postcapillary venular and epithelial permeability. This results in mucosal edema and subsequent influx of neutrophils, eosinophils, and macrophages during late-phase reaction. These newly recruited and activated inflammatory cells (PMN, lymphocytes, and macrophages) generate histamine-releasing factors (HRFs),[3] while eosinophils secrete MBP and free radicals (O_2^-). HRFs, MBP, and O_2^- activate mast cells and continue the cycle of histamine secretion as well as the generation of other mediators (PAF, 5-HPETE, 5-HETE, O_2^-, lipid radicals, and interleukins) (Table 5). Many of these mediators (for example, epithelin, 5-HPETE, and PAF) may act as priming or amplifying factors in the pathogenesis of asthma, inflammation, and induction of airway hyperreactivity.[46,47] The H_1-receptor antagonists, which are also capable of inhibiting the activation of inflammatory cells (epithelial cells, endothelial cells, mast cells, eosinophils, T-lymphocytes, and macrophages), should be effective in both the early- and late-phase reactions in asthmatics.

H_1-Receptor antagonists produce bronchodilatation and attenuate aspirin-, antigen-, and exercise-induced bronchoconstriction. These observations support an important role for histamine in the pathogenesis of the allergic diseases of total airways (rhinitis and asthma).[38-44]

Histamine has been reported to stimulate the synthesis/release of $PGF_{2\alpha}$, thromboxane

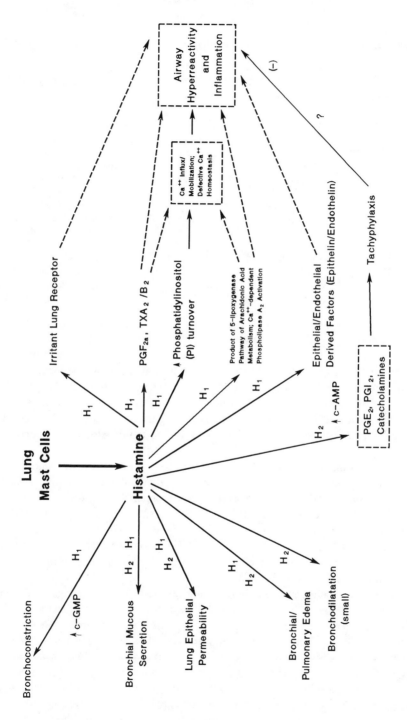

FIGURE 1. Summary of the direct and indirect effects of histamine in the lung. (−) = Antinflammatory, or protective or modulatory effects.

TABLE 5
Possible Interactions between Inflammatory Cells and Their Mediators in the Pathogenesis of Asthma

Pulmonary inflammatory cells	Main mediators	Proposed role in asthma
Alveolar macrophage	O_2^-, lysosomal enzymes	Inflammation
	PAF; leukotrienes	Airway hyperreactivity
	HRFs[a] (histamine releasing factors)	
	Others	
T-Cells (lymphocytes)	Interleukins[a]	IgE production
	Lymphokines[a]	Chemotaxis
B-Cells (lymphocytes)	Cytokines[a]	
	HRF,[a] others	
Mast cells/basophils	Histamine, leukotrienes, 5-LO products, PGD$_2$, others	Edema; cellular influx; mucus secretion; bronchoconstriction
PMN	O_2^-; lysosomal enzyme	
Platelets	PF$_4$ and others	Eosinophil chemotaxis
Eosinophils	MBP,[a] EPO[a]	Epithelial irritation/damage
	LTC$_4$, O_2^-[a]	
	Others	
Epithelial cells	Epithelin	Enhancement of airway hyperreactivity to histamine/other mediators?
Endothelial cells	Endothelin	Edema; airway hyperreactivity?

[a] Histamine-releasing activity, which possibly plays an important role in the development of inflammation and airway hyperreactivity in late phases of asthma

A_2/B_2, products of lipoxygenase pathways.[5,13,33-35] It may stimulate the synthesis/secretion of endothelial- and epithelial-derived factors (epithelin, endothelin). It also stimulates the breakdown of phosphatidylinositol (PI turnover)[7] and increases Ca^{2+} influx/mobilization in airways and increases cGMP as well as stimulates lung irritant receptors. These biochemical and pharmacological effects of histamine could lead to the development of airway hyperreactivity (Figure 1).

In addition to the activation of histamine receptors in the respiratory smooth muscles, bronchial glands, epithelial and endothelial cells, microvasculature, and other inflammatory cells (alveolar macrophages, T-lymphocytes, eosinophils, neutrophils), histamine is also capable of stimulating cholinergic "irritant" receptors. Furthermore, its interaction with other mediators, such as epithelin, endothelin, PF$_4$, PAF, lymphokines (cytokines, interleukins), O_2^-, lipid radicals, 5-HETE, 5-HPETE, leukotrienes, and chemotactic factors, could produce a complex chain of biochemical and pharmacological events in the pathogenesis of rhinitis and asthma (Table 5).

H_2-receptor blockade enhances allergic lung responses in guinea pigs[5] and potentiates histamine-induced bronchoconstriction in asthmatics in some studies.[23] Gastric H_2-histamine receptor function is depressed in asthmatic sheep, which exhibit remarkable bronchial hyperreactivity.[45] Whether or not an H_2-histamine receptor functional defect exists in leukocytes (lymphocytes, eosinophils, PMN, mast cells, basophils) and the airways of asthmatics remain to be established. In actively sensitized guinea pig lung an increased ability of histamine to release TXA$_2$ was considered due to a possible interconversion of H_2 into H_1-receptors.[33]

The adequate blockade of H_1-receptor-mediated responses (bronchoconstriction, microvascular, epithelial permeability, bronchial secretion, and irritant lung receptor activation, etc.)[38-44] by newer/safer H_1-blockers may unmask H_2-receptor-mediated, possibly anti-inflammatory (protective?) effects of histamine, such as inhibition of neutrophil lysosomal enzyme release, allergic histamine secretion, lymphokine release, T-lymphocyte-mediated

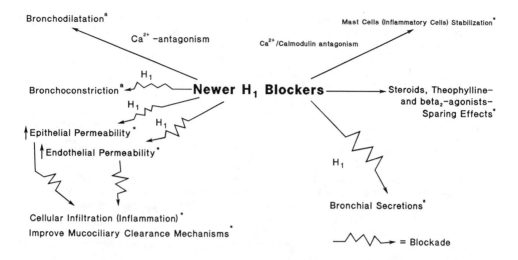

FIGURE 2. Possible antiasthmatic[a] and anti-inflammatory* activities of newer H_1-receptor antagonists. Many of their activities may extend beyond histamine-receptor antagonism.

cytotoxicity, and increase in cAMP in the lung tissues.[5] The possibilities of the modulatory role of H_2-histamine receptors in asthmatics remain controversial.[6,23] In addition, the activation of histamine H_2-receptors may stimulate mucus secretion and produce increased capillary and epithelial permeability and thus could play some role in the pathogenesis of allergic manifestations in the lungs. This anticipated beneficial clinical effect of H_2- and H_3-agonists in allergic lung diseases remains to be established.

III. ANTIHISTAMINES IN ASTHMA

Earlier H_1-blockers were contraindicated in asthmatics. Some "classical" H_1-blockers dried airway secretion and produced bronchoconstriction in some asthmatics. However, several newer H_1-receptor blockers have been reported to be safe, nonsedating, and effective in rhinitis and asthma.[38-44]

We conclude that the newer H_1-receptor blockers, which are not only capable of blocking histamine H_1-receptors, but also exert nonspecific activities, i.e., inhibition of the activation of inflammatory cells perhaps by modulating Ca^{2+}/calmodulin-dependent steps (influx/mobilization/utilization of Ca^{2+}) in target cells (epithelium, airway smooth muscles, and inflammatory cells), may be a good substitute for steroids, theophyline, and β_2-agonists in the management and treatment of asthma and other obstructive lung diseases (Figure 2).

ACKNOWLEDGMENTS

The authors wish to thank Carolyn Denham for her secretarial assistance.

REFERENCES

1. **Kay, A. B.,** Provoked asthma and mast cells, *Am. Rev. Respir. Dis.,* 135, 1200, 1987.
2. **Holgate, S. T., Hardy, C., Howarth, P. H., Robinson, C., Church, M. K., and Asius, R. M.,** Bronchial mucosal mast cells and their implications in the pathogenesis of asthma, *Bull. Eur. Physiopathol. Respir.,* 22, 39, 1986.

3. **Kaliner, M.,** Asthma and mast cell activation, *J. Allergy Clin. Immunol.,* 83, 510, 1989.
4. **Aviado, D. M. and Sadavongvivad, C.,** Pharmacological significance of biogenic amines in the lungs: histamine, *Br. J. Pharmacol.,* 38, 366, 1970.
5. **Chand, N.,** Distribution and classification of airway histamine receptors: the physiological significance of histamine H$_2$-receptors, *Adv. Pharmacol. Chemother.,* 17, 103, 1980.
6. **Eiser, N. M., Mills, J., Snashall, P. D., and Guz, A.,** The role of histamine receptors in asthma, *Clin. Sci.,* 60, 363, 1981.
7. **Joad, J. and Casale, T. B.,** Histamine and airway caliber, *Ann. Allergy,* 61, 1, 1988.
8. **Ash, A. S. F. and Schild, H. O.,** Receptors mediating some actions of histamine, *Br. J. Pharmacol. Chemother.,* 27, 427, 1966.
9. **Black, J. W., Duncan, W. A. M., Durant, C. J., Ganellin, C. R., and Parsons, E. M.,** Definition and antagonism of histamine H$_2$-receptors, *Nature,* 236, 385, 1972.
10. **Brimblecombe, R. W., Duncan, W. A. M., Durant, G. J., Emmett, J. C., Ganellin, C. R., and Parsons, M. E.,** Cimetidine — a non-thiourea H$_2$-receptor antagonist, *J. Int. Med. Res.,* 3, 86, 1975.
11. **Ganellin, C. R., Durant, G. J., and Emmett, J. C.,** Some chemical aspects of histamine H$_2$-receptor antagonists, *Fed. Proc., Fed. Am. Soc. Exp. Biol.,* 35, 1924, 1976.
12. **Durant, G J., Ganellin, C. R., and Parsons, M. E.,** Dimaprit, [S-]3-(N,N-dimethyla-mino)propyl[isothiourea]. A highly specific histamine H$_2$-receptor agonist. Part 2. Structure-activity considerations, *Agents Actions,* 7, 39, 1977.
13. **Mitchell, H. W.,** The effect of inhibitors of arachidonic acid metabolism on drug-induced contractions in isolated tracheal smooth muscle of the pig, *Br. J. Pharmacol.,* 75, 129, 1982.
14. **Bradley, S. L. and Russell, J. A.,** Distribution of histamine receptors in isolated canine airways, *J. Appl. Physiol.,* 54, 693, 1983.
15. **Douglas, J. S., Duncan, P. G., and Mukhopadhyay, A.,** The antagonism of histamine-induced tracheal and bronchial muscle contraction by diphenhydramine: effect of maturation, *Br. J. Pharmacol.,* 83, 697, 1984.
16. **Duncan, P. G., Brink, C., Adolphson, R. L., and Douglas, J. S.,** Cyclic nucleotides and contraction/relaxation in airway muscle: H$_1$ and H$_2$ agonists and antagonists, *J. Pharmacol. Exp. Ther.,* 215, 434, 1980.
17. **Chand, N. and Eyre, P.,** Spasmolytic action of histamine in airway smooth muscle of horse, *Agents Actions,* 8, 191, 1978.
18. **Eyre, P.,** Pulmonary histamine H$_1$ and H$_2$ receptor studies, in *Asthma II Physiology, Immunopharmacology and Treatment,* Austen, K. F. and Lichtenstein, L., Eds., Academic Press, New York, 1977, 164.
19. **Chand, N., Dhawan, B. N., Srimal, R. C., Rahmani, N. H., Shukla, R. K., and Altura, B. M.,** Reactivity of airway smooth muscles to bronchoactive agents in langur monkeys, *J. Appl. Physiol.,* 50, 513, 1981.
20. **Chand, N., DeRoth, L., and Eyre, P.,** Relaxant response to 5-hydroxytryptamine on goat trachea mediated by D-tryptamine receptor, *Br. J. Pharmacol.,* 66, 331, 1979.
21. **Chand, N., Dhawan, B. N., Srimal, R. C., Rahmani, N. H., Shukla, R. K., and Altura, B. M.,** Reactivity of tracheal, bronchi, and lung strips to histamine and carbachol in rhesus monkeys, *J. Appl. Physiol.,* 49, 729, 1980.
22. **Kenakin, T. P. and Beek, D.,** A quantitative analysis of histamine H$_2$-receptor-mediated relaxation of rabbit trachea, *J. Pharmacol. Exp. Ther.,* 220, 353, 1982.
23. **Hofman, J., Michalska, I., Rutkowski, R., and Chyrek-Borowska, S.,** The role of H$_2$-receptors in bronchial reactivity in atopic asthma, *Agents Actions,* 23, 370, 1988.
24. **Chand, N. and DeRoth, L.,** Dual histamine receptor mechanism of guinea-pig lung, *Pharmacology,* 19, 185, 1979.
25. **Wieczorek, W. J. and D'Mello, A.,** Effect of drug-induced tone on the ability of histamine H$_2$ receptor agonists to relax guinea-pig tracheal chain, *J. Pharm. Pharmacol.,* 34, 269, 1982.
26. **Ishikawa, S. and Sperelakis, N.,** A novel class (H$_3$) of histamine receptors on perivascular nerve terminals, *Nature,* 327, 158, 1987.
27. **Anderson, W. H., Krzanowski, J. J., Polson, J. B., and Szentivanyi, A.,** The effect of prostaglandin E$_2$ on histamine-stimulated calcium mobilization as a possible explanation for histamine tachyphylaxis in canine tracheal smooth muscle, *Naunyn-Schmiedeberg's Arch. Pharmacol.,* 322, 72, 1983.
28. **Watanabe, T., Duncan, R., Lockey, R. F., and Krzanowski, J. J., Jr.,** Histamine tachyphylaxis in young dog airway — compared with adult dog, *Arch. Int. Pharmacodyn. Ther.,* 295, 204, 1988.
29. **Williams, J. C., Conaty, J. M., and Townshend-Piala, P.,** On the mechanism of histamine-induced bronchodilation in conscious guinea-pigs, *Agents Actions,* 15, 285, 1984.
30. **Kikuchi, Y., Okayama, H., Okayama, M., Sasaki, H., and Takishima, T.,** Interaction between histamine and vagal stimulation on tracheal smooth muscle in dogs, *J. Appl. Physiol.,* 56, 590, 1984.
31. **Gertner, A., Bromberger-Barnea, B., Traystman, R., and Menkes, H.,** Airway reactivity in the periphery of the lung in mongrel dogs: male and female differences, *Am. Rev. Respir. Dis:,* 126, 1020, 1982.

32. **Maggi, C. A., Santicioli, P., Evangelista, S., and Meli, A.,** The effect of urethane on histamine-induced contraction of guinea-pig tracheal smooth muscle, *Experientia,* 38, 1474, 1982.

33. **Berti, F. Folco, C., Nicosia, S., Omini, C., and Pasargiklian, R.,** The role of histamine H_1- and H_2- receptors in the generation of thromboxane A_2 in perfused guinea-pig lungs, *Br. J. Pharmacol.,* 65, 629, 1979.

34. **Higgs, G. A.,** The mechanism of indomethacin-induced airway hyper-reactivity, *Br. J. Pharmacol.,* 85, 223P, 1985.

35. **Mitchell, H. W.,** Pharmacological studies into cyclo-oxygenase, lipoxygenase and phospholipase in smooth muscle contraction in the isolated trachea, *Br. J. Pharmacol.,* 82, 549, 1984.

36. **Doupnik, C. A.,** Airway smooth muscle hyperresponsiveness induced by a factor(s) released from guinea pig tracheal epithelial cells, *Am. Rev. Respir. Dis.,* 139, A615, 1989.

37. **Lee, H.-K.,** Endothelin-induced Ca^{2+}-dependent membrane excitability in ferret bronchial smooth muscle, *Am. Rev. Respir. Dis,* 139, A468, 1989.

38. **Eiser, N. M.,** Histamine receptors in the bronchi, *Eur. J. Respir. Dis.,* 128, 21, 1983.

39. **Holgate, S. T. and Finnerty, J. P.,** Antihistamines in asthma, *J. Allergy Clin. Immunol.,* 83, 537, 1989.

40. **Perhach, J. L., Chand, N., Diamantis, W., Sofia, R. D., and Rosenberg, A.,** Azelastine — a novel oral antiasthma compound with several modes of action, in *Allergy and Asthma, New Trends and Approaches to Therapy,* Kay, A. B., Ed., Blackwell Scientific, Oxford, 1989, 236.

41. **Rossoni, G., Omini, C., Folco, G. C., Visano, T., Brunelli, G., and Berti, F.,** Bronchodilating activity of mequitazine, *Arch. Int. Pharmacodyn, Ther.,* 268, 128, 1984.

42. **Rafferty, P. and Holgate, S. T.,** Terfenadine (seldane) is a potent and selective histamine H1 receptor antagonist in asthmatic airways, *Am. Rev. Respir. Dis.,* 136, 181, 1987.

43. **Clissold, S. P., Sorkin, E. M., and Goa, K. L.,** Loratadine, a preliminary review of its pharmacodynamic properties and therapeutic efficacy, *Drugs,* 37, 42, 1989.

44. **Sly, R. M. et al.,** The use of antihistamine in patients with asthma, *Am. Acad. Allergy Immunol.,* 82, 481, 1988.

45. **Gonzalez, H. and Ahmed, T.,** Suppression of gastric H_2-receptor mediated function in patients with bronchil asthma and ragweed allergy, *Chest,* 89, 491, 1986.

46. **Chand, N., Mahoney, T. P., Jr., Diamantis, W., and Sofia, R. D.,** Induction of airway hyperreactivity to cold provocation by BAY K-8644 and chemical mediaotrs in ferret trachea, *Am. Rev. Respir. Dis.,* 137, 419, 1988.

47. **Chand, N., Mahoney, T. P., Diamantis, W., and Sofia, R. D.,** The amplifier role of platelet activating factor (PAF), other chemical mediators and antigen in the induction of airway hyperreactivity to cold, *Eur. J. Pharmacol.,* 123, 315, 1986.

Chapter 12

MECHANICAL PROPERTIES OF AIRWAY SMOOTH MUSCLE

C. Y. Seow

TABLE OF CONTENTS

I.   Introduction 272

II.   Conceptual Mechanical Model of Muscle 273

III.   Time-Dependent Smooth-Muscle Mechanical Properties 273
        A.   Time-Dependent Force-Velocity Relations 273
        B.   Time-Dependent Series Elasticity 278

IV.   Length-Dependent Smooth-Muscle Mechanical Properties 284
        A.   Length-Dependent Maximum Shortening Velocity 284
        B.   Length-Dependent Series Elasticity 286

V.   Alteration in Mechanical Properties of Airway Smooth Muscle in Canine Asthmatic
        Model 286

VI.   Conclusion 293

Acknowledgments 293

References 295

I. INTRODUCTION

The basics of airway smooth-mucle mechanics, such as length-tension and tension-velocity relations, have been thoroughly described in some reviews,[1-3] including recent ones.[4-6] This chapter emphasizes new developments in the research of airway smooth-muscle mechanics in recent years. Our understanding of smooth-muscle contraction has been derived in many aspects from our knowledge about the contractile properties of striated muscle. Books and review articles on striated-muscle mechanics[7-12] therefore are useful in providing a good background for studying smooth-muscle mechanics. Airway smooth muscle shares many common features with other smooth muscles. Familiarity with the mechanical properties of smooth muscle in general[13-18] should also benefit our understanding of the properties of airway smooth muscle.

Surprisingly little is known about the physiological role airway smooth muscle plays.[19] Speculation on its functions include: maintenance of ventilation/perfusion balance; reduction of anatomic dead space; and stabilization of airways during forced expiration. Solid experimental evidence is still needed to substantiate the above speculations. The role of airway smooth muscle in producing the respiratory distress of asthma, however, seems unambiguous.[20-24] Because of this, studies of airway smooth muscle constitute an important part of asthma research.

Regulation of smooth-muscle contraction is different from that of striated muscle. To interpret mechanical data from smooth-muscle studies in the light of striated muscle, caution is needed. Activation of actomyosin ATPase activity in smooth muscle requires phosphorylation of the 20,000-Da myosin light chain[25] by myosin light-chain kinase, which is in turn activated by binding to calcium-calmodulin complex.[26] Dillon et al.[27] first showed in vascular smooth muscle that both myosin phosphorylation and shortening velocity increased rapidly during the initial phase of contraction. The values of both parameters peaked before the isometric tension reached plateau, then decreased to about 50% of their respective peak values during the sustained phase of contraction. Kamm and Stull[28] observed the same phenomenon in bovine trachealis. These observations have led Dillon et al.[27] to propose that dephosphorylation of attached cross bridges produced the so-called "latch" bridges that are characterized by their low cycling rate and hence the ability to maintain tension with low energy cost. The kinetic model proposed by Hai and Murphy[29] suggests that calcium-calmodulin activation of myosin light-chain kinase alone may be necessary and sufficient to explain the cycling and latch bridges. The spatial-temporal model proposed by Rasmussen et al.,[30] however, suggests that the initial transient rise in cytosolic calcium is responsible for the activation (via calcium-calmodulin complex) of a subset of phosphoproteins including the 20,000-Da myosin light chain, and results in the formation of the phosphorylated, cycling cross bridges. The sustained phase of smooth-muscle contraction, on the other hand, is thought to be brought about by the interaction of calcium with diacylglycerol, to cause the association of protein kinase C with the plasma membrane. Activation of protein kinase C in turn phosphorylates another subset of phosphoproteins, including some cytoskeletal proteins, and somehow prolongs the contraction in the absence, or reduced phosphorylation, of myosin light chain. Phosphorylation of cytoskeletal proteins presumably could change the mechanical properties of the cytoskeleton and result in maintenance of tension without or with little participation of the cross bridges.

In addition to the above two models, several mechanisms[31-34] have been proposed to explain the "latch" phenomenon, that is, tension maintenance with reduced phosphorylation and cycling rate of the cross bridges. There are controversies with regard to the mechanisms underlying the latch state in smooth-muscle contraction, whereas the existence of the latch state itself is well accepted.[27,35-38] Through mechanical experiments[35,36] we have confirmed the presence of "latch" bridges in canine trachealis, a preparation used in the studies that make up the bulk of the work upon which this chapter is based. Studies on the changes of mechanical properties of smooth muscle during contraction (both isometric and isotonic) are important for elucidating the subcellular mechanism of contraction. Some of the conventional methods used in studies of striated-muscle mechanics have been shown to be inappropriate for smooth muscle. For instance, the finding that the force-velocity relation in smooth muscle is time dependent[36] suggests that the conventional method (i.e., the isotonic afterloaded method) for obtaining force-velocity curve is invalid, because the time variable is not held constant during the measurement. The time- and length-dependent muscle properties such as maximum shortening velocity, stiffness, and maximum amount of shortening are emphasized in this chapter. The alteration of the properties in sensitized canine trachealis is also discussed.

II. CONCEPTUAL MECHANICAL MODEL OF MUSCLE

Figure 1A depicts idealized tension and length records of a quick-release experiment. Before the quick release, the muscle is developing a tetanic force P_0. After the release, it is no longer held at constant length, but at constant force P. Figure 1B depicts a four-component conceptual model of muscle. The components are defined functionally; their possible anatomical counterparts in the muscle will be discussed in later sections. The parallel elastic component (PEC) acts in parallel with the part of the muscle which generates force, the contractile element (CE). Together, the PEC and the series elastic component (SEC) account for the passive tension properties of muscle. Quick-release experiments have provided direct evidence of the existence of a SEC, as shown in Figure 1A. The rapid change in length which accompanies the sharp change in load is consistent with the mechanical definition of a spring in which force is purely a function of spring length. It is assumed that the CE is damped by a viscous element (VE) and cannot change its length instantaneously. The quick elastic recoil after quick release, therefore, is thought to stem entirely from the SEC. The model has proven very useful in analyzing the pure mechanical features of muscle and it will be referred to frequently in the following sections.

III. TIME-DEPENDENT SMOOTH-MUSCLE MECHANICAL PROPERTIES

The "latch" bridge phenomenon observed in smooth-muscle contraction[27,35-38] suggests that to characterize smooth-muscle force-velocity and length-velocity relations, one extra dimension has to be added, that is, time (after onset of stimulation). The "time" variable probably reflects the time course of change in phosphorylation and dephosphorylation of a certain subset of phosphoproteins, and also the delivery of energy for force and shortening generation by hydrolysis of ATP during smooth-muscle contraction.

A. TIME-DEPENDENT FORCE-VELOCITY RELATIONS

Figure 2 shows typical force-velocity curves for canine tracheal smooth muscle measured by quick-release technique (Figure 1) at the early (2 s) and late (8 s) phases of electrically elicited contraction of canine trachealis. The force-velocity data were fitted with the hyperbolic Hill equation. Clearly, the force-velocity characteristics are different at different point in time during the isometric contraction. Kamm and Stull[28] observed the same time dependency of the force-velocity relations in bovine trachealis. Similar observation was made in arterial smooth muscle by Dillon et al.[27] It appears that the time-dependent change in the values of the force-velocity parameters occurs in contraction of all types of smooth muscle. Therefore, the velocity predicted by the Hill equation should not be a function of load alone, but also of time. A more generalized Hill equation (at least for smooth muscle) should be

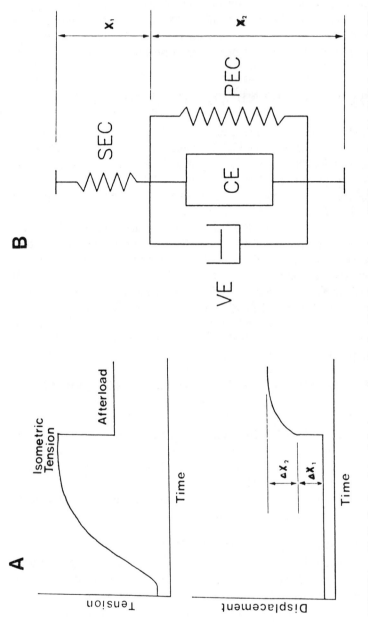

FIGURE 1.   (A) Idealized tension and displacement records of a quick-release experiment. (B) Conceptual model of muscle. ΔX_1 and ΔX_2 represent displacements (after quick release) of X_1 and X_2, respectively. SEC, series elastic component; PEC, parallel elastic component; CE, contractile element; VE, viscous element.

275

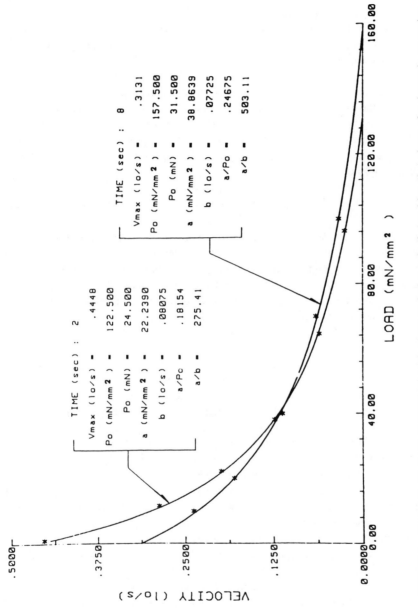

FIGURE 2. Force-velocity curves measured by quick-release method at early (2 s) and late (8 s) phases of an isometric contraction. (From Seow, C. Y. and Stephens, N. L., *Am. J. Physiol.*, 251(20), C362, 1986. With permission.)

$$V(P,t) = b(t)[P_0(t) - P]/[P + a(t)] \tag{1}$$

where V is the shortening velocity; P is the load on muscle; $P_0(t)$ is the maximum isometric tension at *time t*; and a(t) and b(t) are the time functions of the Hill constants a and b. By obtaining force-velocity curves at 1-s intervals throughout the contraction, the time behavior of the functions $P_0(t)$, a(t), and b(t) can be delineated, as shown in Figures 3 and 4 for canine trachealis. Constant b probably is a true constant, with respect to load and time. Constant a is constant with respect to load (because of the observed close fit of the force-velocity data to the Hill equation); however, it is not constant with respect to time (Figure 3). The maximum shortening velocity (V_{max}) of the muscle is also shown in Figure 4. It shows a characteristic (for smooth muscle) transient increase during the early phase of contraction. In contrast to V_{max}, $P_0(t)$ increases monotonically (Figure 4).

In muscular contraction, the force generated by the cross bridges is counterbalanced by the external load. If the external load (P) is less than the force generated by the cross bridges (P_0), muscle shortening will occur. The magnitude of the shortening velocity (V) will depend on the load (P) on muscle. If the shortening velocity is not constant with respect to time, acceleration (*a*) of the center of mass of the muscle will also occur. A simple mathematical description of the mechanical events therefore is

$$P_0 = P + \alpha V + \beta a \tag{2}$$

where α and β are coefficients: α possesses the same unit as the coefficient of viscosity; β possesses the same unit as mass. In fact, β is the equivalent mass of the muscle. If the muscle strip is fixed at one end and free to shorten at the other, as it is in most *in vitro* experimental setups, β is exactly one half of the mass of the muscle. The magnitude of the inertial force (βa), however, is negligible in isolated muscle in contraction.[36,39] Therefore, the term βa can be neglected, and Equation 2 becomes

$$P_0 = P + \alpha V \tag{3}$$

P_0, P, and V are all experimentally determinable; therefore, the value of the coefficient α can also be obtained experimentally ($\alpha = [P_0 - P]/V$). If we treat the muscle as a "black box", and apply a force step ($P_0 - P$) to the muscle, the resulting velocity (V) can be measured. The correlating factor between the force step and velocity is α, and it is a property of the "black box". This is analogous to electrical resistance correlating voltage drop and current, or flow resistance correlating pressure drop and flow velocity of fluid through a pipe. It is logical then to call α the internal resistance to shortening. In smooth muscle the internal resistance is a function of time. This can be seen clearly in Figure 4. Especially in the region where P_0 is constant (from 6 to 10 s), the change of α with time can be demonstrated unambiguously. For instance, quick release of the muscle from P_0 to zero load at 6 s results in a shortening velocity of 0.28 (l_0/s) $\pm$ 0.07 (l_0 is the optimum muscle length). The same quick release at 10 s results in a significantly ($p < 0.05$) reduced shortening velocity of 0.22 (l_0/s) $\pm$ 0.06. Since the force step ($P_0 - P$) is the same, according to Equation 3, the change in V with time is due to the change in α with time. If indeed the slowing down of the cycling rate of the cross bridges is due to the formation of latch bridges,[27,29] then the increase in internal resistance (α) with time is a direct reflection of the impeding effect of the latch bridges.

As mentioned earlier, α can be measured experimentally. When values of α at different loads are plotted as a function of load, a straight line is obtained. An arbitrary linear function for α is

$$\alpha = (a + P)/b \tag{4}$$

277

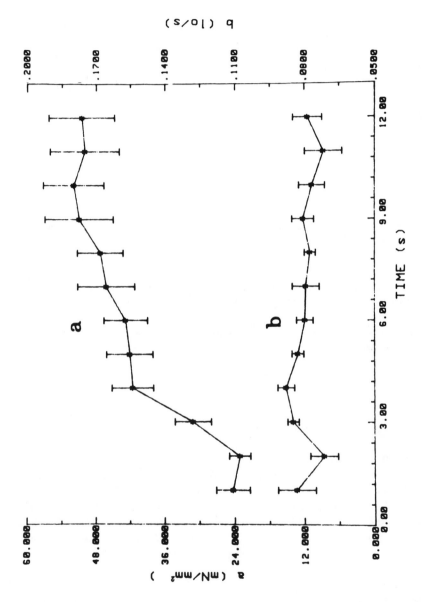

FIGURE 3. Hill's constants a and b as function of time. Means ± SE are shown; n = 5. (From Seow, S. Y. and Stephens, N. L., *Am. J. Physiol.*, 251(20), C362, 1986. With permission.)

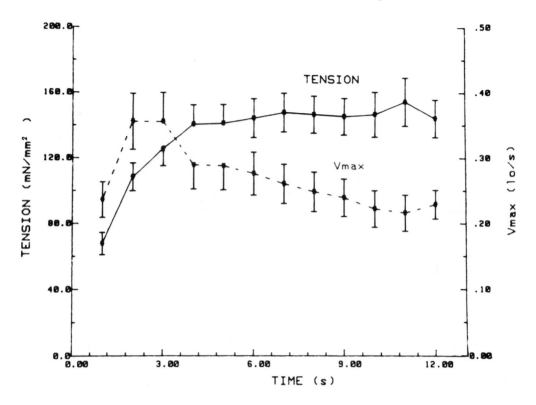

FIGURE 4.   Isometric tension and maximum velocity as functions of time. Means ± SE are shown; n = 5. (From Seow, C. Y. and Stephens, N. L., *Am. J. Physiol.,* 251(20), C362, 1986. With permission.)

where a and b are constants. Substitute α in Equation 3 with Equation 4, and Equation 3 becomes the Hill equation:

$$P_0 = P + [(a + P)/b]V \qquad (5)$$

When muscle is shortening against zero load (P = 0), the internal resistance is a/b. Figure 5 shows a/b as a function of time. It reveals a progressive increase in the internal resistance with time.

The four-component model presented in Figure 1B is capable of simulating the complex time behavior of the force-velocity relations in smooth muscle. The "viscous" force αV (from Equation 3) can be represented by the force stemming from the VE. The coefficient of viscosity for the VE, of course, has to be a function of both load and time, instead of being a constant. It should be pointed out that the force-velocity behavior of a muscle is not governed by the simple "mechanical dashpot", but rather (or mainly) by biochemical processes (that are both load- and time-dependent) that control the cross-bridge cycle.

B. TIME-DEPENDENT SERIES ELASTICITY

Stiffness of the SEC of muscle is thought to be directly proportional to the number of attached cross bridges.[40-48] The stress-strain curve for the SEC can be obtained by the quick-release method (Figure 1). Knowing the amount of elastic recoil (ΔX_1 in Figure 1A) and the corresponding force step, a stress-strain curve can be constructed.[48] The curve is exponential in shape.[48-51] An equation widely used to describe the curve is

$$\sigma = (E_0/A)(e^{A\epsilon} - 1) \qquad (6)$$

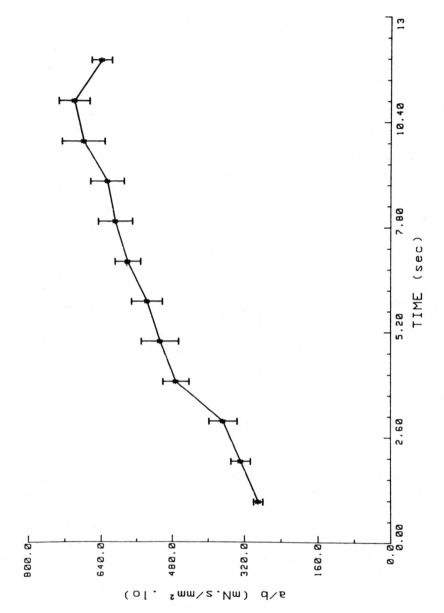

FIGURE 5. Internal resistance to shortening under zero external load (a/b) as a function of time. Means ± SE are shown; n = 5. (From Seow, C. Y. and Stephens, N. L., *Am. J. Physiol.*, 251(20), C362, 1986. With permission.)

where σ is the stress in the SEC, ϵ is the strain of the SEC (normalized to l_0), E_0 is the initial elastic modulus, and A is a constant. Studies[40,49-51] have shown that the SEC stiffness and the stress are linearly related. A linear equation describing the relationship is

$$d\sigma/d\epsilon = E_0 + A\sigma \qquad (7)$$

where $d\sigma/d\epsilon$ is the stiffness. By defining that $\epsilon = 0$ when $\sigma = 0$, Equation 7 can be integrated to give Equation 6.

Figure 6 shows typical stress-strain curves of canine trachealis obtained at different times in contraction and also at rigor and resting conditions. It is clear that the SEC is more compliant at resting condition than that at rigor condition. This is believed to be a reflection of the fact that the number of attached cross bridges is less in resting than in rigor muscle. The stress-strain curves obtained at different times are different, and the variation in stiffness is within the limits of the stiffness set by the resting (lower limit) and rigor (upper limit) muscle. This is in agreement with X-ray diffraction studies of striated muscle, in which it is found that "the changes in structure that occur when a relaxed muscle is activated are in the direction of those changes that occur when a relaxed muscle goes into rigor".[52]

Stiffness is defined as the slope of the stress-strain curve. From Figure 6 it is clear that the curves are not linear. Therefore, the stiffnesses are different at different stress levels. To compare stiffnesses, a common stress level has to be specified. Figure 7 shows the constant-stress stiffness as a function of muscle-contraction time. The preload on muscle (dashed line shown in Figure 6) was chosen as the constant stress level for calculating the $A\sigma$ values in Figure 7. According to Equation 7, the total stiffness equals E_0, which is stress-independent, plus $A\sigma$, which depends on stress linearly. For canine trachealis contracting at or near l_0, the initial elastic modulus (E_0) is small (Figure 7), and remains constant throughout contraction. Constant A (the slope of the stiffness-stress curve) therefore is the only important parameter that characterizes the SEC stiffness.

Constant A, however, is not constant with respect to time, nor is isometric tension constant throughout the time course of contraction (Figure 7). The continuous measurement of the dynamic SEC stiffness using high-frequency length perturbations therefore involves a changing value of A with time and a changing P_0 with time. The dynamic stiffness can be described by the modified Equation 7:

$$d\sigma/d\epsilon = E_0 + A(t) \cdot P_0(t) \qquad (8)$$

where $A(t)$ is the time function of A. The instantaneous isometric tension $P_0(t)$ is the load on the SEC when muscle is contracting isometrically. By plotting the dynamic stiffness [$E_0 + A(t)P_0(t)$] and the isometric tension [$P_0(t)$] vs. time (Figure 8), a shift to the left of the dynamic stiffness curve compared to the isometric tension curve is found. Similar results have been found in skeletal muscle[41,42] and smooth muscle.[46,53] Their interpretation is that a long-lived state exists between cross-bridge attachment and force generation. Data shown in Figure 8 seem to confirm the existence of such a state in canine trachealis. However, the change of $A(t)$ value during contraction is at least partly responsible for the leftward shift of the dynamic stiffness curve. Mathematically speaking, it is the time dependence of constant A that prevents the superimposition of the stiffness and isometric tension curves (Figure 8). If we assume that A is constant with respect to time, then the dynamic stiffness [$E_0 + A P_0(t)$; note that $A(t)$ is replaced by A] is proportional to the isometric tension $P_0(t)$. By selecting the proper scales, the two curves can be made to superimpose. In our experiment it is the fact that $A(t)$ is greater early in contraction compared with the $A(t)$ at the plateau of contraction, that results in the left-shift of the dynamic stiffness curve. As mentioned earlier, since the value of E_0 is relatively small and time independent, constant A directly

281

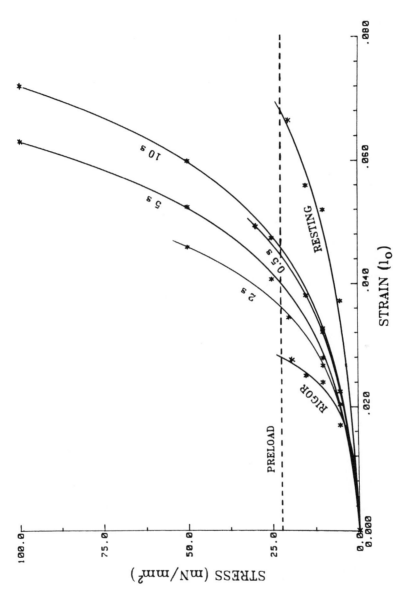

FIGURE 6. Stress-strain curves of the series elastic component from a single experiment. Equation 6 was used to fit the data. Labels on the curves indicate state of muscle under which the curves were obtained. Time (in seconds) labeled on the curves indicates time in contraction when the curve was obtained. Dashed line indicates stress level (preload in this case) at which stiffnesses of SEC were compared. Constant-stress stiffness was obtained by measuring slopes of stress-strain curves at intersections of the broken line and the curves; l_0, optimum muscle length. (From Seow, C. Y. and Stephens, N. L., *J. Appl. Physiol.*, 62(4), 1556, 1987. With permission.)

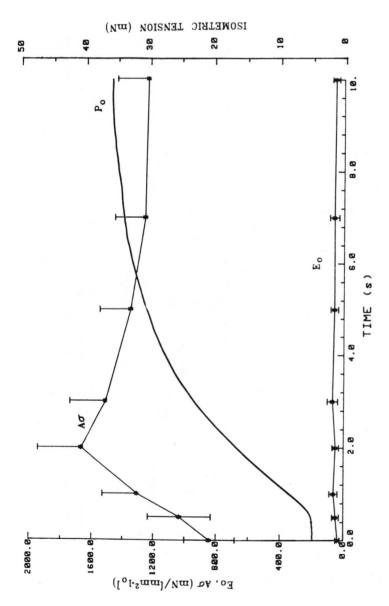

FIGURE 7.   SEC stiffness is broken down into two components: E_0 (initial elastic modulus, stress independent) and $A\sigma$ (stress dependent, where A is slope and σ is stress) and both are plotted against time. Means ± SE are shown. $n = 4$. Isometric tension curve (solid line with no SE bars) is plotted to illustrate time relationship of stages in contraction. (From Seow, C. Y. and Stephens, N. L., *J. Appl. Physiol.*, 62(4), 1556, 1987. With permission.)

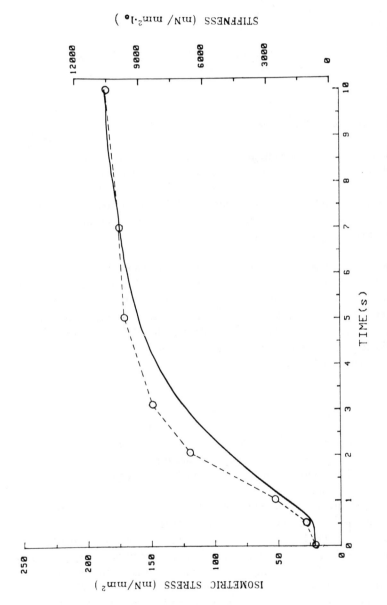

FIGURE 8. Isometric stress curve (solid line) and the associated dynamic stiffness curve (broken line). The circles are Stiffnesses at various times calculated from Equation 7, based on the mean values of E_0 and A from four experiments. The stress (σ) at corresponding times are obtained from the isometric stress curve shown in the figure (solid line). Note that unlike the stiffness curve shown in Figure 7, stiffness here is obtained at different stress levels. (From Seow, C. Y. and Stephens, N. L., *J. Appl. Physiol.*, 62(4), 1556, 1987. With permission.)

reflects the SEC stiffness (at any stress level), which could be directly related to the number of attached cross bridges. Therefore, the shift to the left of the stiffness curve could partly be due to the fact that the number of attached cross bridges is greater early in contraction than at plateau.

The V_{max} (Figure 4) and constant-stress stiffness $[E_0 + A\sigma]$ (Figure 8) vary in a very similar fashion with time. Studies[27,28] have shown that shortening velocity and myosin light-chain phosphorylation vary in a similar manner with time. These findings, together with our observation, suggest that myosin phosphorylation, maximum shortening velocity, and stiffness of muscle are intimately related.

IV. LENGTH-DEPENDENT SMOOTH-MUSCLE MECHANICAL PROPERTIES

Smooth muscle has a greater physiological shortening capacity than do skeletal or cardiac muscle.[1,18] For striated muscle, under normal physiological condition, there is no need for it to shorten much below its *in situ* length. In smooth muscle, a physiological working length range is difficult to define. In airway and vascular smooth muscle, from a pathological point of view, it is the behavior of the muscle at short lengths that seems to be important. For instance, asthma and essential hypertension in animals models seem to be associated with an increased ability of the smooth muscle to shorten.[22,24,54,55] Characterization of smooth-muscle mechanical properties as a function of muscle length therefore has meaningful physiological (or pathophysiological) implications.

A. LENGTH-DEPENDENT MAXIMUM SHORTENING VELOCITY
In muscle contraction, shortening per se results in reduction of shortening velocity of the muscle.[56-60] In skeletal muscle it is found that at sarcomere length <1.65 μm (about 75% of optimum sarcomere length) the velocity of shortening decreases linearly with length.[58] In cardiac muscle the zero-load velocity is reduced if the length is less than about 87% of l_0.[56] For the multicellular preparation of canine trachealis (Figure 9), the decrease of zero-load velocity with reduced muscle length is gradual, and can be fitted with a parabolic function of the form

$$V_0(l) = V_{max}\{1 - [(1 - l)/(1 - l_{min})]^2\} \qquad (9)$$

where $V_0(l)$ is the zero-load velocity at muscle length l, V_{max} is the zero-load velocity at l_0, l_{min} is the minimum muscle length or the maximally contracted length under zero load. The two important parameters that determine the velocity-length curve therefore are V_{max} and $l_{min.}$

The mechanisms underlying the decrease in shortening velocity at $l < l_0$ could be many. One well-observed phenomenon is shortening inactivation. This has been described in skeletal,[61] cardiac,[56,62] and smooth muscles.[63] The reduced tension due to shortening inactivation could affect the shortening velocity. Reduction in tension at short muscle length could also result from the fact that the muscle is operating on the ascending phase of the length-tension curve of the muscle. This could also reduce the shortening velocity if there is an internal load. An internal viscoelastic load in actively shortening cat papillary muscle is well described by Chiu et al.[57] A recent study by Harris et al.[64] provides some evidence of internal load in single smooth-muscle cells. A study by Gunst[59] on the effect of length history on contractile behavior of tracheal smooth muscle shows that the initial muscle length and the shortening process per se affect the rate and the magnitude of force redevelopment. This suggests that different V_0-length-time surfaces would be obtained if contraction started at different initial lengths.

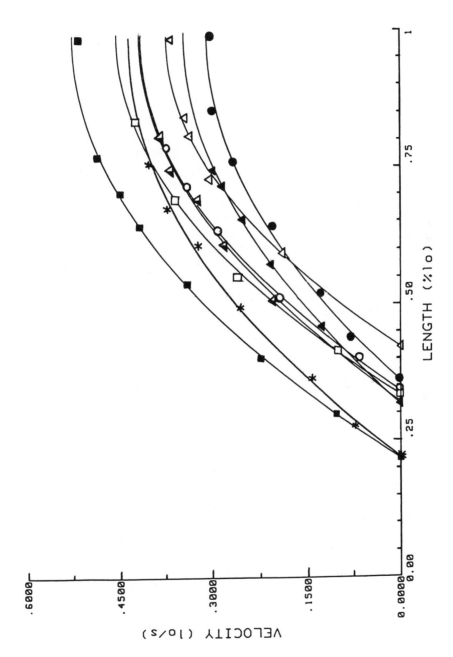

FIGURE 9. Zero-load velocity as a function of muscle length. Curves were all obtained at 5 s after stimulation. Data were fitted with Equation 9. Each symbol represents data from different experiments. (From Seow, C. Y. and Stephens, N. L., *J. Appl. Physiol.*, 64(5), 2053, 1988. With permission.)

Figure 10 shows $V_0 - l$ curves obtained at different times after onset of contraction. In contrast to V_{max}, l_{min} is relatively time independent. This probably indicates that the maximum amount of shortening produced by a muscle is largely determined by the physical properties of passive components of the muscle; for instance, the stiffness of the parallel elastic component, but not the degree of activation of the contractile element. Changes in l_{min} associated with pathological alterations in smooth-muscle function such as those found in the canine asthmatic and rat essential hypertension models[22,24,54,55] therefore probably involve alterations in noncontractile components of the muscle, such as cytoskeletal proteins.

B. LENGTH-DEPENDENT SERIES ELASTICITY

As mentioned before, stiffness of the SEC is directly related to the number of attached cross bridges. It seems, however, that there are a number of factors that also affect the stiffness; for example, tension in the SEC, as evidenced in Figure 6. Muscle length is another factor that affects the stiffness. To correctly use the SEC stiffness as an index of the number of attached cross bridges, it is important to understand the relations among stiffness, tension, and length. Figure 11 shows stress-strain curves of the SEC at different muscle lengths. It is clear that the SEC is stiffer at shorter lengths. The same equation (Equation 6) is used to fit all the curves, but with different constants (E_0 and A). Analysis of the stress-strain curves such as the ones shown in Figure 11 reveals that stiffness of the SEC obtained at a constant stress level is directly proportional to the reciprocal of the SEC length (Figure 12). This suggests that the apparent stiffness increase with decreasing muscle length is likely to be due to the diminution of the SEC length itself during muscle shortening. No evidence has been found in either smooth or striated muscle to indicate that the number of attached cross bridges increases as muscle shortens below l_0. On the contrary, evidence gathered from length-tension studies[65-68] indicates that tension decreases at short muscle lengths, suggesting that the number of attached cross bridges decreases when muscle shortens below its optimum length.

Theoretical relationship between the various sources of series compliance and the apparent muscle stiffness has been well described by Ford et al.[69] for striated muscle. The description is probably valid for smooth muscle if one accepts that the sliding-filament, cycling-cross bridge mechanism is also responsible for smooth-muscle contraction. At $l < l_0$, the extensibility of the thin filament is critical in determining the behavior of the apparent SEC stiffness with respect to muscle length. If the nonoverlap portion of the thin filaments contributes to the series compliance of the muscle, then as the muscle shortens, an apparent increase in muscle stiffness would be observed due to the diminution of the nonoverlap portion. A shorter SEC will produce a smaller length response when it is subjected to a constant load step. (The muscle appears to be stiffer). It follows that the SEC stiffness must be inversely proportional to the SEC length. The finding[70] that the SEC stiffness is highly correlated to 1/[SEC length] suggest that the thin filaments may be an important source of the series compliance in smooth muscle. By applying force perturbations, ΔP (with constant amplitude), to a muscle during an isotonic contraction,[70] it is found that the amplitude of the resulting length response, ΔL, decreases as the muscle shortening increases. This is consistent with the notion that in canine trachealis the SEC stiffness increases with decreasing length. (Stiffness of the SEC can be estimated by the ratio $\Delta P/\Delta L$). The physiological implications of the increased SEC stiffness with reduced muscle length may be important. This increased stiffness may be instrumental in stabilizing the narrowed airways.

V. ALTERATION IN MECHANICAL PROPERTIES OF AIRWAY SMOOTH MUSCLE IN CANINE ASTHMATIC MODEL

Antonissen et al.[22] were the first to report that airway smooth-muscle function is mechanically altered in (ovalbumin) sensitized dogs. Typical force-velocity curves obtained

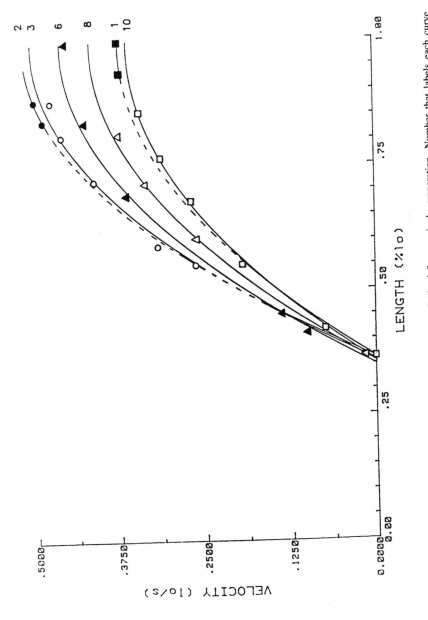

FIGURE 10. Family of zero-load velocity vs. length curves obtained from a single preparation. Number that labels each curve indicates time (in seconds) after onset of stimulation when the data were obtained. Note that early in contraction there was not enough time for muscle to produce an adequate amount of shortening, and therefore V_0 data at short muscle length could not be obtained. The broken line indicates the portion of the curve that was technically impossible to measure (---). (From Seow, C. Y. and Stephens, N. L., *J. Appl. Physiol.*, 64(5), 2053, 1988. With permission.)

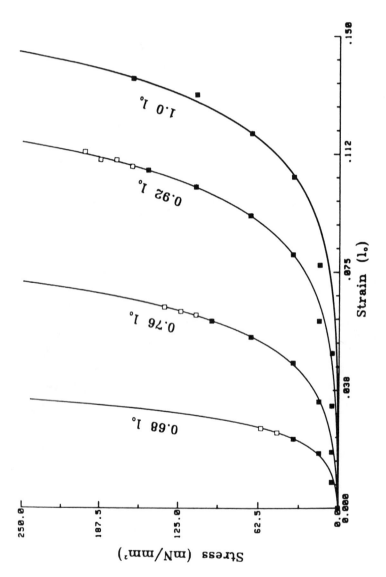

FIGURE 11. Stress-strain curves of the SEC obtained at different muscle lengths. The curves were all obtained at 10 s after contraction. Muscle lengths at which curves were obtained were labeled on curves; ■, data obtained from quick releases; □, data obtained from quick stretches. Data were fitted with Equation 6. (From Seow, C. Y. and Stephens, N. L., *Am. J. Physiol.*, 256(25), 1989. With permission.)

289

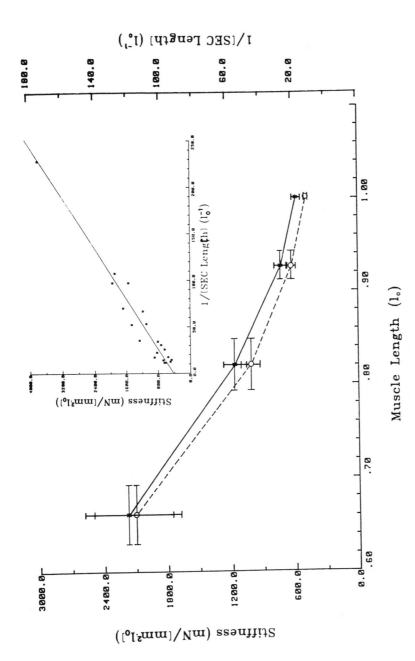

FIGURE 12. Constant-stress stiffness (solid line) and 1/[SEC length] (broken line) as functions of muscle length obtained 10 s after onset of stimulation. Means ± SE are shown. n = 5. Correlation of stiffness and reciprocal of SEC length is shown in the inset. Correlation coefficient (r) is 0.945. (From Seow, C. Y. and Stephens, N. L., *Am. J. Physiol.*, 256(25), 1989. With permission.)

from a paired (littermate) experiment are shown in Figure 13. The major alteration in the force-velocity characteristics in sensitized trachealis is the increased velocity of shortening, especially at light loads. There is no significant difference in P_0 (elicited by electrical stimulation) and a/P_0 (an index of the curvature of the force-velocity curve) between sensitized and control muscles.[22] A more recent study[24] on the same subject further reveals that the shortening velocity of sensitized tissue is only affected (increased) at the early stage of contraction where normally cycling bridges (as opposed to the ''latch'' bridges[27] operating in the late or sustained phase of contraction) are active. Since the early cross bridges are activated by phosphorylation of the myosin light chain,[27] this finding suggests that the myosin phosphorylation may be altered in sensitized muscle.

A more relevant muscle parameter related to the increased airway resistance seen in asthmatics is probably the amount of shortening, but not the velocity of shortening. Figure 14 shows that the amount of shortening under various loads produced by sensitized trachealis is greater than that produced by the control. This mechanical alteration in sensitized muscle may be important in developing and maintaining bronchoconstriction in the animal.

Myofibrillar ATPase activity in ragweed-sensitized canine tracheal smooth muscle is found to be significantly higher than in the control.[71] This may explain the increased shortening velocity found in the muscle. The cause of this increase in ATPase activity is uncertain. There is no statistically significant difference in myosin isozymes band pattern between proteins obtained from the sensitized and control trachealis muscles.[72] Therefore, the difference in isozyme distribution cannot account for the increased ATPase activity seen in sensitized muscle. Preliminary measurements of myosin light-chain (20,000 Da) phosphorylation[73a] show that phosphorylation is increased in sensitized trachealis. If the increase is significant, this could be the underlying mechanism responsible for the increased myofibrillar ATPase activity. Myosin phosphorylation is influenced by factors such as myosin light-chain kinase activity, phosphatase activity, and intracellular calcium-calmodulin concentration. Alterations in any one of the factors could potentially change the mechanical properties of the muscle.

Figure 15 shows the length-velocity curves from sensitized and control trachealis muscles. The zero-load velocity is higher for the sensitized muscle compared to the control at any muscle length. This mechanical alteration can be simulated by the mechanical model shown in Figure 1. If we assume that when muscle shortens under zero load the amount of shortening is limited by the stiffness of the PEC (under compression), then by changing the PEC stiffness the extent of shortening can be altered. By stretching a passive tracheal muscle strip beyond its resting length, the strip will return to its original length if it is released. Also, if the muscle is stimulated under zero load and thus shortens to its minimum length, it will return to its original length when the stimulus is removed. Similar phenomena are also observed in single smooth-muscle cells.[73] These observations seem to suggest that there is an anatomical counterpart in the muscle that functions as the PEC in the model. The mechanical property of the extracellular matrix that the smooth-muscle cells are embedded in is probably important in determining the stiffness of the PEC. The effect of intracellular components on the PEC stiffness cannot be neglected either. The recent finding that the length-dependent internal load is present in single smooth-muscle cells[64] indicates the importance of intracellular components in influencing the PEC stiffness. The intracellular structure that is mechanically capable of resisting both tensile and compressive stress is probably the cytoskeleton, a protein network that consists mostly of intermediate filaments. The observation that the amount of shortening is greater in sensitized muscle compared to the control, whereas the isometric tensions are the same for both muscles,[22,24] has led us to speculate that a more compliant PEC in the sensitized muscle may be responsible for the increased ability of the muscle to shorten. An answer to this speculation can come from direct measurement of stiffness of the PEC under compressive stress. Unfortunately, at the

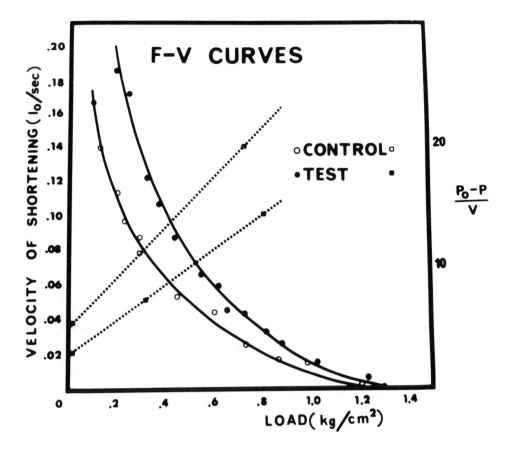

FIGURE 13. Force-velocity curves obtained from a pair of sensitized and control tracheales. Linearized from (broken lines) shows that the relationships are hyperbolic. (From Antonissen, L. A., Mitchell, R. W., Kroeger, E. A., Kepron, W., Tse, K. S., and Stephens, N. L., *J. Appl. Physiol.*, 46(4), 681, 1979. With permission.)

present time there is no satisfactory method for the direct measurement. An indirect method used by us[72] is a combination of force-velocity and length-velocity measurements. Force-velocity relations can be described by the hyperbolic equation (a form of the Hill equation)

$$V = a(V_{max} - bP/a)/(a + P) \qquad (10)$$

and length-velocity relations are described by Equation 9. Since velocity from the force-velocity curve is obtained at l_0, length effect on the velocity is minimal (Figure 9), and since velocity from the length-velocity curve is obtained at zero external load, the force that reduces velocity is entirely from the internal source. The magnitude of the internal force associated with a certain length can be estimated by the zero-load shortening velocity of the muscle at that length, assuming that the internal force is of the same magnitude as the force that is predicted from the force-velocity curve, and that is associated with the same velocity. Mathematically, this is equivalent to combining Equations 9 and 10 by eliminating the velocity term:

$$l = (1 - l_{min})[1 - a(V_{max} - bP/a)/(V_{max}(a + P))]^{1/2} \qquad (11)$$

where l is the CE length, and (from Figure 1) it also is the PEC length. Equation 12 therefore describes the length (l) and tension (P) relations of the PEC. The use of the equation is

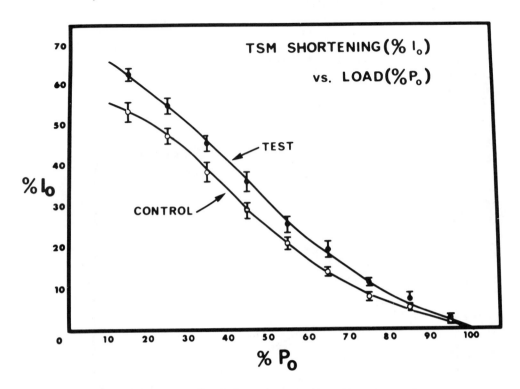

FIGURE 14.   Shortening of sensitized and control tracheales under various loads. Means ± SE are shown. n = 11 for sensitized; n = 9 for control. (From Antonissen, L. A., Mitchell, R. W., Kroeger, E. A., Kepron, W., Tse, K. S., and Stephenson, N. L., *J. Appl. Physiol.*, 46(4), 681, 1979. With permission.)

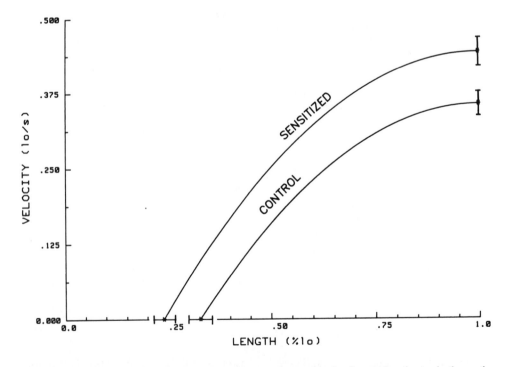

FIGURE 15.   Zero-load velocity vs. muscle-length curves for sensitized and control canine tracheal smooth muscle. The curves are parabolic in shape (Equation 9). The V_{max} and l_{min} values are from our previous report.[24]

TABLE 1
V_{max}, a, b, and l_{min} Values for Sensitized and Control Trachealis

	V_{max} (l_0/s)	a (mN/mm^2)	b (l_0/s)	l_{min} (l_0)
Sensitized	0.32 ± 0.01[a]	54.7 ± 5.5	0.118 ± 0.039[a]	0.32 ± 0.02[a]
Control	0.26 ± 0.03	52.1 ± 9.3	0.082 ± 0.013	0.256 ± 0.03

Note: The values were obtained at 8 s (plateau phase) in contraction by quick-release method. The number of experiments was 5. Ragweed-sensitized dogs and their littermate controls were used.

[a] Significantly different from control, $p < 0.05$.

limited by the assumptions mentioned above. The length-tension curve for the PEC thus can be obtained from the force-velocity constants V_{max}, a, b, and the minimum (shortened) length l_{min}. Values of these parameters are listed in Table 1 for sensitized and control trachealis. Figure 16 shows the compression-tension curves of the PEC for sensitized and control muscles using the mean values provided in Table 1. The PEC of the sensitized muscle is more compliant, as suggested by the greater compression of the PEC of the sensitized muscle, at the same tension level, compared to that of the control. This increase in compliance of the PEC may account for the increased amount of shortening (with no increase in P_0) observed in sensitized tracheal muscle.

VI. CONCLUSION

The time-dependent mechanical properties of airway smooth muscle are likely to be related to the unique regulatory features of smooth muscle, that is, phosphorylation and dephosphorylation of the myosin light chain. The length-dependent mechanical properties are probably related directly to the structural rearrangement of the muscle components at different lengths, or indirectly, to the change in the degree of activation of the contractile apparatus due to the length-dependent structural change. A complete understanding of the mechanical behavior of airway smooth muscle cannot be achieved unless all variables that affect the behavior are identified and their relationships with the muscle behavior and among themselves are characterized. Characterization of the alterations in mechanical properties of sensitized airway smooth muscle is important because of the role airway smooth muscle plays in asthma. Airway resistance is inversely proportional to the fourth power of the diameter of the airway. A slight change in the diameter (due to shortening of the airway smooth muscle) therefore could result in a drastic increase in airway resistance. The increased amount of shortening found in sensitized trachealis, though a moderate increase, cannot be overlooked. Although the mechanical alterations found in sensitized muscle may involve changes in the contractile components, as suggested by the increased myofibrillar ATPase activity, the mechanism underlying the increased ability of the muscle to shorten may not be related to the cross bridges, as suggested by the increased compliance of the PEC found in sensitized tissue.

ACKNOWLEDGMENTS

I would like to thank the editors, D. K. Agrawal and R. G. Townley, for allowing me the opportunity to write the chapter. Also I would like to thank Dr. N. L. Stephens (in whose laboratory most of the above-mentioned experiments were conducted) for critically

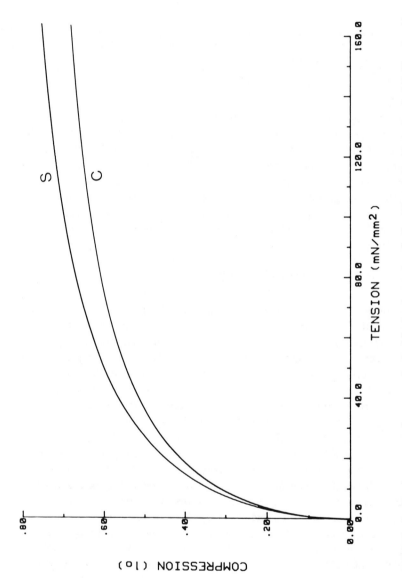

FIGURE 16. Tension-compression curves for sensitized and control tracheales. The relationship is described by Equation 11. Mean values of V_{max}, a, b, and l_{min} (from Table 1) are used to plot the curves; S, sensitized: C, control. Shortening (compression) is in the upward direction.

reading the manuscript. Most of the work presented in this chapter is supported by grants from the MRC of Canada and the Council for Tobacco Research.

REFERENCES

1. **Stephens, N. L.,** Physical properties of contractile system, in *Methods in Pharmacology. Smooth Muscle,* Daniel, E. E. and Paton, D. M., Eds., Plenum Press, New York, 1975, 265.
2. **Stephens, N. L.,** Airway smooth muscle: biophysics, biochemistry and pharmacology, in *Asthma: Physiology, Immunopharmacology, and Treatment,* Austen, K. F. and Lichtenstein, L. M., Eds., Academic Press, New York, 1977, 147.
3. **Stephens, N. L. and Kroeger, E. A.,** Ultrastructure, biophysic and biochemistry of airway smooth muscle, in *Lung Biology in Health and Disease. Physiology and Pharmacology of the Airways,* Nadel, J. A., Ed., Marcel Dekker, New York, 1980, 31.
4. **Stephens, N. L. and Hoppin, F. G., Jr.,** Mechanical properties of airway smooth muscle, in *The Respiratory System. III. Mechanics of Breathing, Part 1,* Macklem, P. T. and Mead, J., Eds., Waverly Press, Baltimore, 1986, 17.
5. **Stephens, N. L.,** Airway smooth muscle, *Am. Rev. Respir. Dis.,* 135, 960, 1987.
6. **Stephens, N. L., Nathaniel, V., Kepron, W., Mitchell, R. W., Seow, C. Y., and Kong, S.-K.,** Theory: anatomy and physiology of respiratory smooth muscle tone, in *Drug Therapy for Asthma: Research and Clinical Practice,* Jenne, J. W. and Murphy, S., Eds., Marcel Dekker, New York, 1987, 1.
7. **Hill, A. V.,** *First and Last Experiments in Muscle Mechanics,* Cambridge University Press, London, 1970.
8. **Close, R. I.,** Dynamic properties of mammalian skeletal muscle, *Physiol. Rev.,* 52, 129, 1972.
9. **McMahon, T. A.,** *Muscle, Reflexes, and Locomotion,* Princeton University Press, Princeton, NJ, 1984.
10. **Woledge, R. C., Curtin, N. A., and Homsher, E.,** *Energetics Aspects of Muscle Contraction,* Academic Press, Orlando, FL, 1985.
11. **Huxley, A. F.,** *Reflections on Muscle,* Princeton University Press, Princeton, NJ, 1980.
12. **Eisenberg, E. and Hill, T. L.,** Muscle contraction and free energy transduction in biological systems, *Science,* 227, 999, 1985.
13. **Axelsson, J.,** Mechanical properties of smooth muscle, and the relationship between mechanical and electrical activity, in *Smooth Muscle,* Bülbring, E., Brading, A. F., Jones, A. W., and Tomita, T., Eds., Williams & Wilkins, Baltimore, 1970, 289.
14. **Murphy, R. A.,** Contractile system function in mammalian smooth muscle, *Blood Vessels,* 13, 1, 1976.
15. **Rüegg, J. C.,** Smooth muscle tone, *Physiol. Rev.,* 51, 201, 1971.
16. **Somlyo, A. P. and Somlyo, A. V.,** Vascular smooth muscle. I. Normal structure, pathology, biochemistry, and biophysics, *Pharmacol. Rev.,* 20, 197, 1968.
17. **Twarog, B. M.,** Aspects of smooth muscle function in molluscan catch muscle, *Physiol. Rev.,* 56, 829, 1976.
18. **Murphy, R. A.,** Mechanics of vascular smooth muscle, in *The Cardiovascular System. II. Vascular Smooth Muscle,* Bohr, D. F., Somlyo, A. P., and Sparks, H. V., Jr., Eds., Waverly Press, Baltimore, 1980, 13.
19. **Otis, A. B.,** A perspective of respiratory mechanics, *J. Appl. Physiol.,* 54, 1183, 1983.
20. **Akasaka, K., Konno, K., and Ono, Y.,** Electromyography study of bronchial smooth muscle in bronchial asthma, *Tohoku J. Exp. Med.,* 117, 55, 1975.
21. **Souhrada, M. and Souhrada, J. F.,** Reassessment of electrophysiological and contractile characteristics of sensitized airway smooth muscle, *Respir. Physiol.,* 46, 17, 1981.
22. **Antonissen, L. A., Mitchell, R. W., Kroeger, E. A., Kepron, W., Tse, K. S., and Stephens, N. L.,** Mechanical alterations of airway smooth muscle in a canine asthmatic model, *J. Appl. Physiol.,* 46, 681, 1979.
23. **Kong, S. K., Shiu, R. P. C., and Stephens, N. L.,** Studies of myofibrillar ATPase in ragweed sensitized canine pulmonary smooth muscle, *J. Appl. Physiol.,* 60(1), 92, 1986.
24. **Stephens, N. L., Morgan, G., Kepron, W., and Seow, C. Y.,** Changes in crossbridge properties of sensitized airway smooth muscle, *J. Appl. Physiol.,* 61(4), 1492, 1986.
25. **Sobieszek, A. and Small, J. V.,** Relation of the actin-myosin interaction in vertebrate smooth muscle: activation via a myosin light chain kinase and the effect of tropomyosin, *J. Mol. Biol.,* 112, 559, 1977.
26. **Dabrowska, R., Sherry, J. M. F., Aromatorio, D., and Hartshorne, D. J.,** Modulator protein as a component of the myosin ligh chain kinase, *Biochemistry,* 17, 253, 1978.
27. **Dillon, P. F., Aksoy, M. O., Driska, S. P., and Murphy, R. A.,** Myosin phosphorylation and t crossbridge cycle in arterial smooth muscle, *Science,* 211, 495, 1981.

28. **Kamm, K. E. and Stull, J. T.,** Myosin phosphorylation, force, and maximal shortening velocity in neurally stimulated tracheal smooth muscle, *Am. J. Physiol.,* 249(18), C238, 1985.

29. **Hai, C.-M. and Murphy, R. A.,** Cross-bridge phosphorylation and regulation of latch state in smooth muscle, *Am. J. Physiol.,* 254(23), C99, 1988.

30. **Rasmussen, H., Tacuwa, Y., and Park, S.,** Protein kinase C in the regulation of smooth muscle contraction, *FASEB J.,* 1, 177, 1987.

31. **Butler, T. M., Siegman, M. J., and Moores, S. U.,** Slowing of cross-bridge cycling in smooth muscle without evidence of an internal load, *Am. J. Physiol.,* 251(20), C945, 1986.

32. **Hoar, P. E., Pato, M. D., and Kerrick, W. G.,** Myosin light chain phosphotase—effect on the activation and relaxation of gizzard smooth muscle skinned fibers, *J. Biol. Chem.,* 260, 8760, 1985.

33. **Moreland, R. S. and Murphy, R. A.,** Determinants of Ca^{2+}-dependent stress maintenance in skinned swine carotid media, *Am. J. Physiol.,* 251(20), C892, 1986.

34. **Walsh, M. P.,** Caldesmon, a major actin- and calmodulin-binding protein of smooth muscle, in *Regulation and Contraction of Smooth Muscle,* Siegman, M. J., Somlyo, A. P., and Stephens, N. L., Eds., Alan R. Liss, New York, 1987, 119.

35. **Stephens, N. L., Kagan, M. L., and Packer, C. S.,** Time dependence of shortening velocity in tracheal smooth muscle, *Am. J. Physiol.,* 251(20), C435, 1986.

36. **Seow, C. Y. and Stephens, N. L.,** Force-velocity curves for smooth muscle: analysis of internal factors reducing velocity, *Am. J. Physiol.,* 251(20), C362, 1986.

37. **Siegman, M. J., Butler, T. M., Moores, S. U., and Davies, R. E.,** Crossbridges: attachment, resistance to stretch and viscoelasticity in resting mammalian smooth muscle, *Science,* 191, 383, 1976.

38. **Uvelius, B.,** Shortening velocity, active force and homogeneity of contraction during electrically evoked twitches in smooth muscle from rabbit urinary bladder, *Acta Physiol. Scand.,* 106, 481, 1979.

39. **Buchthal, F. and Rosenfalck, P.,** Elastic properties of striated muscle, in *Tissue Elasticity,* Remington, J. W., Ed., Waverly Press, Baltimore, 1957, 73.

40. **Bressler, B. H. and Clinch, N. F,** Crossbridges as the major source of compliance in contracting skeletal muscle, *Nature,* 250, 221, 1975.

41. **Cecchi, G., Griffiths, P. J., and Taylor, S.,** Muscular contraction: kinetics of crossbridge attachment studied by high frequency stiffness measurements, *Science,* 217, 70, 1980.

42. **Ford, L. E., Huxley, A. F., and Simmons, R. M.,** Tension transient during the rise of tetanic tension in frog muscle fibre, *J. Physiol.,* 372, 595, 1986.

43. **Ford, L. E., Huxley, A. F., and Simmons, R. M.,** The relation between stiffness and filament overlap in stimulated frog muscle fibres, *J. Physiol.,* 311, 219, 1981.

44. **Huxley, A. F. and Simmons, R. M.,** Mechanical properties of the crossbridges of frog striated muscle, *J. Physiol.,* 218, 59, 1971.

45. **Julian, F. J. and Sollins, M. R.,** Variation of muscle stiffness with force at increasing speeds of shortening, *J. Gen. Physiol.,* 66, 287, 1975.

46. **Kamm, E. K. and Stull, J. T.,** Activation of smooth muscle contraction: relation between myosin phosphorylation and stiffness, *Science,* 232, 80, 1986.

47. **Meiss, R. A.,** Dynamic stiffness of rabbit mesotubarium smooth muscle: effect of isometric length, *Am. J. Physiol.,* 234(3), C14, 1978.

48. **Seow, C. Y. and Stephens, N. L.,** Time dependence of series elasticity in tracheal smooth muscle, *J. Appl. Physiol.,* 62(4), 1556, 1987.

49. **Herlihy, J. T. and Murphy, R. A.,** Force-velocity and series elastic characteristics of smooth muscle from the hog carotid artery, *Circ. Res.,* 34, 461, 1974.

50. **Stephens, N. L. and Kromer, U.,** Series elastic component of tracheal smooth muscle, *Am. J. Physiol.,* 220, 1890, 1971.

51. **Warshaw, D. M. and Fay, F. S.,** Cross-bridge elasticity in single smooth muscle cells, *J. Gen. Physiol.,* 82, 157, 1983.

52. **Squire, J.,** *The Structural Basis of Muscular Contraction,* Plenum Press, New York, 1981, 523.

53. **Dillon, P. F. and Murphy, R. A.,** Tonic force maintenance with reduced shortening velocity in arterial smooth muscle, *Am. J. Physiol.,* 242(11), C102, 1982.

54. **Kepron, W., James, J. M., Kirk, B., Sehon, A. H., and Tse, K. S.,** A canine model for reaginic hypersensitivity and allergic bronchoconstriction, *J. Allergy Clin. Immunol.,* 59, 64, 1977.

55. **Packer, C. S. and Stephens, N. L.,** Force-velocity relationships in hypertensive arterial smooth muscle, *Can. J. Physiol. Pharmacol.,* 63, 669, 1985.

56. **Brutsaert, D. L., Claes, V. A., and Sonnenblick, E. H.,** Effect of abrupt load alterations on force-velocity-length and time relation during isotonic contractions of heart muscle: load clamping, *J. Physiol.,* 216, 319, 1971.

57. **Chiu, Y., Ballow, E. W., and Ford, L. E.,** Velocity transients and viscoelastic resistance to active shortening in cat papillary muscle, *Biophys. J.,* 40, 121, 1982.

58. **Edman, E. A. P.,** The velocity of unloaded shortening and its relation to sarcomere length and isometric force in vertebrate muscle fibres, *J. Physiol.,* 291, 143, 1979.
59. **Gunst, S. J.,** Effect of length history on contractile behavior of canine tracheal smooth muscle, *Am. J. Physiol.,* 250(19), C134, 1986.
60. **Seow, C. Y. and Stephens, N. L.,** Velocity-length-time relations in canine tracheal smooth muscle, *J. Appl. Physiol.,* 64(5), 2053, 1988.
61. **Taylor, S. R. and Rudel, R.,** Striated muscle fibers: inactivation of contraction induced by shortening, *Science,* 167, 882, 1970.
62. **Jewell, B. R. and Blinks, J. R.,** Drugs and mechanical properties of heart muscle, *Annu. Rev. Pharmacol.,* 8, 113, 1968.
63. **Stephens, N. L., Mitchell, R. W., and Brutsaert, D. L.,** Shortening inactivation, maximum force potential, relaxation, contractility, in *Smooth Muscle,* Stephens, N. L., Ed., Marcel Dekker, New York, 1984, 91.
64. **Harris, D., Yamakawa, M., and Warshaw, D.,** Evidence for an internal load in single smooth muscle cells, *Biophys. J.,* 55(2), 69a, 1989.
65. **Close, R. I.,** The relations between sarcomere length and characteristics of isometric twitch contractions of frog sartorius muscle, *J. Physiol.* 220, 745, 1972.
66. **Edman, K. A. P.,** The relation between sarcomere length and active tension in isolated semitendinosus fibers of the frog, *J. Physiol.,* 183, 407, 1966.
67. **Ramsey, R. W. and Street, S. F.,** The isometric length-tension diagram of isolated skeletal fibers of the frog, *J. Cell Comp. Physiol.,* 15, 11, 1940.
68. **Stephens, N. L., Kroeger, E. A., and Mehta, J. A.,** Force-velocity characterization of respiratory airway smooth muscle, *J. Appl. Physiol.,* 26, 685, 1969.
69. **Ford, L. E., Huxley, A. F., and Simmons, R. M.,** The relation between stiffness and filament overlap in stimulated frog muscle fibres, *J. Physiol.,* 311, 219, 1981.
70. **Seow, C. Y. and Stephens, N. L.,** Changes of tracheal smooth muscle stiffness during an isotonic contraction, *Am. J. Physiol.,* 256(25), 1989.
71. **Kong, S.-K., Shiu, R. P. C., and Stephens, N. L.,** Studies of myofibrillar ATPase in ragweed-sensitized canine pulmonary smooth muscle, *J. Appl. Physiol.,* 60(1), 92, 1986.
72. **Stephens, N. L., Kong, S. K., and Seow, C. Y.,** Mechanisms of increased shortening of sensitized airway smooth muscle, in *Mechanisms in Asthma: Pharmacology, Physiology, and Management,* Armour, C. L. and Black, J. L., Eds., Alan R. Liss, New York, 1988, 231.
73. **Warshaw, D. M., McBride, W. J., and Work, S. S.,** Corkscrewlike shortening in single smooth muscle cells, *Science,* 236, 1457, 1987.
73a. **Kong, S. K. and Stephens, N. L.,** unpublished observations.

INDEX

A

Acetylcholine (ACh)
    dosage-response curve of canine bronchial strips, 136
    effect of epithelium removal, 134—135
    spasmodic effects, 83—85
Action potentials and K$^+$ channel blockade, 74—75
Adenosine 3′:5′ cyclic monophosphate, see cAMP
Adenosine 5′-triphosphate (ATP)
    in bronchial challenge testing, 173
    relaxant effects, 82
Adrenergic innervation of airways, 230—232
Adrenergic receptor classification, 232—233
α-Adrenoreceptors, see Alpha-receptors
β-Adrenoreceptors, see Beta-receptors
Afferent receptors
    pulmonary and bronchial C-fiber endings, 206—214
    rapidly adapting (irritant), 194—206
    significance in pulmonary function, 182—187
    slowly adapting (stretch), 186—194
Agonist/antagonist effects, 57—60, 82—90, see also Functional antagonism
Agonist effects and sample preparation, 112, 114—115
Airway conductance measurement, 154—157
Airway response
    allergen challenge testing, 175—176
    bronchial asthma and, 168
    clinical methods of evaluation, 168—176
    factors influencing, 169—171
    indications for testing, 168—169
    measurement, 157—159, 169
    pharmacologic challenge testing, 172—173
    physiologic challenge testing, 173—175
Airway smooth muscle
    conceptual model of mechanics, 273
    mechanical properties
    conceptual model, 273
    length-dependent, 284—286
    time-dependent, 273—284
    structure, 10—31
Allergen challenge testing, 175—176
Allergic diseases and histamine receptors, 264—267
Alpha-receptors, 245—246
Alveolar ducts, 11
Alveolar macrophage β-adrenoreceptors, 238—239
Alveolar-wall interstitial cells, 114
Aminophylline, 88
Amiodipine, 104
Anesthetics and receptor activity, 215—216
Animal studies, methodology for *in vivo*, 148—164
Antihistamines in asthma, 267
Arachidonic acid metabolites and contractility, 138—139

Asthma
    antihistamines in, 267
    canine model mechanical alterations, 286—293
ATP, see Adenosine 5′-triphosphate

B

Basement membrane, 17—20
BAY K 8644, 99, 100
Benidipine, 104
Beta-blockers, 193, 241—242, 244
Beta-receptors
    agonists, 85—87
    on alveolar macrophages, 238—239
    antagonists, see β-blockers
    epithelial, 237
    epithelium removal and, 135
    functional antagonism and, 120
    glandular, 237—238
    mast cell, 238
    pulmonary
    in bronchial asthma, 239—243
    glucocorticoid effects, 243—245
    tracheopulmonary, 236—237
Bovine lung parenchymal strips, 114
BRL 34915, see Cromakalin
BRL 38277, 102, 104
Bronchi 4—6
Bronchial airway structure, 4—10
Bronchial asthma
    airway response and, 168
    antihistamines in, 267
    cholinergic receptors and, 235—236
    pulmonary β-adrenoreceptors in, 245—246
Bronchial hyperresponsiveness, 230
Bronchial mucosa, 4
Bronchial tissue sample preparation, 112—113
Bronchial wall, 4
Bronchioles, 7—9, see also specific types
Bronchomotor tone, 183—185
Bupivacaine, 215—216

C

Ca^{2+}, 40—41, 49—50, 85
Ca^{2+} agonists, 90
Ca^{2+} channel blockers, 90, 98—99, 103, 105
Ca^{2+} channels, 79, 98
    receptor-operated, 98—100
    voltage-sensitive, 100
Calmodulin, 41—42
cAMP, 51, 241
cAMP-dependent protein kinase, 51—53
Canine asthmatic model mechanical alteration, 286—293
Canine tracheal smooth muscle, 15—17, 20, 23, 27—29, 31—33

Capsaicin and chemoreflex in C-fiber endings, 212—213
Carbachol response in human lung parenchymal strips, 115
Central integration of pulmonary receptors, 214—215
C-fiber endings, 206—214
cGMP, 53—56, 234—235
Chemical stimulation
    C-fiber endings, 211
    irritant receptors, 199—205
    pulmonary stretch receptors, 191—192
Chimeric molecules, 103
Chloride channels, 79, 98
Cholinergic modulation, 80—81, 233—234
Cholinergic receptors, 234—236
Chromakalin, 88
Clinical indications for inhalation challenge, 169
Clinical measurement of airway response, 168—176
Cold-air hyperventilation testing, 173—175
Contractile agents and epithelium-derived relaxing factor, 130
Contractile apparatus, 26—31, 41
Contractile/relaxant pathway integration, 57—60
Contraction, 40—44, 58
Corticosteroids, 244
Cromakalin (BRL 34915), 78, 101, 103—104
Cyclic nucleotide-mediated relaxation, 50—57
Cyclic nucleotide phosphodiesterases, 56—57

D

Darodipine, 104
Data analysis, 151—153, 155—156
DeVilbiss Jet Nebulizer Model 646, 170
1,2-Diaglycerol, 44—45, 47—49
1,2-Diaglycerol/protein kinase C pathway, 47—49, 85
Diazoxide, 102
Dihydropyridines, 104
Diltiazem, 99, 103
Diverticula in bronchial mucosa, 5
Dogs, see Canine entries
Dose response curve, 159
Drug inhibition, 213—214, see also Agonist/antagonist effects
Drug response, see also specific drugs
    in airway tube preparations, 116—117
    anatomic regional differences, 113
    isotonic vs. isometric, 116
    in lung strip preparations, 114—115
Dynamic compliance measurement *in vivo*, 158—159

E

Electrophysical studies of epithelium-derived relaxing factor, 133—134
Electrophysiological properties and behavior
    exogenous effects
        relaxant agents, 85—90

spasmogens, 82—85
general, 70—75
ion channels, 75—80
modulation of electrical activity, 80—82
EMD 52692, 102
Epithelial β-receptors, 237
Epithelium-derived relaxant factor, 80—82, 120—122, 138—143
Eupneic breathing, 187, 195, 207
Excitation-contraction coupling, 18—20, 97
Exercise challenge testing, 174, 236
Exogenous relaxants, 85—90
Exogenous spasmogens, 82—85

F

Feline lung parenchymal strips, 113—114
Felodipine, 104
Force-velocity relations, 273—278
Franidipine, 104
Functional antagonism, 57—60, 118—120
Functional residual capacity measurement, 153—154

G

Gallopamil, 99
Gap junctions, 21—25
Glandular β-receptors, 237—238
Glucocorticoids, 243—245
Golgi apparatus, 26
G-protein receptor coupling, 45—46
Guanosine 3':5' cyclic monophosphate, see cGMP
Guinea pigs
    airway response measurement, 160—161
    sphincter papillae, 19
    taenia coli, 22
    tracheal response to osmotic stimuli, 139—141
    tracheobronchial tube preparations, 116—117

H

Hackenbrock's classification of mitochondria, 26
Hering-Breur stretch reflex, 182—183
Hexamethonium, 235
Histamine
    effect of epithelium removal, 134—135
    in pharmacologic challenge testing, 172—173
    preparation for bronchial challenge, 171
Histamine H1 receptor agonists, 83—85
Histamine receptors
    in allergic airway diseases, 264—267
    distribution and classification, 261—264
    possible mechanisms of action, 264
HOE 166, 105
5-Hydroxytriptamine (5HT)
    effect of epithelium removal, 134—135
    response in human lung parenchymal strips, 115

I

Innervation, 31—33
Inositol (1,4,5)-triphosphate, 44, 46—47
Intercellular communications, 21—25
In vitro functional evaluation
  alternative airway preparations, 117—118
  epithelium-modulated airway responsiveness, 120—122
  functional antagonism, 118—120
  isometric/isotonic measurements compared, 115—117
  lung parenchymal strip as peripheral airway model, 113—115
  standard central airway preparations, 112—113
In vivo measurement in animals
  airway response, 157—159
  functional residual capacity and specific lung compliance, 153—154
  resistance and dynamic compliance, 149—153
  respiratory flow resistance and dynamic lung compliance, 149—153
  selection of method, 159—164
  specific airway conductance, 154—157
Ion channel-modulating drugs, 103—106, see also specific drugs
Ion channels, 75—80, 97—98, see also specific types
Ipratroprium, 216, 236
Irritant receptors, 194—206
  chemical stimulation, 199—205
  in eupneic breathing, 195
  location, 194—195
  mechanical stimulation, 195—198
  reflex effects, 205—206
Isometric vs. isotonic measurements, 115—117
Isoprenaline, 86—87
Isoprotenerol, 134—137
Isradipine, 104

K

K$^+$ channel activators, 88—90, 102—105
K$^+$ channels, 74—78, 98, 100—102

L

Latch bridge theory, 42—44
Length-dependent mechanical properties, 284—286
Leukotrienes, 85, 173
Local anesthetics, 215—216, see also specific drugs
Lung compliance measurement *in vivo,* 149—153, 158—159
Lung parenchymal strip as peripheral airway model, 113—115
Lungs, β-receptors in, 236—237, 239—243
Lysosomes, 26

M

Mast cells, 234, 238
Maximum shortening velocity, 284—286
MCI-176, 105
MDL 12,330A, 105
Mechanical properties
  alteration in canine asthmatic model, 286—293
  conceptual model, 273
  length-dependent, 284—286
  time-dependent, 273—284
Mechanical stimulation
  of C-fiber endings, 207—210
  irritant receptors, 195—198
  pulmonary stretch receptors, 187—191
Membrane structure, 15—20
Methacholine, 171—173
Methylxanthines, 88
Microscopic features, 14
Minoxidil, 102
Mitochondria, 25—31
Monkeys, airway response measurement, 163
Mucosa, 3—5
Multiunit and single-unit properties, 13—15
Muscarinic agonists, 83—85
Muscle bundle morphology, 14
Muscle contraction, see Contraction
Muscle relaxation, see Relaxation, cyclic-nucleotide mediated
Muscle tone
  biochemical regulation
    contractile/relaxant pathway integration, 57—60
    contraction, 40—44
    cyclic nucleotide-mediated relaxation, 50—57
    signal transduction, 44—51
  bronchomotor reflex, 183—185
Musculus transversus tracheae, 3, 14
Myosin light-chain kinase, 42—43
Myosin light-chain phosphorylation, 42—44

N

Na$^+$ channel blockers, 97
Na$^+$ channels, 97
Neurotransmitters, 80—82
Nexuses, see Gap junctions
Nicorandil, 89—90, 102
Nifedipine, 99, 103, 104
Niguldipine, 104
Nilvadipine, 104
Nisoldipine, 104
Nitrendipine, 104
Nitroglycerin and Ca^{2+} response, 55
Nitroprusside and Ca^{2+} response, 56
Nonadrenergic, noncholinergic neuroregulation, 81—82
Noradrenergic regulation, 81
Norepinephrine response in human lung parenchymal strips, 115
Nucleus and nuclear membrane, 31

O

Osmotic stimuli and epithelium-derived relaxation, 139—140

P

Parenchymal smooth muscle, 9—10
Paries membranaceous, 14
Passive electrical properties, 70—72
Pathological stimulation of C-fiber endings, 210—211
PDEs (cyclic nucleotide phosphodiesterases), 56—57
Pharmacologic challenge testing of airway response, 172—173
Phosphatidylinositol turnover, 46—49
Phosphoinositol 4,5-biphosphate (PIP$_2$), 46—47
Physiologic antagonism, see Functional antagonism
Physiologic challenge testing, 173—175
Pinacidil, 102
Pinocytic vesicles, 18
Platelet-activating factor, 173, 239—243
Portal vein smooth muscle cell, 30
Potassium channels, see K$^+$ channels
Potassium chloride spasmogenic effects, 82—83
Propanolol, 87, 193, 240—241
Prostaglandin D$_2$, 173
Prostaglandin E$_2$, 138—139
Protein kinases
  cAMP dependent, 43—44, 47—49, 51—53, 234
  cGMP dependent, 55
Pulmonary function and afferent receptors, 182—187
Pulmonary receptors, 214—216, see also Afferent receptors
Pulmonary reflex effects
  receptors with intravagal afferent fibers
    pulmonary and bronchial C-fiber endings, 206—213
    rapidly adapting (irritant) receptors, 194—206
    slowly adapting (pulmonary stretch) receptors, 186—194
  significance of afferent receptors, 182—187
  studies of reflex integration, 213—216
Pulmonary reflexes, drug inhibition, 213—214
Pulmonary stretch receptors, 186—194
  chemical stimulation, 191—192
  in eupneic breathing, 187
  location, 186—187
  mechanical stimulation, 187—191
  reflex actions, 192—194
Purines and inhibitory response, 81—82

R

Rapidly adapting (irritant) afferent receptors, 194—206
Rats, airway response measurement, 162
Receptor-operated Ca^{2+} channels, 49—50, 98—100

Recording and analysis of data, 151—153, 155—156
Rectification, 72
Relaxant/contractile pathway integration, 57—60
Relaxants, exogenous, 85—90
Relaxation, cyclic-nucleotide mediated, 50—57
Respiratory broncioles, 7—9
Respiratory resistance measurement *in vivo*, 149—153, 158—159
Resting membrane potential, 70
Ro 31-6930, 102
RP 49356, 102

S

Sample preparation, 113—115
Sarcolemma, 15—17
Sarcoplasmic reticulum, 18
Series elasticity
  length-dependent, 286—293
  time-dependent, 278—284
Serotonergic receptor effect of epithelium removal, 135
Sheep, airway response measurement, 163—164
Signal transduction, 44—50, see also Agonist/antagonist effects
SKF 96365, 99
Skinned muscle cells, 118
Skin test correlation with bronchial challenge, 175
Slowly adapting afferent receptors, 186—194, see also Pulmonary stretch receptors
Sodium channels, see Na$^+$ channels
Sodium cromoglycate, 213—216
Spasmogens
  exogenous, 82—85
  selection and functional antagonistic effects, 119
Spontaneous activity, 72—74
Stretch receptors, see Pulmonary stretch receptors
Structure
  of airways
    bronchial airways, 4—10
    trachea, 2—3
  airway smooth muscle, 10—13
    contractile apparatus, 26—31
    Golgi apparatus and lysosomes, 26
    human vs. other, 34
    innervation, 31—33
    intercellular communications, 21—25
    membranes, 15—20
    mitochondria, 25—26
    multiunit and single-unit properties, 13—15
    nucleus and nuclear membrane, 31

T

TA 3090, 99
Terminal bronchioles, 7
Tetraethylammonium spasmogenic effects, 82—83
(+)-Tetrandine, 105
Tetrodotoxin, 80—81
Time-dependent mechanical properties, 273—284

Trachea
  β-receptors in, 236—237
  structure, 2—3
Tracheal mucosa, 3
Tracheal tissue sample preparation, 112
Tracheopulmonary β-receptors, 236—237
Transpulmonary pressure measurement, 149—161
Tropomyosin regulation, 40
Tunica fibrosa tracheae, 3

U

Ultrasonic nebulization, 170, 175

V

Vagal influences on pulmonary function, 182—185,
  see also Afferent receptors
Vasoactive intestinal peptide system, 31—32,
  81—82
Verapamil, 99, 112, 103
Voltage-dependent Ca^{2+} channels, 49—50, 83, 98,
  101